SELECTED TOPICS IN OPTICAL COHERENCE TOMOGRAPHY

Edited by **Gangjun Liu**

Selected Topics in Optical Coherence Tomography
Edited by Gangjun Liu

Published by InTech

Janeza Trdine 9, 51000 Rijeka, Croatia

Publishing Process Manager Romana Vukelic

Technical Editor Teodora Smiljanic

Cover Designer InTech Design Team

Additional hard copies can be obtained from orders@intechopen.com

Selected Topics in Optical Coherence Tomography, Edited by Gangjun Liu
p. cm.
ISBN 978-953-51-0034-8

For EU product safety concerns:
IN TECH d.o.o., Prolaz Marije Krucifikse Kozulić 3, 51000 Rijeka, Croatia, info@intechopen.com or visit our website at intechopen.com.

Meet the editor

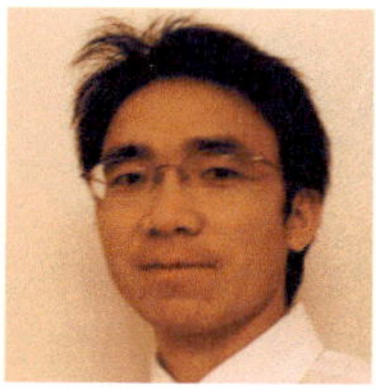

Dr Gangjun Liu received a BS degree in Electrical Engineering from the Xi'an Jiao Tong University in 1998, and a PhD degree in Optics from the Shanghai Jiao Tong University in 2003. He worked as an Engineer at STMicroelectronics, Singapore, from 2004 until 2007, when he joined the Beckman Laser Institute and Medical Clinic, University of California, Irvine, where he is currently an assistant specialist. He has authored or co-authored more than 50 papers in peer-reviewed scientific journals and conference proceedings. His research interests are in the area of biophotonics.

Contents

Preface

Optical coherence tomography (OCT) is an interferometric technique based on optical coherent gating. In OCT, imaging contrast originates from the sample inhomogeneous scattering properties that are linearly dependent on the sample's refractive indices. OCT offers axial resolution of 2-15 μm and penetration depth around 2 mm. Since its invention in the late 1980s and early 1990s, OCT has experienced explosive growth in both technology and application.

With the development of Fourier domain OCT, the A-line rate and the sensitivity of the OCT systems have been improved dramatically in the past few years. The potentials of OCT for real time, in-vivo diagnostic, surgery guidance and monitoring applications have been recognized. In recent years, we have seen an increase in the number of research groups, as well as industry companies, involved in the OCT system development and application. OCT was first used clinically in ophthalmology, for the imaging and diagnosis of retinal disease. Recently, it has been applied to image subsurface structure in skin, vessels, oral cavities, as well as respiratory, urogenital and gastrointestinal tracts. The application of OCT will continue to penetrate more exciting fields in the near future.

This book contains different exciting topics in the OCT fields, written by experts from all over the world. Technological developments, as well as clinical and industrial applications are covered. Some interesting topics, like the ultrahigh resolution OCT, the functional extension of OCT and the full field OCT are reviewed, and the applications of OCT in ophthalmology, cardiology and dentistry are also addressed. I believe that a broad range of readers, such as students, researchers and physicians will benefit from this book.

I would like to thank all who made this project possible. Firstly, my sincere gratitude goes to the InTech staff for inviting me to participate as Editor and for providing assistance with the editing process, especially to Ms. Romana Vukelic for her professional assistance throughout the entire process. I also thank all the authors for generously sharing their knowledge and experience with the readers, and for the time they have taken to write these chapters. Most importantly, on behalf of the authors and myself, we hope that the readers will download, read and benefit from this book.

Gangjun Liu
Beckman Laser Institute,
University of California,
Irvine, California
USA

Part 1

OCT Techniques

1

Full-Field Optical Coherence Microscopy

Arnaud Dubois
Laboratoire Charles Fabry, UMR 8501
Institut d'Optique, CNRS, Univ Paris Sud 11
Palaiseau
France

1. Introduction

Optical coherence tomography (OCT) is a well-established optical imaging technique with micrometer-scale resolution. OCT is based on low-coherence interferometry to measure the amplitude of light backscattered by the sample being imaged [1-4]. The most significant impact of OCT is in ophthalmology for *in situ* examination of the pathologic changes of the retina [5-8] and measurement of the dimensions of the anterior chamber of the eye [9, 10]. OCT has also been established in a variety of other biomedical applications [11] and for material characterization [12, 13].

Optical Coherence Microscopy (OCM) is an OCT technique where high numerical aperture optics are used to achieve higher transverse spatial resolution. OCM generates *en face* rather than cross-sectional images with the transverse resolution of a microscope. Two general approaches for OCM have been reported to date. The first approach is based on the principle of point-scanning imaging developed in confocal microscopy [13-15]. The second approach involves full-field illumination and detection. Also sometimes termed Full-Field Optical Coherence Tomography (FF-OCT), Full-Field Optical Coherence Microscopy (FF-OCM) is an alternative technique to scanning OCM, based on white-light interference microscopy [16-18]. FF-OCM produces tomographic images in the *en face* orientation by arithmetic combination of interferometric images acquired with an area camera and by illuminating the whole field of view using a low-coherence light source [19-23]. The major interest of FF-OCM lies in its high imaging resolution in both transverse and axial directions, far higher than the resolution of conventional OCT, using a simple and robust experimental arrangement [24, 25]. Two extensions to the FF-OCM technique were recently proposed to provide additional information on the spectroscopic or birefringence properties of the sample being imaged [26, 27].

This chapter reports on the latest developments of the FF-OCM technology. Tomographic images can be acquired in two distinct spectral regions, centered at 750 nm and 1250 nm using two different cameras and a halogen lamp as illumination source. The principle of operation is explained and the system characteristics are reported in details, including the detection sensitivity and spatial resolution. Some limitations of the technique due to sample motion are studied theoretically and experimentally. A few images of biological samples are shown to illustrate the imaging capabilities.

2. The FF-OCM technique

2.1 Instrumentation

FF-OCM is typically based on the Linnik interference microscope configuration [19, 28]. The experimental arrangement is represented schematically in Figure 1. It consists of a Michelson interferometer with identical microscope objectives placed in both arms. Light is split into the reference and sample arms by a broadband beam splitter, with a variation of the ratio transmission/reflection less than 10% in the entire wavelength region of interest (700 - 1600 nm). The polished surface of an $Y_3Al_5O_{12}$ (YAG) crystal is placed in the reference arm of the Linnik interferometer in the focal plane of the microscope objective. This reference surface in contact with the immersion medium of the microscope objectives (water) provides a reflectivity $R_{ref} \sim 2.5\%$. A 100 W tungsten halogen lamp is incorporated in a Köhler system to provide uniform illumination of the microscope objective fields with spatially incoherent broadband light. The interferometric images delivered by the Linnik microscope are projected onto two camera arrays, a silicon-based CCD camera (Model 1M15 from Dalsa, 15 Hz, 1024×1024 pixels, 12 bits, called "Si camera" in this chapter) with a maximal sensitivity at the wavelength of ~ 750 nm and an InGaAs area scan camera (Model SU320MS from Sensors Unlimited, 25 Hz, 320×256 pixels, 12 bits, called here "InGaAs camera") with a maximal sensitivity at ~ 1300 nm. 2×2 pixel binning is applied with the Si camera to increase the dynamic range of the detection, and hence the detection sensitivity as will be explained later. This 2×2 pixel binning is performed numerically after each image acquisition. A dichroic mirror with high reflectivity (>98%) in the 650-950 nm band and high transmission (>85%) in the 1100 -1500 nm is used to separate both spectral bands before detection. Water-immersion microscope objectives (Olympus, 10×, numerical aperture of 0.3) are used to minimize dispersion mismatch in the interferometer arms as the imaging depth in the sample increases, and to reduce light reflection from the sample surface. The length of the interferometer reference arm can be varied without modifying the focus on the reference surface by translating together all the elements placed in this arm using a motorized axial translation stage. Another motorized axial translation stage is used to translate the objective in the sample arm so that the focus plane and the coherence plane always match. This adjustment is performed automatically by entering the proper value of the refractive index of the sample in the graphical interface of the FF-OCM system software.

2.2 Principle of operation

The tomographic signal in FF-OCM is extracted by calculating the amplitude of the interference signal using the principle of phase-shifting interferometry [17-21]. We use here a two-step phase-shifting method, *i.e.* The tomographic image is obtained by combination of only two interferometric images (two frames), the phase being shifted between each of them [25, 29].

The reference surface is attached to a piezoelectric actuator (PZT) to make it oscillate between two positions distant of a quarter of the illumination center wavelength divided by the refractive index of water, *i.e.* 0.14 µm when the Si camera is used and 0.23 µm when the InGaAs camera is used. The change of position of the reference mirror thus generates a phase-shift in the interferometer of about π. An adjustable number N of pairs of phase-

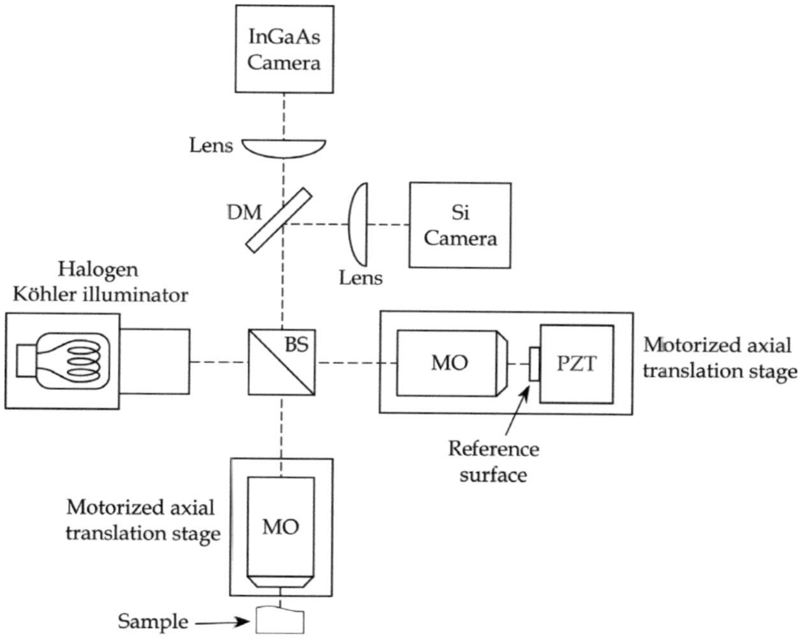

Fig. 1. Schematic of the experimental set-up of FF-OCM. MO, microscope objective; BS, beam-splitter cube; DM, dichroic mirror; PZT, piezoelectric actuator.

opposed interferometric images can thus be acquired by both cameras. The images corresponding to the same phase are summed up, which yields a single pair of frames that can be written as

$$E_1 = \left\{ \sum_{n=0}^{N-1} \left[\int_{2nT}^{(2n+1)T} I_1 dt \right] \right\}, \; E_2 = \left\{ \sum_{n=0}^{N-1} \left[\int_{(2n+1)T}^{(2n+2)T} I_2 dt \right] \right\}. \tag{1}$$

where T is the integration time of the camera in use. The irradiance (or intensity) I_1 and I_2 received by each pixels of the camera are (K being a proportionality coefficient):

$$\begin{cases} I_1(x,y,z) = K\left\{R_{sample}(x,y,z) + R_{ref} + 2\gamma(z)\sqrt{R_{sample}(x,y,z)R_{ref}}\cos\left[\phi(x,y,z)\right]\right\}, \\ I_2(x,y,z) = K\left\{R_{sample}(x,y,z) + R_{ref} + 2\gamma(z)\sqrt{R_{sample}(x,y,z)R_{ref}}\cos\left[\phi(x,y,z)+\pi\right]\right\}. \end{cases} \tag{2}$$

The squared difference of the pair of accumulated frames,

$$\left(E_1 - E_2\right)^2 = 16K^2N^2T^2R_{ref}\gamma^2(z)R_{sample}(x,y,z)\cos^2\left[\phi(x,y,z)\right], \tag{3}$$

is proportional to the three-dimensional reflectivity distribution of the sample $R_{sample}(x,y,z)$ multiplied by the coherence function $\gamma^2(z)$. It corresponds to an image of the reflecting or backscattering structures of the sample located in a slice, perpendicular to the optical axis, of width equal to the coherence length (width of the coherence function). This image corresponds to an *en face* tomographic image of the sample at depth z.

One can see from Eq. (3) that the tomographic image contains a term with the optical phase ϕ. A combination of more than two frames would be required to separate the amplitude and the phase [19-23]. However, due to the size and distribution of the structures in most samples being imaged, interference fringes are generally not visible in the tomographic images. We have adopted a method with only two frames to maximize the processing speed. A tomographic image can be produced at a maximum rate equal to half the camera frame rate, *i.e.* 7.5 Hz with the Si camera and 12.5 Hz with the InGaAs camera. However, in practice it is necessary to accumulate several interferometric images to improve the detection sensitivity, as will be shown later. The tomographic images are then produced at a frequency on the order of 1 Hz.

3. System characteristics

3.1 Detection sensitivity

Detection sensitivity is a key system parameter in OCT that affects the imaging contrast and penetration depth. Several possible sources of noise have to be considered for the determination of the detection sensitivity in FF-OCM. In addition to the shot noise induced by the fundamental photon noise, other kinds of noise originating from the cameras may not be negligible such as the electrical noise, including the read out noise and the dark noise. Assuming the well of the camera pixels to be full upon maximal illumination, and neglecting the relative intensity noise, it has been shown [19, 21, 22, 30] that the minimal detectable reflectivity can be written as

$$R_{min} = \frac{\left(R_{inc} + R_{ref}\right)^2}{4NR_{ref}} \left(\frac{1}{\xi_{sat}} + \frac{\eta^2}{\xi_{sat}^2} \right). \tag{4}$$

The parameter ξ_{sat} denotes the full-well-capacity of the camera pixels, and η the noise-equivalent electrons representing the total electrical noise. One can see from Eq. (4) that increasing the full-well-capacity decreases the value of R_{min} (*i.e.* the sensitivity is improved). The full-well-capacity can be increased by custom adjustment of the camera gain setting. However, since increasing the gain also generally causes the electrical noise of the camera to increase in the same proportion (η and ξ_{sat} are proportional) [22, 30], one can see from Eq. (4) that the sensitivity is limited. Besides, a larger full-well-capacity requires a more powerful light source, which constitutes a technological limit. At last, the illumination power that can be tolerated by the sample is also limited, especially when the sample is a biological medium.

One can also see from Eq. (4) that the detection sensitivity depends on the amount of incoherent light, through the parameter R_{inc}. This parameter represents the proportion of incoherent light (light that does not interfere), resulting essentially from backscattering and backreflection by structures within the sample present outside the coherence volume. The detection sensitivity is maximized (R_{min} is minimized) when R_{inc} is minimal. For that purpose, all the optical components are antireflection coated and the beam-splitter is slightly tilted to avoid specular reflections. We have measured that the incoherent light coming from the setup without sample represents a reflectivity of $R_{inc} \sim 0.5\%$. When a biological sample is imaged, the reflection on the sample surface is minimized by index matching, achieved by using water-immersion objectives. The incoherent light coming from typical biological samples and collected by the microscope objective does not exceed a few percents. The reference mirror reflectivity R_{ref} has also an influence on the detection sensitivity. By calculating the derivative of Eq. (4) with respect to R_{ref}, one can easily establish that the optimal value of R_{ref} is reached when $R_{ref} = R_{inc}$, which is approximately the case in practice ($R_{ref} = 2.5\%$).

At last, Equation (4) indicates that the detection sensitivity can be improved with image accumulation (parameter N). The benefit of image accumulation is illustrated in Figure 2. A mouse embryo embedded in an agarose gel was imaged with different accumulation numbers. The signal-to-noise ratio in the images is clearly improved when the accumulation number is increased. Since accumulating images increases the acquisition time, this way of improving the detection sensitivity is however limited if the sample is likely to move during this time. *In vivo* imaging, in particular, may be incompatible with image accumulation. A study of artifacts in FF-OCM induced by sample motion will be presented in section 4.

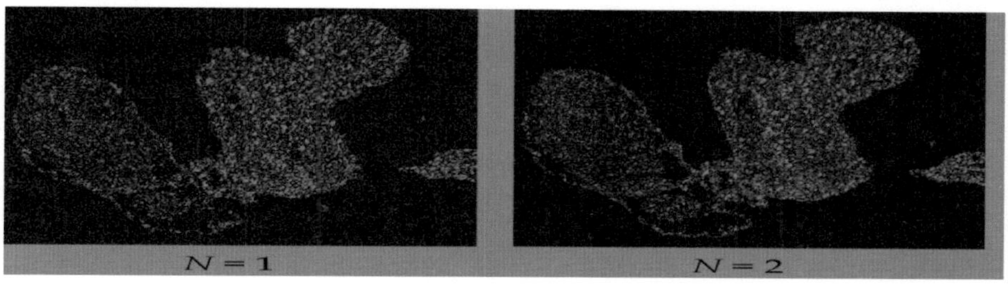

Fig. 2. FF-OCM images of a mouse embryo, *in vitro*, for different numbers N of accumulated images, using the Si camera.

Measurements of the detection sensitivity were carried out. A glass plate was used as low reflectivity sample. The results are summarized in Figure 3 showing the value of $R_{\min}$ in logarithmic scale as a function of the number N of images accumulated by each camera. One can see that a detection sensitivity on the order of - 90 dB is achievable with an accumulation of 10 images using the Si camera and 30 images using the InGaAs camera, which represents an acquisition time of ~ 1 s and 2 s for the Si and InGaAs cameras respectively. The straight lines correspond to the sensitivity calculated with Eq. (4) by taking $R_{ref} = 2.5\%$ and $R_{inc} = 0.5\%$ for both cameras. For the Si camera, we considered a full-well-capacity $\xi_{sat} = 1\times10^6$ (with 2×2 pixel binning) and a noise-equivalent electrons $\eta = 0$; for the InGaAs camera, these parameters were $\xi_{sat} \sim 8\times10^5$ and $\eta = 400$. The theory is in agreement with the experiment for the Si camera, whereas a discrepancy is observed for the InGaAs camera, which may be explained by the presence of additional noise not taken into account in the model and (or) optical aberrations of the microscope objectives at these large wavelengths.

3.2 Wavelength and imaging penetration depth

Detection sensitivity affects the imaging contrast and therefore the imaging penetration depth. For a given sensitivity, however, the imaging penetration depth may depend on the illumination wavelength. The propagation of light in biological media is affected by two wavelength-dependant attenuation mechanisms: scattering and absorption. Scattering is due to the presence of structures within the sample creating refractive index heterogeneities.

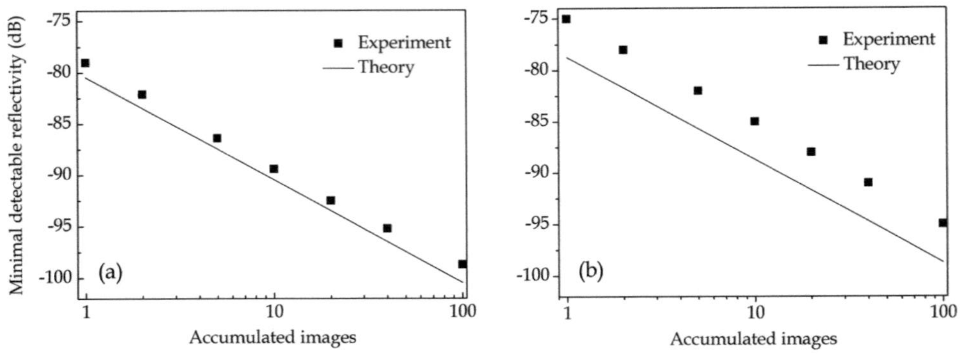

Fig. 3. Detection sensitivity of FF-OCM as a function of image accumulation using the Si camera (a) and the InGaAs camera (b).

The intensity of light scattered by these particles depends strongly on their size and nature. A general tendency of scattering is a decrease of its intensity when wavelength increases [31, 32]. Absorption of light in biological media is dominated by the absorption water. This absorption is minimal at the wavelength of ~ 500 nm and globally increases with wavelength [33]. The optimal wavelength to maximize the OCT imaging penetration depth results from the best trade-off between scattering and absorption. Previous works have shown better imaging penetration depth in highly scattering tissues for OCT operating in the 1300 nm wavelength region compared to 800 nm [34, 35]. Similar results were also observed in FF-OCM [36].

The effect of scattering on the imaging penetration depth was studied in FF-OCM by imaging a highly contrasted sample placed behind a scattering medium. We considered as sample a mask for photolithography made of metallic structures deposited on a glass substrate. The scattering medium was a 3 mm-thick layer of 4% Intralipid solution commonly used to simulate scattering by biological media [37, 38]. Figures 4 shows *en face* tomographic images in the plane of the glass surface through the scattering layer, obtained with both cameras with the same detection sensitivity (by adjustement of the accumulation number N). The metallic structures of the sample are perfectly revealed by using the InGaAs camera, whereas they are almost completely obscured by the scattering medium when imaged with the Si camera because of much stronger scattering.

When a biological sample is imaged, however, the situation is quite different because the intensity of light backscattered by the structures inside the sample is also wavelength-dependent, which was not the case with the sample considered here. Reduced scattering permits longer propagation distances of useful light, but on the other hand weakens the signal resulting from backscattering by small particles.

3.3 Axial resolution

In conventional OCT, the axial response is governed by the coherence function $\gamma(z)$ equal to the Fourier transform of the effective source power spectrum [3]. Since this technique produces cross-sectional images (B scans), a large depth of focus is generally required, which imposes

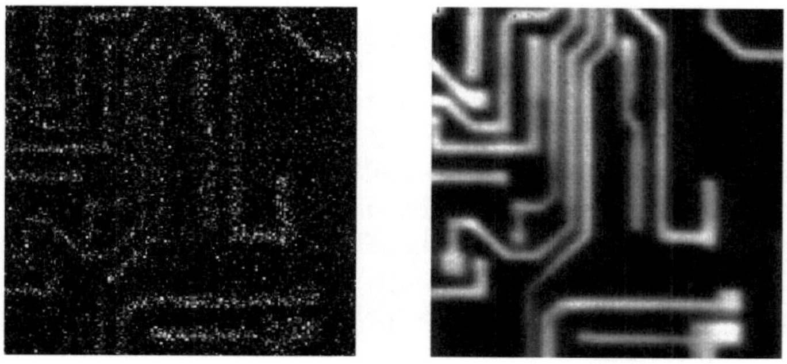

(a) (b)

Fig. 4. FF-OCM images, using the Si camera (a) and the InGaAs camera (b), of a mask for photolithography through a layer of 3 mm thick Intralipid solution.

the use of low numerical aperture optics. FF-OCM acquires images in the *en face* orientation like a conventional microscope, which permits the use of microscope objectives of relatively high numerical aperture (*NA*). In that case, the axial response is determined not only by the coherence function but also by the depth of focus. Assuming a Gaussian-shaped effective spectrum, the theoretical axial resolution of FF-OCM can be defined, at the surface of the sample, as [19]

$$\Delta z = \left[\frac{NA^2}{n_{im}\lambda} + \frac{n_{im}\pi}{2\ln 2}\left(\frac{\Delta\lambda}{\lambda^2}\right) \right]^{-1}, \tag{5}$$

where n_{im} is the refractive index of the objective immersion medium, λ the center wavelength and $\Delta\lambda$ the full-width at half maximun (FWHM) of the effective optical spectrum given by the product of the light source, the spectral transmission of the system optical components including the sample and the immersion medium themselves, and the spectral response of the camera in use.

The set-up described here is characterized by a relatively modest numerical aperture ($NA = 0.3$) and a very broadband light source (halogen lamp); the axial resolution is then essentially imposed by the temporal coherence in both detection bands. The theoretical axial resolution with the Si camera was calculated to be equal to 0.75 µm (λ = 750 nm, $\Delta\lambda$ = 250 nm). With the InGaAs camera, the absorption by the immersion medium (water) limits the effective spectral range above 1400 nm (although the spectral response of the InGaAs camera extends to 1700 nm). Considering an effective spectrum of width $\Delta\lambda$ = 400 nm centered at λ = 1250 nm, the theoretical axial resolution is 1.3 µm. The use of dry microscope objectives would yield a theoretical axial resolution of 0.9 µm because of a broader effective spectrum. However, it would severely degrade as the imaging depth in the sample increases because of dispersion mismatch in the interferometer [24]. From a certain depth, the axial resolution with dry objectives would even be weaker than the one obtained with immersion objectives. A configuration with water-immersion objectives was therefore favored to minimize dispersion mismatch and also reduce the reflection of light at the surface of the sample. The degradation of axial resolution with depth is then weak, but cannot be totally avoided because of refractive index inhomogeneities in the sample that are at the origin of the image contrast.

We have measured the interferogram response of our FF-OCM system with both cameras using a glass plate as sample (see Figure 5). The coherence function that comprises the interference fringes looks Gaussian with the Si camera. In comparison with broadband sources used in ultrahigh-resolution OCT, such as ultra-short femtosecond lasers or supercontinuum fiber lasers [39, 40], a thermal light source provides a smoother spectrum that does not contain spikes or emission lines that could cause side lobes in the coherence function and create artifacts in the images. The coherence function measured with the InGaAs camera, in contrast with the Si camera, has some wings resulting from dips in the effective spectrum due to water absorption [29, 33, 36]. The experimental FWHM of the coherence function was found to be 0.8 μm for the Si camera and 1.5 μm for the InGaAs camera, close to the theoretical values.

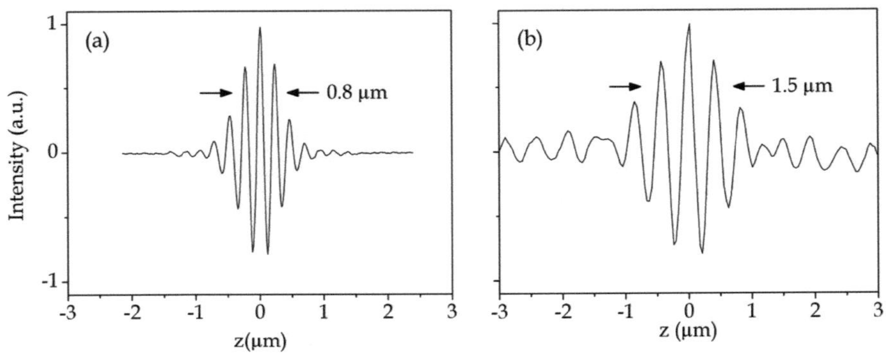

Fig. 5. Interferogram response measured with the Si camera (a) and the InGaAs camera (b). The width (FWHM) of the interferogram envelope is indicated.

3.4 Transverse resolution

The transverse resolution of an imaging system is commonly defined as the width of the transverse point-spread function (TPSF). When the optical system is diffraction-limited (*i.e.* bare of any optical aberration), the TPSF is the well-known Airy function. In that case an expression of the theoretical transverse resolution is

$$\Delta r = \frac{\lambda}{2NA}. \tag{6}$$

The previous equation gives theoretical diffraction-limited resolutions of 1.3 μm and 2.1 μm for the FF-OCM system using the Si camera and the InGaAs camera respectively, when microscope objective with numerical aperture of NA = 0.3 are employed.

We have measured the FWHM of the experimental TPSF of our FF-OCM system indirectly by recording an intensity profile across a cleaved mirror. Theoretically, the response is the convolution of a perfect edge and the experimental TPSF and a rectangular function that simulates the image sampling by the camera pixels. We considered here a Gaussian-shaped TPSF. Simulations were carried out to fit the experimental data by adjusting the TPSF width. The results are presented in Table 1. The experimental transverse resolutions are 1.4 μm and

2.7 μm for the Si and InGaAs cameras respectively. The degradation between experimental and theoretical transverse resolution for the InGaAs setup is attributed to optical aberrations of the microscope objectives that are not optimized in the spectral region detected by the InGaAs camera. Their transmission drops from 81% at 800 nm to 59% at 1200 nm. Moreover, optical aberrations are not well corrected, which degrades the image contrast and resolution.

	Theoretical	Experimental
Δr (μm) Si camera	1.3	1.4
Δr (μm) InGaAs camera	2.1	2.7

Table 1. Transverse resolution Δr associated to each camera. Microscope objectives with a numerical aperture of 0.3 were employed.

4. Sample motion artifacts

Artifacts resulting from motion of the sample being imaged occur in nearly all biomedical imaging modalities [41-43], including OCT [44]. Great efforts have been made to eliminate these artifacts since they may severely degrade the image quality and cause misinterpretations. In this section, we propose a theoretical and experimental study of motion artifacts in FF-OCM [45]. We distinguish the effect of signal loss and the effect of spurious signal apparition.

4.1 Loss of signal

Optical systems based on interferometry are generally very sensitive to vibrations. Due to the short wavelength of optical waves, path length variations of only a few tens of nanometers may generate significant phase changes, which may cause a blurring of the detected interference signal if the integration time of the detector is not short enough.

In FF-OCM, sample motions along the axial direction generate changes of the optical path length of the interferometer sample arm. In contrast, motions along the transverse direction do not change the optical path length. Assuming monochromatic illumination at wavelength λ and axial displacement of the sample at constant speed v, the optical phase in the interferometer varies linearly with time as

$$\phi(t) = \frac{4\pi n}{\lambda} vt, \tag{7}$$

where n denotes the refractive index of the immersion medium. The tomographic image obtained from the squared difference of two phase-opposed accumulated interferometric images can then be written as

$$\begin{aligned}(E_1 - E_2)^2 &= 4K^2\gamma^2 R_{sample} R_{ref} \left\{ \sum_{n=0}^{N-1} \left[\int_{2nT}^{(2n+2)T} \cos\left(\frac{4\pi n}{\lambda} vt \right) dt \right] \right\}^2 \\ &= 16K^2\gamma^2 N^2 T^2 R_{sample} R_{ref} \times B(v),\end{aligned} \tag{8}$$

where

$$B(v) = \left[\frac{\sin\left(\frac{8\pi n}{\lambda} vNT \right)}{\left(\frac{8\pi n}{\lambda} vNT \right)} \right]^2 . \quad (9)$$

One can see from the previous equations that the variation of the amplitude of the tomographic signal with axial speed of the sample is described by the function $B(v)$. One can define the maximal tolerable speed v_{max} as the first zero of the function $B(v)$, *i.e.*

$$v_{\max} = \frac{\lambda}{8nNT} . \quad (10)$$

The maximal tolerable speed corresponds to a displacement of the sample of $\lambda/4n$ during the total acquisition time (equal to $2NT$), which corresponds to an optical path length change of $\lambda/2n$ or a phase change of π. Theoretical values of v_{max} calculated with Eq. (10) are reported in Table 2 for both cameras for different accumulation numbers N.

Accumulations N	1	2	5	10	20
$v_{\max}$ (µm/s) Si camera	1.05	0.53	0.21	0.10	0.05
$v_{\max}$ (µm/s) InGaAs camera	2.94	1.47	0.59	0.29	0.15

Table 2. Maximal tolerable axial speed of the sample for both cameras. These theoretical values are obtained by computation of Eq. (10) with [T = 67 ms, λ = 750 nm] for the Si camera , and [T = 40 ms, λ = 1250 nm] for the InGaAs camera. The immersion medium is water (n = 1.33).

We also performed measurements of the amplitude of the tomographic signal as a function of axial speed of the sample. For this experiment, a mirror mounted on a piezoelectric actuator was used as a sample. The position of the mirror at zero voltage applied to the piezoelectric coincided with the focal plane of the microscope objective. Figure 6 shows how the amplitude of the tomographic signal decreases as a function of the mirror axial speed for accumulations of 1, 2 and 3 pairs of images. A very good agreement is observed between the experimental data and the theoretical curves based on Eq. (9).

In conclusion, the present FF-OCM technique is not appropriate for imaging samples whose axial motion is faster than 1µm/s typically. *In vivo* imaging may therefore be difficult with this technique. For example the speed of blood flow is a few hundreds of µm/s. Physiological motions such as the cardiac motion may even reach 100 mm/s. For these kinds of applications, a shorter acquisition time is definitely required. High speed systems have been proposed [45-49], making *in vivo* imaging possible. However, the detection sensitivity of these systems is quite low. A real benefit would be to use a camera such that the ratio ξ_{sat}/T is larger. The reduction of acquisition time, without loss of sensitivity, would then be approximately inversely proportional to the increase of this ratio, provided that the

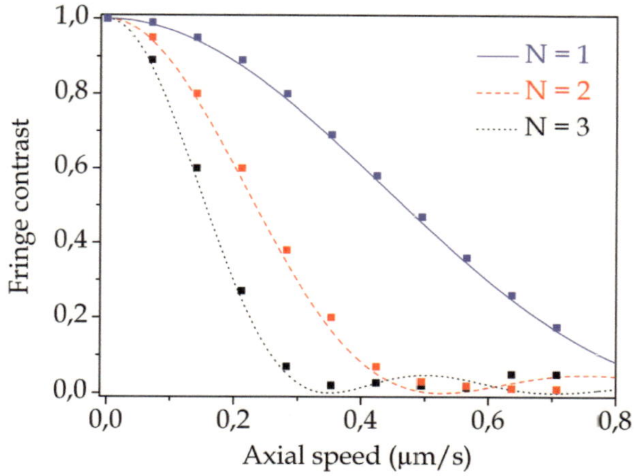

Fig. 6. Fringe contrast as a function of axial speed of the sample using the Si camera, for different accumulation numbers *N*. Comparison between experimental data (squares) and theory (lines).

brightness of the light source can be sufficiently increased to fill the pixel wells and that the sample can tolerate a higher illumination power.

4.2 Spurious signal

FF-OCM images are obtained by combination of interferometric images (frames) acquired sequentially in time. The tomographic signal in FF-OCM is generated by the variation of the interferometric signal amplitude induced by the phase-shift introduced between these successive frames by the reference surface oscillation. However, the intensity of light upon each pixel of the cameras may also vary if the backscattering structures of the sample move transversally. This variation of intensity generates a spurious signal, which superimposes on the tomographic signal and may cause misinterpretations of the tomographic images. Axial motion of the sample has much less influence on this spurious signal, since it only causes a defocus, which does not change significantly the intensity of light received by each pixel.

We performed numerical simulations to evaluate the effect of continuous transverse motion of the sample during the integration time of the camera. We considered as a sample a particle smaller than the optical wavelength. The image of this particle on the camera array detector is assumed to be an Airy pattern of dimension determined by the center wavelength and the numerical aperture of the microscope objective (see Eq. (6)), and also the magnification of the complete imaging system. The principle of the simulation is to calculate the variation of intensity on the CCD pixels induced by a transverse displacement of the particle. We consider that the motion of the particle becomes visible when the resulting intensity variation is greater than the minimal detectable reflectivity R_{min} given by Eq. (4). Figure 7 shows the evolution of the maximal tolerable transverse speed of the particle as a function of its reflectivity for different accumulation numbers. For example, for a particle with equivalent reflectivity of 10^{-5} and an accumulation of 5 pairs of images, transverse motion at speed lower than ~ 100 μm/s is not visible. The effect of transverse motion is clearly less severe than the effect of axial motion. Artifacts resulting from transverse motion can even be completely removed if the frames are acquired simultaneously and not sequentially in time. For that purpose, instantaneous phase-shifting interferometry was successfully applied in FF-OCM, at the price of an increase in system complexity, calibration and cost [45, 46, 48, 50].

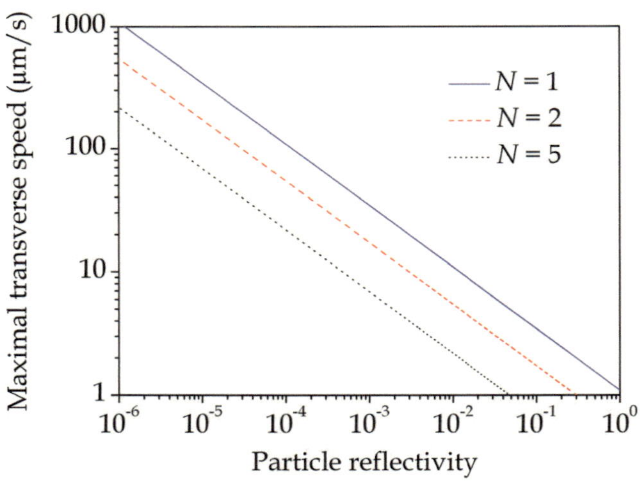

Fig. 7. Theoretical maximal transverse speed of a particle versus its reflectivity, using the Si camera. The calculations were done for different accumulation numbers *N*.

5. Illustration of imaging capabilities

The imaging capability of FF-OCM in the biomedical field has been extensively reported. Cellular-level resolution images of various ophthalmic tissues [51], embryos and plants [24, 25, 52, 53] have been published. A few other examples obtained with the FF-OCM technique described in this chapter are presented in this section. All the biological samples considered here are biopsy tissues. They were imaged *ex vivo*, with a drop of physiological serum inserted between the microscope objective and the samples. The microscope objectives, with numerical aperture of 0.3, had a working distance of 3.3 mm. The experimental procedure consisted of acquiring a stack of tomographic images at successive depths in constant steps of 0.7 μm. Sections in arbitrary orientations could then be computed for display. All the images are presented in logarithmic scale using different colormaps.

Cross-sectional images of rabbit cornea, obtained with both cameras, are presented in Figure 8. Two layers corresponding to the choroid and the sclera of the cornea can be distinguished. As expected, deeper structures can be imaged by using the InGaAs camera. The spatial resolution, however, is better at shorter wavelengths using the Si camera.

Another example of tissue imaged with FF-OCM is presented in Figure 9. The sample consisted of a piece of cartilage removed from a pig shoulder. Two sections in orthogonal orientations (cross-sectional and *en face*) show the distribution of isogenous groups within the cartilage tissue. The territorial and interterritorial matrices are clearly visible. Within the cartilage matrix, cells are located in spaces called lacunae filled by chondrocyte. In *ex vivo* cartilage, however, the cells frequently shrink and even fall out. Only empty spaces, where the chondrocytes once sat, are probably observed here.

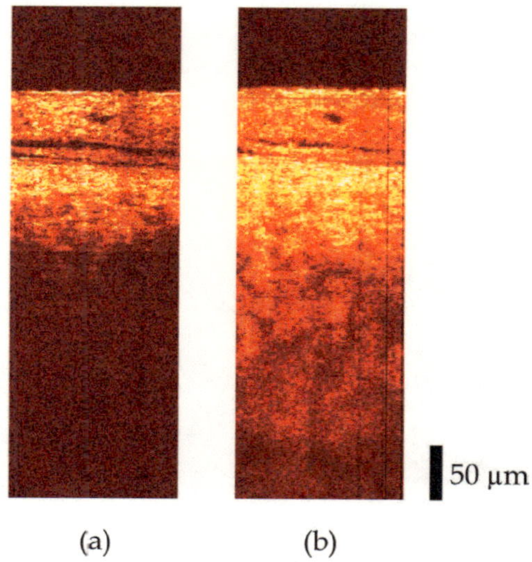

Fig. 8. FF-OCM images of rabbit cornea, *in vitro*, obtained with the Si camera (a) and the InGaAs camera (b). These cross-sectional (XZ) tomographic images are computed from a stack of 800 *en face* tomographic images.

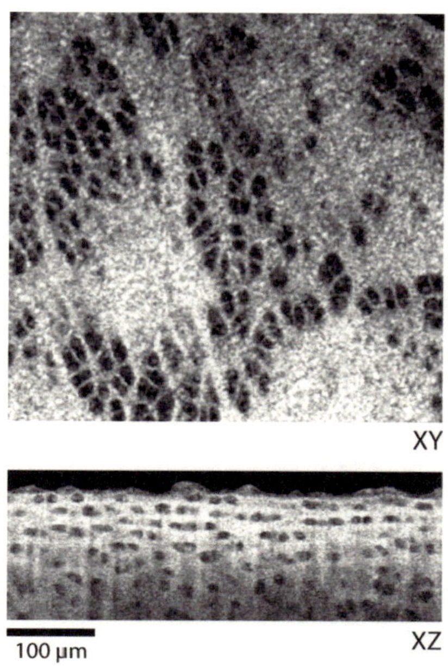

Fig. 9. FF-OCM images, in orthogonal views, of pig cartilage from a biopsy conducted in the region of the shoulder.

A cross-sectional image of human skin obtained with FF-OCM is shown in Figure 10. The skin sample was imaged immediately after a punch biopsy performed in the region of the forearm. The cross-sectional view allows for the visualization of different layers. The epidermis and dermis layers, in particular, can be clearly distinguished. Theses layers are separated by the papillary region. The reticular region in the dermal layer contains small blood vessels, lymph and nerves, fine collagen and elastic fibers. The epidermis layer is composed of several thinner layers including the stratum corneum, the stratum granulosum, the stratum spinosum and the stratum basale.

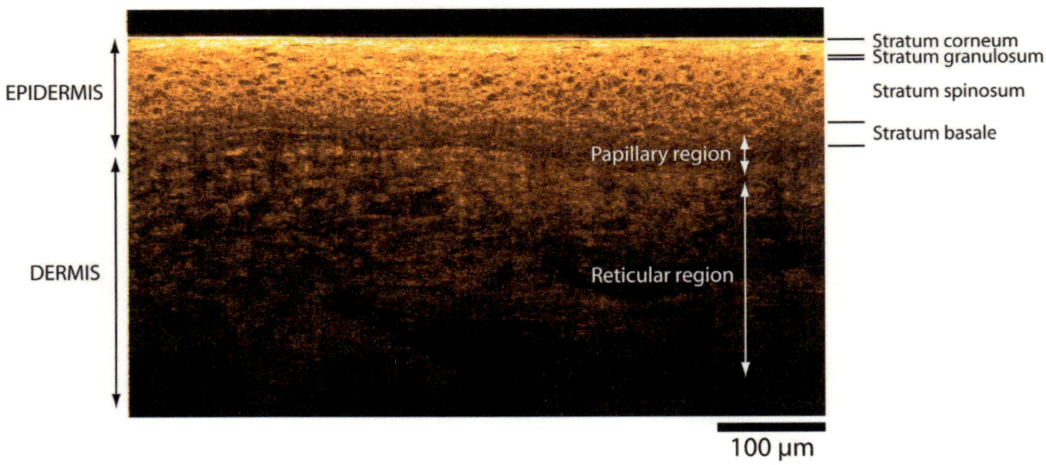

Fig. 10. FF-OCM cross-sectional image of human skin in the forearm region.

6. Conclusion

FF-OCM is an alternative technique to conventional scanning OCM that provides ultrahigh-resolution images using a simple tungsten-halogen lamp, instead of a sophisticated laser-based source. We have demonstrated here a system capable of imaging in two distinct spectral regions, which is relevant depending on whether one wish to favor the imaging penetration depth or the spatial resolution. With a spatial resolution approaching that of microscopy, this technology has the potential to replace conventional methods used for histology. *In vivo* imaging is still difficult with FF-OCM because of the appearance of artifacts resulting from sample motion. With the constant advances in the technologies of cameras and light sources, one can reasonably think that the acquisition speed of FF-OCM will be considerably improved in a near future. FF-OCM would then become a powerful tool for ultrahigh-resolution *in vivo* imaging without any contrast agent, making *in situ* examination possible without the need for histological processing of tissues.

7. Acknowledgment

This work would not have been possible without the invaluable contribution of postdoctoral associates and PhD students, including Delphine Sacchet, Gael Moneron, Kate Grieve, Julien Moreau, Elvire Guiot, Wilfrid Schwartz, and Laurent Vabre. I acknowledge the fruitful collaborations with multidisciplinary research teams and the company LLTech. I thank the ophthalmologists Jean-François Legargasson, Michel Paques, Manuel Simonutti, and José Sahel of the "Laboratoire de Physiopathologie Cellulaire et Moléculaire de la Rétine" at "Institut National de la Santé et de la Recherche Médicale", and of the Ophthalmology Department, at the "Fondation Ophthalmologique Rothschild" in Paris. We are grateful to the physicists François Lacombe, Marie Glanc, Pierre Léna, from the "Observatoire de Paris", Ruikang Wang and Ying Yang from Cranfield University (UK). I thank the biologists Jérôme Collignon and Aitana Perea-Gomez, at "Institut Jacques Monod", Jean-François Riou at "Université Pierre et Marie Curie" in Paris, Luc Fetler at "Institut Pasteur" in Paris, Martine Boccara at "Génoplante" in Evry. Lastly, I am particularly grateful to Claude Boccara for our impassioned discussions.

This research has been supported by the "Centre National de la Recherche Scientifique (CNRS)" and the French Research Ministry ("Ministère de la Recherche").

8. References

[1] Huang, D.; Swanson, E.A.; Lin, C.P.; Schuman, J.S.; Stinson, W.G.; Chang, W.; Hee, M.R.; Flotte, T.; Gregory, K.; Puliafito, C.A. & Fujimoto J.G. (1991). Optical Coherence Tomography. *Science*, Vol.254, pp. 1178-1181

[2] Fujimoto, J.G.; Brezinski, M.E.; Tearney, G.J.; Boppart, S.A.; Bouma, B.E.; Hee, M.R.; Southern, J.F. & Swanson E.A. (1995). Optical biopsy and imaging using optical coherence tomography. *Nature Medicine*, Vol.1, pp. 970-972

[3] Fercher, A.F. (1996). Optical coherence tomography. *Journal of Biomedical Optics*, Vol.1, pp. 157-173

[4] Tearney, G.J.; Bouma, B.E.; Boppart, S.A.; Golubovic, B.; Swanson, E.A. & Fujimoto, J.G. (1996). Rapid acquisition of in-vivo biological images by use of optical coherence tomography. *Optics Letters*, Vol.21, pp. 1408-1410

[5] Swanson, E.A.; Izatt, J.A.; Hee, M.R.; Huang, D.; Lin, C.P.; Schuman, J.S.; Puliafito, C.A.; Fujimoto, J.G. (1993). In-vivo retinal imaging by optical coherence tomography. *Optics Letters*, Vol.18, pp. 1864-1866

[6] Wojtkowski, M.; Leitgeb, R.; Kowalczyk, A.; Bajraszewski, T. & Fercher, A.F. (2002). In-vivo human retinal imaging by Fourier domain optical coherence tomography. *Journal of Biomedical Optics*, Vol.7, pp. 457-463

[7] Hitzenberger, C.K.; Trost, P.; Lo, P.W. & Zhou, Q. (2003). Three-dimensional imaging of the human retina by high-speed optical coherence tomography, *Optics Express*, Vol.11, pp. 2753-2761

[8] Nassif, N.; Cense, B.; Park, B.H.; Yun, S.H.; Chen, T.C.; Bouma, B.E.; Tearney G.J., & de Boer, J.F. (2004). In-vivo human retinal imaging by ultrahigh-speed spectral domain optical coherence tomography. *Optics Letters*, Vol.29, pp. 480-482

[9] Izatt, J.A.; Hee, M.R.; Swanson, E.A.; Lin, C.P.; Huang, D.; Schuman, J.S.; Puliafito C.A. & Fujimoto, J.G. (1994). Micrometer-scale resolution imaging of the anterior eye in vivo with optical coherence tomography, *Archives of Ophthalmology*, Vol.112, pp. 1584-1589

[10] Trefford, S. & Desmond, F. (2008). Optical Coherence Tomography of the Anterior Segment. *Ocular Surface*, Vol.6, pp. 117-127

[11] Fujimoto, J.G. (2003). Optical coherence tomography for ultrahigh resolution in vivo imaging. *Nature Biotechnology*, Vol. 21, pp. 1361-1367

[12] Desmond, C.A.; Stenger, J.; Gorczynska, I; Lie, H.; Teri, H.; Spronk, R.; Wolohojian, S., Khandekar, N.; Jiang, J.Y.; Barry, S.; Cable, A.E.; Huber, R. & Fujimoto J.G. (2007). Comparison of three-dimensional optical coherence tomography and high resolution photography for art conservation studies. *Optics Express*, Vol.15, pp. 15972-15986

[13] Wiesauer, K.; Pircher, M.; Götzinger, E.; Bauer, S.; Engelke, R.; Ahrens, G.; Grützner, G.; Hitzenberger, C. & Stifter, D. (2005). En face scanning optical coherence tomography with ultra-high resolution for material investigation. *Optics Express*, Vol.13, pp. 1015-1024

[14] Izatt, J.A.; Hee, M.R.; Owen, G.M.; Swanson, E.A. & Fujimoto J.G. (1994). Optical coherence microscopy in scattering media. *Optics Letters*, Vol.19, pp. 590-592

[15] Podoleanu, A.G.; Dobre, G.M. & Jackson, D.A. (1998). En face coherence imaging using galvanometer scanner modulation. *Optics Letters*, Vol.23, pp. 147-149

[16] Caber, P.J. (1993). Interferometric profiler for rough surfaces. *Applied Optics*, Vol.32, pp. 3438-3441

[17] Larkin, K.G. (1996). Efficient nonlinear algorithm for envelope detection in white light interferometry, *Journal of the Optical Society of America A*, Vol.13, pp. 832-843

[18] Kino, G.S. & Chim, S.C. (1990). Mirau correlation microscope, *Applied Optics*, Vol. 29, pp. 3775-3783

[19] Dubois, A.; Vabre, L.; Boccara, A.C. & Beaurepaire, E. (2002). High-resolution full-field optical coherence tomography with a Linnik microscope. *Applied Optics*, Vol.41, pp. 805-812

[20] Vabre, L.; Dubois, A. & Boccara, A.C. (2002). Thermal-light full-field optical coherence tomography. *Optics Letters*, Vol.27, pp. 530-532

[21] Laude, B.; De Martino, A.; Drévillon, B.; Benattar, L. & Schwartz, L. (2002). Full-field optical coherence tomography with thermal light. *Applied Optics*, Vol. 41, pp. 6637-6645

[22] Oh, W.-Y.; Bouma, B. E.; Iftimia, N.; Yelin, R. & Tearney, G.J. (2006). Spectrally-modulated full-field optical coherence microscopy for ultrahigh-resolution endoscopic imaging. *Optics Express*, Vol.14, pp. 8675-8684

[23] Sato, M.; Nagata, T.; Niizuma, T.; Neagu, L.; Dabu, R. & Watanabe, Y. (2007). Quadrature fringes wide-field optical coherence tomography and its applications to biological tissues. *Optics Communications*, Vol.271, pp. 573-580

[24] Dubois, A.; Grieve, K.; Moneron, G.; Lecaque, R.; Vabre, L. & Boccara, A.C. (2004). Ultrahigh-resolution full-field optical coherence tomography. *Applied Optics*, Vol.43, pp. 2874-2882

[25] Dubois, A.; Moneron, G.; Grieve, K. & Boccara, A.C. (2004). Three-dimensional cellular-level imaging using full-field optical coherence tomography. *Physics in Medicine and Biology*, Vol.49, pp. 1227-1234

[26] Dubois, A.; Moreau, J. & Boccara, A.C. (2008). Spectroscopic ultrahigh-resolution full-field optical coherence microscopy. *Optics Express*, Vol.16, pp. 17082-17091

[27] Moneron, G.; Boccara, A.C. & Dubois, A. (2007). Polarization-sensitive full-field optical coherence tomography. *Optics Letters*, Vol.32, pp. 2058-2060

[28] Gale, D.M.; Pether M.I. & Dainty, J.C. (1996). Linnik microscope imaging of integrated circuit structures. *Applied Optics*, Vol.35, pp. 131-148

[29] Dubois, A.; Moneron, G. & Boccara, A.C. (2006). Thermal-light full-field optical coherence tomography in the 1.2 micron wavelength region. *Optics Communications*, Vol.266, pp. 738-743

[30] Oh, W.Y.; Bouma, B.E.; Iftimia, N.; Yun, S.H.; Yelin, R. & Tearney G.J. (2006). Ultrahigh-resolution full-field optical coherence microscopy using InGaAs camera. *Optics Express*, Vol.14, pp. 726-735

[31] Parsa, P.; Jacques, S.L. & Nishioka, N.S. (1989). Optical properties of rat liver between 350 and 2200 nm. *Applied Optics*, Vol. 28, pp. 2325-2330

[32] Schmitt, J.M.; Knuttel, A.; Yadlowsky, M. & Eckhaus, M.A. (1994). Optical coherence tomography of a dense tissue: statistics of attenuation and backscattering. *Physics in Medicine and Biology*, Vol.39, pp. 1705-1720

[33] Hale, G.M.; Querry, M.R. (1973). Optical constants of water in the 200 nm - 200 μm wavelength region. *Applied Optics*, Vol. 12, pp. 555-563

[34] Pan, Y. & Farkas D. L. (1998). Noninvasive imaging of living human skin with dual-wavelength optical coherence tomography in two and three dimensions. *Journal of Biomedical Optics*, Vol.3, pp. 446-455.

[35] Aguirre, A.D.; Nishizawa, N.; Seitz, W.; Ledere, M.; Kopf, D. & Fujimoto, J.G. (2006). Continuum generation in a novel photonic crystal fiber for ultrahigh resolution optical coherence tomography at 800 nm and 1300 nm. *Optics Express*, Vol.14, pp. 1145-1160

[36] Sacchet, D.; Moreau, J.; Georges, P. & Dubois, A. (2008). Simultaneous dual-band ultra-high resolution full-field optical coherence tomography. *Optics Express*, Vol.16, pp. 19434-19446

[37] Van Staveren, H.G.; Moes, C.J.M.; Van Marle, J.; Prahl, S.A. & Van Gemert, M.J.C. (1991). Light scattering in Intralipid-10% in the wavelength range of 400-1100 nanometers. *Applied Optics*, Vol.30, pp. 4507-4515

[38] Flock, S.T.; Jacques, S.L.; Wilson, B.C; Star, W.M. & Van Gemert, M.J.C. (1992). Optical properties of Intralipid: a phantom medium for light propagation studies. *Lasers in Surgery and Medicine*, Vol. 12, pp. 510-519

[39] Drexler, W.; Morgner, U.; Kärtner, F.X.; Pitris, C.; Boppart, S.A.; Li, X.D.; Ippen, E.P. & Fujimoto, J.G. (1999). In-vivo ultrahigh-resolution optical coherence tomography. *Optics Letters*, Vol. 24, pp. 1221-1223

[40] Wang, Y.; Zhao, Y.; Nelson, J.S.; Chen, Z. & Windeler, R.S. (2003). Ultrahigh-resolution optical coherence tomography by broadband continuum generation from a photonic crystal fiber. *Optics Letters*, Vol.28, pp. 182-184

[41] Alfidi, R. J.; MacIntyre, W. J. & Haaga, R. (1976). The effects of biological motion in CT resolution. *American Journal of Radiology*, Vol.127, pp. 11-15

[42] Wood, M.L. & Henkelman, R.M. (1985). NMR image artifact from periodic motion. *Medical Physics*, Vol.12, pp. 143-151

[43] Nadkarni, S.K.; Boughner, D.R.; Drangova, M. & Fenster, A. (2001). In vitro simulation and quantification of temporal jitter artifacts in ECG-gated dynamic three-dimensional echocardiography. *Ultrasound in Medicine & Biology*, Vol.27, pp. 211-222

[44] Yun, S.H.; Tearney, G.; De Boer, J. & Bouma, B. (2004). Motion artifacts in optical coherence tomography with frequency-domain ranging, *Optics Express*, Vol.12, pp. 2977-2998

[45] Sacchet, D.; Brzezinski, M.; Moreau, J.; Georges, P. & Dubois, A. (2010). Motion artifact suppression in full-field optical coherence tomography. *Applied Optics*, Vol.49, pp. 1480-1488

[46] Moneron, G.; Boccara, A.C & Dubois, A. (2005). Stroboscopic ultrahigh-resolution full-field optical coherence tomography, *Optics Letters*, Vol.30, pp. 1351-1353

[47] Grieve, K. ; Dubois, A. ; Simonutti, M. ; Pâques, M. ; Sahel, J. ; Le Gargasson, J.F. & Boccara A.C. (2005). In vivo anterior segment imaging in the rat eye with high speed white light full-field optical coherence tomography. *Optics Express*, Vol.13, pp. 6286-6295

[48] Hrebesh, M.S.; Dabu, R. & Sato, M. (2009). In vivo imaging of dynamic biological specimen by real-time single-shot full-field optical coherence tomography. *Optics Communications*, Vol.282, pp. 674-683

[49] Watanabe, Y. & Sato, M. (2008). Three-dimensional wide-field optical coherence tomography using an ultrahigh-speed CMOS camera. *Optics Communications*, Vol.281, pp. 1889-1895

[50] Akiba, M.; Chan, K.P. & Tanno, N. (2003). Full-field optical coherence tomography by two-dimensional heterodyne detection with a pair of CCD cameras. *Optics Letters*, Vol.28, pp. 816-818

[51] Grieve, K.; Paques, M.; Dubois, A.; Sahel, J.; Boccara, A.C. & Le Gargasson, J.F. (2004). Ocular tissue imaging using ultrahigh-resolution full-field optical coherence tomography. *Investigative Ophthalmology & Visual Science*, Vol.45, pp. 4126-413

[52] Boccara, M.; Schwartz, W.; Guiot, E.; Vidal, G.; De Paepe, R.; Dubois, A. & Boccara, A.C. (2007). Early chloroplastic alterations analysed by optical coherence tomography during harpin-induced hypersensitive response. *The Plant Journal*, Vol.50, pp. 338-346

[53] Perea-Gomez, A.; Moreau, A.; Camus, A.; Grieve, K.; Moneron, G.; Dubois, A.; Cibert, C. & Collignon, J. (2004). Initiation of gastrulation in the mouse embryo is preceded by an apparent shift in the orientation of the anterior-posterior axis. *Current Biology*, Vol.14, pp. 197-207

2

Doppler OCT and OCT Angiography for *In Vivo* Imaging of Vascular Physiology

Vivek J. Srinivasan[1], Aaron C. Chan[2] and Edmund Y. Lam[2]
[1]MGH/MIT/HMS Athinoula A. Martinos Center for Biomedical Imaging, Department of Radiology, Massachusetts General Hospital, Harvard Medical School, Charlestown, Massachusetts
[2]Department of Electrical and Electronic Engineering, The University of Hong Kong, Pokfulam Road,
[1]U.S.A.
[2]Hong Kong

1. Introduction

Optical imaging methods (Grinvald et al., 1986; Villringer and Chance, 1997; Wilt et al., 2009) have had a significant impact on the field of neuroimaging and are now widely used in studies of both cellular and vascular physiology and pathology. Currently, *in vivo* optical imaging modalities can be broadly classified into two groups: macroscopic methods using diffuse light (optical intrinsic signal imaging (Grinvald et al., 1986), laser Doppler imaging (Dirnagl et al., 1989), laser speckle imaging (Dunn et al., 2001), diffuse optical imaging (Villringer and Chance, 1997), and laminar optical tomography (Hillman et al., 2004)) which achieve spatial resolutions of hundreds of microns to millimeters, and microscopic methods (two photon and confocal microscopy) which achieve micron-scale resolutions. Two-photon microscopy (Denk et al., 1990), in particular, is widely used in structural and functional imaging at the cellular and subcellular levels. While macroscopic imaging methods using diffuse light can achieve high penetration depths and large fields of view, they do not provide high spatial resolution. While two-photon microscopy achieves subcellular spatial resolution, the imaging speed, penetration depth, and field of view are limited.

Optical Coherence Tomography (OCT) (Huang et al., 1991) possesses a unique combination of high imaging speed, penetration depth, field of view, and resolution and therefore occupies an important niche between the macroscopic and microscopic optical imaging technologies discussed above. Relative to the optical imaging technologies currently used for neuroscience research, OCT has several advantages. Firstly, OCT enables volumetric imaging with high spatiotemporal resolution. OCT volumetric imaging requires tens of seconds to a few minutes. By contrast, volumetric imaging with two-photon microscopy typically requires tens of minutes to a few hours. Secondly, OCT achieves high penetration depth. OCT rejects out-of-focus and multiple scattered light, enabling imaging at depths of greater than 1 mm in scattering tissue. By comparison, conventional two-photon microscopy enables imaging depths of approximately 0.5 mm in scattering tissue. Third, OCT can be performed with long working distance, low numerical aperture (NA) objectives. Because the OCT depth resolution depends on the coherence length of light and not the confocal parameter (depth of field), low NA lenses may be used without sacrificing depth resolution. This contrasts with two-photon microscopy, where high depth resolution and penetration depth in scattering tissue *in vivo* can be achieved only with high-NA water immersion objectives. The use of relatively low NA objectives allows imaging of large fields of view, enabling the synthesis of microscopic and macroscopic information. Fourth, since OCT can measure well-defined volumes using predominantly single scattered light, quantitative assessment of hemodynamic parameters such as blood vessel diameter and blood flow using Doppler algorithms (Chen et al., 1997; Izatt et al., 1997) are possible. Fifth, OCT is performed using intrinsic contrast alone, and does not require the use of dyes or extrinsic contrast agents. This capability is attractive for longitudinal studies where cumulative dye toxicity is a concern.

In this chapter, we describe Doppler OCT and OCT angiography methods for the study of cerebrovascular physiology. We describe OCT technologies and methodologies relevant to *in vivo* imaging of the brain and other organs; with a focus on understanding signal modelling and software algorithms. While the methods and algorithms we describe here are applied to brain imaging, similar techniques can be used to image and quantify vascular physiology in other organ systems.

2. Methods

2.1 OCT Technologies

In conventional "time-domain" OCT, a low coherence light source is used with a Michelson interferometer with a sample arm and a reference arm. The reference path length is varied in time to generate a profile of backscattering or backreflectance vs. depth (Huang et al., 1991), and light is detected with a single photodiode or pair of photodiodes. Since 2003, new Fourier domain OCT detection methods have enabled dramatic increases in sensitivity (Choma et al., 2003; de Boer et al., 2003; Leitgeb et al., 2003) compared to conventional OCT detection methods. These methods are called "Fourier domain" because they detect the interference spectrum and do not require mechanical scanning of the reference path length in time. Fourier domain OCT has two known embodiments. The first embodiment, "spectral / Fourier domain" OCT (Fercher et al., 1995), uses a broadband light source and a high-speed, high resolution spectrometer for detection. The second embodiment, "swept source / Fourier domain" OCT (Golubovic et al., 1997; Yun et al., 2003), uses a frequency tunable light source and a photodiode or pair of photodiodes for detection.

The Doppler OCT and OCT angiography techniques described in this chapter may be applied to any of the OCT embodiments, provided that phase-resolved axial scan information is available. Fourier domain OCT techniques naturally provide this information, if the full complex signal is retained after Fourier transformation. For all the data presented here, we use spectral / Fourier domain OCT (Fercher et al., 1995), which uses a broadband light source and spectrometer. The relative merits of spectral / Fourier domain OCT and swept source OCT for Doppler OCT have been discussed in the literature (Hendargo et al.).

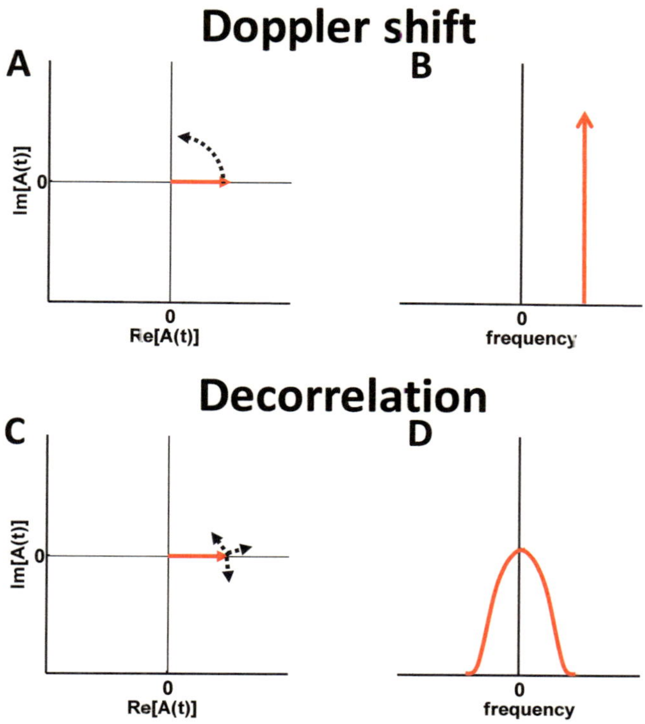

Fig. 1. Qualitative visualization of dynamics in the time and frequency domains. (A-B) Doppler shifting causes a pure rotation of the OCT signal in the complex plane, and leads to a frequency shift of the power spectrum. (C-D) Decorrelation causes random deviations of the OCT signal in the complex plane, and leads to a broadening of the power spectrum. In general, blood flow is accompanied by both Doppler shifts and decorrelation, leading to both shifting and broadening of the power spectrum.

2.2 Theory

The starting point for our discussion is the complex-valued OCT signal, as shown below.

$$A(t)=|A(t)|\exp[j\theta(t)] \tag{1}$$

The complex OCT signal is proportional to the electric field backscattered from scatterers in a voxel. In general, motion of scatterers is accompanied by both 1) Doppler phase shifts (caused by axial translation of a particle) and 2) decorrelation (typically caused by relative translation of a particle and the resolution voxel). Doppler phase shifts can be visualized as rotations of the electric field vector in the complex plane (Fig. 1A-B), while decorrelation can be visualized as random deviations of the electric field vector (Fig. 1C-D). Both Doppler OCT and OCT angiography can be understood from Fig. 1. Doppler OCT measures linear changes in the phase (θ) over time, to infer velocity axial projections. By comparison, OCT angiography generates contrast for moving scatterers based on field deviations in the complex plane.

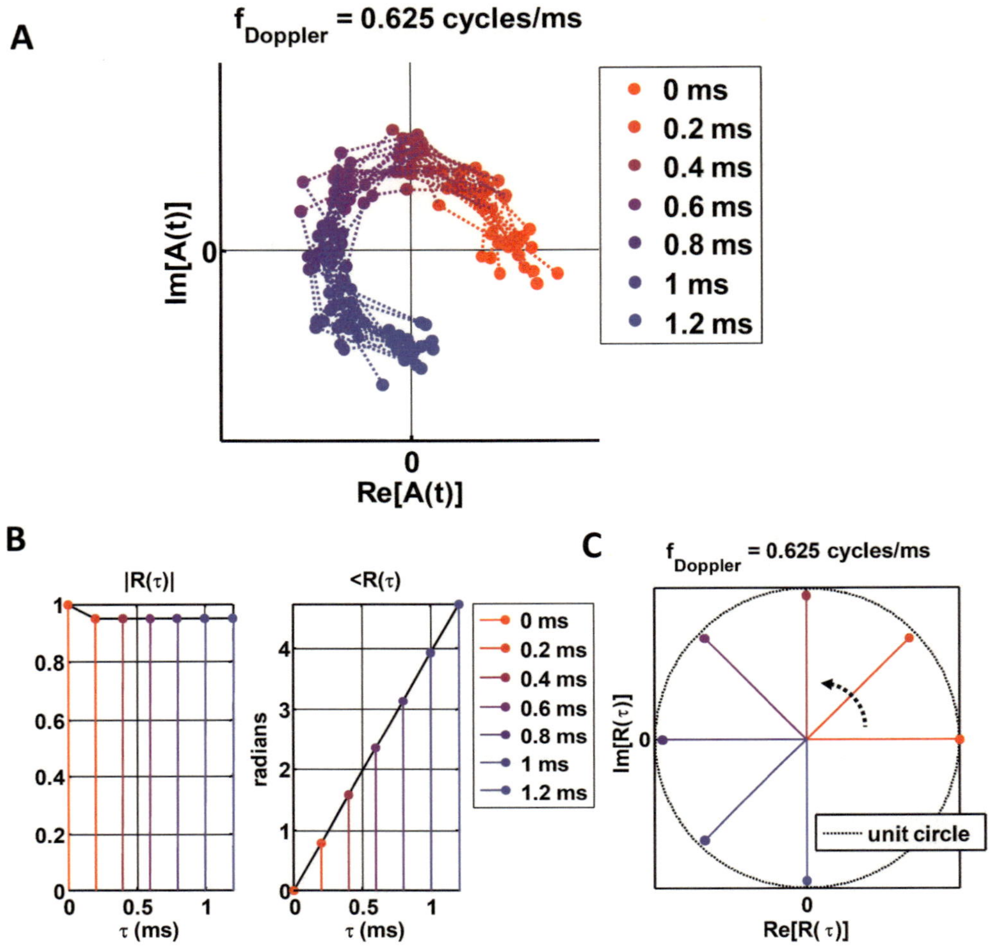

Fig. 2. (A) Visualization of the electric field in the complex plane under additive noise (SNR=$(A_0/\sigma)^2$=20) and Doppler shifting. The model in Eq. (5) was used, with a sampling rate of T=0.2 ms. The phase of the initial time point is set to zero, the amplitude is set to 1, and different time points are color-coded. (B) Magnitude and phase of the normalized autocorrelation function. (C) Rotation of the normalized autocorrelation function in the complex plane. Under additive noise, the distribution spread remains constant over time. For simplicity the effects of static scattering have been neglected (A_s=0 in Eq. (2)), and no decorrelation was assumed.

An additional concept required for the discussion of Doppler OCT and OCT angiography is the notion of a three-dimensional resolution voxel. The complex OCT signal (A) can be described as the superposition of a static scattering component (A_s), a dynamic scattering component (A_d), and additive noise (N) (Srinivasan et al., 2010; Yousefi et al., 2011) within a single voxel defined by the axial (z) and transverse (xy) resolutions, as shown below.

$$A(t)=A_s+A_d(t)+N(t) \tag{2}$$

In OCT, the axial image resolution in tissue, Δz, is inversely proportional to the bandwidth of the light source used for imaging as shown below,

$$\Delta z=\frac{2\ln(2)}{\pi n_{group}}\frac{\lambda_0^2}{\Delta\lambda} \tag{3}$$

where $\Delta\lambda$ is the full width half maximum (FWHM) of the light source, n_{group} is the group refractive index in tissue, and λ_0 is the center wavelength of the light source. The transverse resolution is determined by the numerical aperture of focusing as shown below,

$$\Delta x=\Delta y=\frac{\sqrt{2\ln(2)}\lambda_0}{\pi NA} \tag{4}$$

In the above expression, NA is the numerical aperture, as defined for Gaussian beams.

Doppler OCT estimates the angular frequency of the complex OCT signal, whereas angiography generates contrast for moving scatterers based on deviations in the complex OCT signal. In order to understand how these methods operate, it is instructive to develop and visualize simple stochastic models for the complex OCT signal.

The simplest model for the complex OCT signal, shown in Fig. 2, assumes a rotating complex electric field vector with a pure Doppler shift and additive, white noise. Under these conditions, the complex electric field can be represented by the following expression:

$$\begin{aligned} &A(nT)=\exp(j2\pi f_{Doppler}nT)A_0+N_n \\ &\text{where } N_n \sim N[0,\sigma^2] \text{ and are i.i.d} \end{aligned} \tag{5}$$

In Eq. (5), $f_{Doppler}$ is the Doppler frequency shift, n is a discrete index, and T is the sampling interval. A_0 is a complex constant. The N_n represent a random process. The N_n are zero-mean, independent, and identically distributed complex Gaussian random variables with a variance of σ^2. The axial projection of velocity v_z is related to the Doppler frequency shift $f_{Doppler}$ as follows:

$$v_z=f_{Doppler}\frac{\lambda_0}{2n_{phase}} \tag{6}$$

where n_{phase} is the phase refractive index in tissue and λ_0 is the center wavelength.

While the additive noise model is intuitive and simple, it is also important to realize that Eq. (5) represents an idealized situation. In reality, so-called "decorrelation noise" (Vakoc et al., 2009) is present. Decorrelation is caused by random deviations in the amplitude and phase from the average path of the electric field in the complex plane. Decorrelation can be caused by translation of the probe beam due to transverse scanning, or translation of scatterers due to blood flow. Decorrelation can also be caused by random amplitude and phase fluctuations from red blood cell orientation or shape changes. Decorrelation may additionally be caused by a random distribution of individual red blood cell velocities, or random deviations in the paths of individual red blood cells from uniform translation, which can be modelled as diffusion (Weitz et al., 1989). Decorrelation has a characteristic

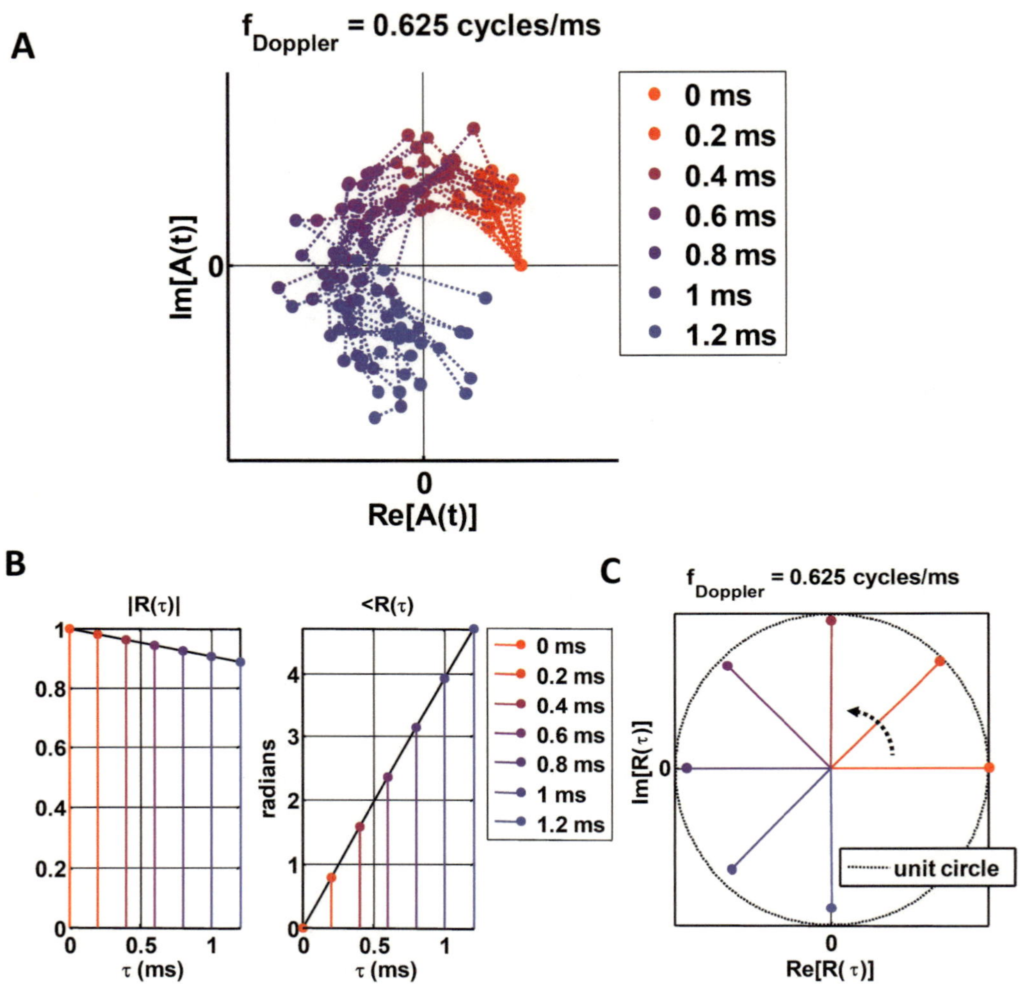

Fig. 3. (A) Visualization of the electric field in the complex plane under both decorrelation and Doppler shifting. The model in Eq. (7) was used, with a sampling rate of T=0.2 ms. The phase of the initial time point is set to zero, the amplitude is set to 1, and different time points are color-coded. (B) Magnitude and phase of the normalized autocorrelation function. (C) Rotation of the normalized autocorrelation function in the complex plane. The distinguishing feature of decorrelation is an increase in the spread of the distribution with time. For simplicity the effects of static scattering and additive noise have been neglected (A_s=0 and N=0 in Eq. (2)).

time scale, known as the decorrelation time, after which the complex amplitude is randomized. In other words, the value of the complex OCT signal at any given time would have no predictive value after the decorrelation time has passed. Under conditions of decorrelation, the complex electric field can be represented by the following model, which represents a Gaussian random process:

$$A[(m+n)T]=\alpha_n \exp(j2\pi f_{Doppler} nT)A[mT]+D_n \quad \text{where } D_n \sim N[0,\Sigma]. \tag{7}$$

The model described in Eq. (7) accounts for both Doppler shifting and decorrelation, and is shown in Fig. 3. The elements of the covariance matrix (Σ_{mn}) can be derived by assuming wide sense stationarity.

$$\Sigma_{mn}=E[D_m D_n^*]= E[|A|^2]\exp[j2\pi f_{Doppler}(m-n)T][\alpha_{m-n}-\alpha_m\alpha_n] \tag{8}$$

In the above equations, α_n is a real coefficient with a magnitude between 0 and 1, with $\alpha_0=1$. The autocorrelation function is given by

$$R[nT]=\frac{E\{A^*[mT]A[(m+n)T]\}}{E\{|A|^2\}}=\alpha_n \exp(j2\pi f_{Doppler} nT) \tag{9}$$

Thus the width of α_n determines the decorrelation time. The right side of Eq. (7) can be viewed as a sum of a deterministic component and a random component, where the first term, $\alpha_n \exp(j2\pi f_{Doppler} nT)A[mT]$, represents the deterministic component, and the second term, D_n, represents the random component. As n increases, α_n decreases, and the random component dominates. Therefore, if nT is much larger than the decorrelation time, A[mT] yields no information about A[(m+n)T]. Finally, we note that is possible to model the effects of static scattering by insertion of a constant term in Eq. (5) or (7); however for simplicity we have not included the effects of static scattering here.

2.3 Motion correction

Bulk axial motion is the dominant motion artefact in Doppler OCT. In general, bulk motion causes both a phase shift (White et al., 2003) and an axial image shift (Swanson et al., 1993). For bulk motion on the order of a wavelength, which in turn is much smaller than the axial resolution, the dominant effect of motion is a phase shift. Either galvanometer jitter, thermal drift, or physiologic motion may cause phase shifts. A number of strategies for bulk motion correction have been proposed (Makita et al., 2006; White et al., 2003). Motion correction techniques ideally use a reference (non-vascular) tissue region that can be analyzed to determine the phase shift due to bulk motion. The simplest method to determine the bulk phase shift between two axial scans is to calculate their complex cross-correlation; however, this approach has the disadvantage that it does not account for Doppler shifts from flowing blood. More sophisticated methods use histogram techniques to estimate the bulk phase shift (Yang et al., 2002).

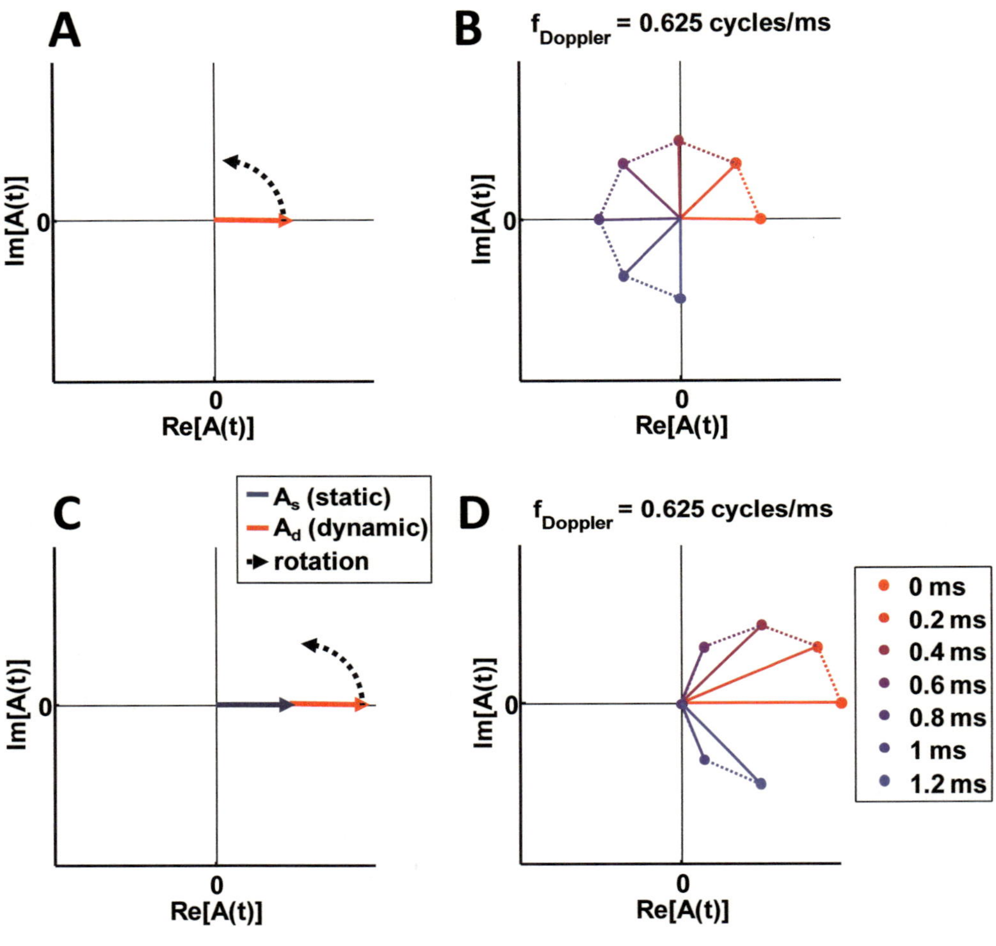

Fig. 4. Static scattering can lead to underestimation of Doppler frequency. (A-B) Visualization of the electric field vector in the complex plane for a pure Doppler shift with no static scattering and no additive noise (A_s=0 and N=0 in Eq. (2)). (C-D) Visualization of the electric field vector in the complex plane for a pure Doppler shift in the presence of static scattering ($A_s \neq 0$ and N=0 in Eq. (2)).

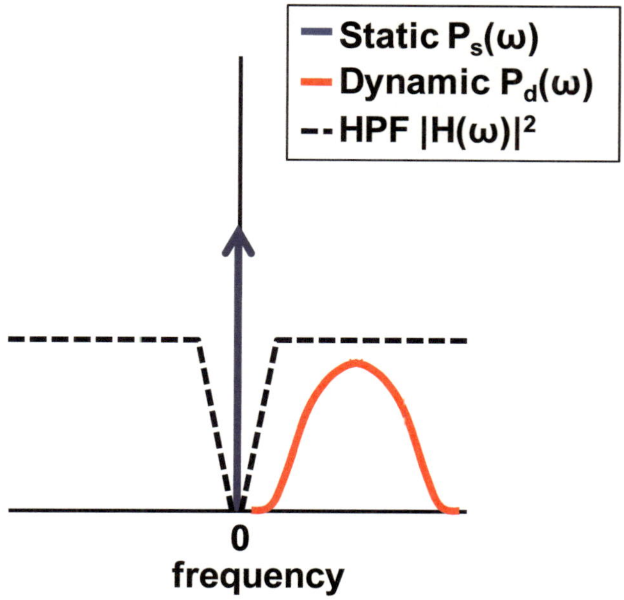

Fig. 5. High-pass filtering is one method to separate static and dynamic scattering components. The static scattering or "D.C." component of the power spectrum is shown in blue, while the dynamic scattering component of the power spectrum is shown in red.

2.4 Isolation of dynamic scattering

Early in the development of high-speed Doppler OCT techniques, the detrimental effect of static scattering on the accuracy of Doppler velocity estimation was recognized. If standard Doppler estimation algorithms are applied in a region with both static and dynamic scattering, the velocity of the dynamic component will be underestimated due to the presence of the static scattering (Ren et al., 2006). This can be seen visually in Fig. 4. Therefore, it is necessary to correctly account for the effects of static scattering in any Doppler estimation procedure. Scattered power from a voxel can be represented as a linear superposition of static and dynamic scattering components (Srinivasan et al., 2010; Tao et al., 2008). In the frequency domain, the power spectrum contains a so-called "D.C" (Tao et al., 2008) or static (Srinivasan et al., 2010) component centered at zero frequency, and a Doppler shifted, broadened component corresponding to dynamic scattering (Srinivasan et al., 2010; Tao et al., 2008; R. K. Wang and An, 2009).

$$P(\omega)=P_s(\omega)+P_d(\omega) \tag{10}$$

Therefore, both the complex OCT signal (Eq. (2)) and the power spectrum (Eq. (10)) can be represented as a superposition of static and dynamic scattering components. If the optical beam is scanned across the tissue, the spectral width of the static scattering component is related to the scanning speed and the transverse resolution (Srinivasan et al., 2010). We will argue that the dynamic scattering component can be estimated by high-pass filtering. Similar filtering techniques can also be found in the ultrasound literature (Bjaerum et al., 2002). Mathematically,

$$A_d(nT) \approx A(nT)*h(nT) \tag{11}$$

In the above equation, h(nT) is the high-pass filter kernel, and * denotes a discrete convolution. Therefore, the power spectrum of the dynamic scattering component is approximately equal to the high-pass filtered power spectrum, as shown below,

$$P_d(\omega) \approx P(\omega) \mid H(\omega) \mid^2 \tag{12}$$

Eq. (12) can also be understood intuitively from Fig. 5. After removal of static scattering, estimation algorithms can be applied to determine the Doppler frequency shift, as described below. We also note here that the high-pass filtering operation to remove static scattering, while simple and intuitive, is an *ad hoc* procedure and may result in biased velocity estimates (Srinivasan et al., 2010). Further work in the area of parametric estimation algorithms could directly account for static scattering in the velocity estimation procedure.

2.5 Doppler frequency estimation

A number of Doppler frequency and velocity estimation algorithms have been proposed. However, to date, a comprehensive comparative study on the properties of different estimators (such as bias and mean squared error) has not been performed. Two particular algorithms in widespread use, the Kasai autocorrelation method (Y. Zhao et al., 2000) and the joint spectral and time domain OCT (STdOCT) approach described by Szkulmowski et. al (Szkulmowski et al., 2008), will be discussed.

The Kasai autocorrelation method, as applied to phase-resolved Doppler OCT, first estimates the autocorrelation at a time lag of one sampling period.

$$\hat{R}(T)=\sum_{n=0}^{N-1} A^*[nT]A[(n+1)T] \tag{13}$$

A Kasai window can be defined, over which the estimation is performed. The Doppler frequency is estimated as the phase of the autocorrelation at a time lag of T divided by T.

$$f_{Kasai}=\frac{\angle\hat{R}(T)}{2\pi T} \tag{14}$$

Recently, the technique of joint Spectral and Time domain OCT was proposed (Szkulmowski et al., 2008). In this technique, a series of axial scans are performed at approximately the same transverse position, yielding a time series. The frequency estimate is then chosen as the point in the power spectrum of the time series with the highest amplitude:

$$\hat{\omega}=\arg\max_{\omega\in[-\pi,\pi]}\left\{\hat{P}(\omega)\right\}$$

$$f_{STdOCT}=\frac{\hat{\omega}}{2\pi T} \tag{15}$$

To compare these two methods, it is instructive to view the frequency domain equivalent of the Kasai method. In order to relate the Kasai autocorrelation method to the power spectrum, the autocorrelation estimate can be defined as follows.

$$\hat{R}(nT)=\sum A^{*}[mT]A[(m+n)T] \tag{16}$$

By the Weiner-Khinchin theorem, the autocorrelation and power spectrum are related by a Fourier transformation. The autocorrelation estimate described in Eq. (16) can be thus be approximately related to a power spectrum estimate, shown below.

$$\hat{P}(\omega) \approx \sum_{n=-\infty}^{n=\infty} \hat{R}[nT]e^{-j\omega n} \tag{17}$$

Therefore, the autocorrelation at a time lag of T can be approximately determined with an inverse discrete-time Fourier transformation as shown below.

$$\hat{R}(T) \approx \frac{1}{2\pi}\int_{-\pi}^{\pi} e^{j\omega}\hat{P}(\omega)d\omega \tag{18}$$

Thus, the angle of the autocorrelation at a time lag of T can be loosely viewed as the weighted circular average of frequencies in the power spectrum, where each frequency ω is represented by a complex phasor $e^{j\omega}$ and weighted by the power spectrum estimate at that frequency. Hence the Kasai autocorrelation can be seen as performing a weighted circular average of digital frequencies in the power spectrum, and estimating the frequency using the argument of the result as shown in Eq. (14). By contrast, the joint STdOCT method chooses the frequency with maximum amplitude in the power spectrum for the estimate. The best velocity estimator for a given situation may depend on the noise characteristics, and the relative contributions of additive noise (Fig. 2) versus decorrelation noise (Fig. 3). We do not present a detailed characterization of the different estimators. Desirable characteristics of a good velocity estimator are "unbiasedness" and efficiency. However, to date a systematic study of velocity estimation algorithms in Doppler OCT has not been performed.

3. OCT Angiography

Angiography techniques aim to visualize the lumens of blood vessels. Red blood cells are the predominant cellular scattering component in blood. Therefore, blood vessels are typically visualized as highly scattering regions in standard OCT intensity images. However, smaller blood vessels such as capillaries may be obscured by surrounding highly scattering tissue. Therefore, in order to achieve high contrast angiograms, the contrast of red blood cells must be enhanced relative to that of surrounding tissue. OCT angiography techniques make use of the fact that red blood cell scattering is dynamic, exhibiting phase or amplitude fluctuations over time, while static tissue scattering is relatively constant over time.

Soon after the development of Doppler OCT in the mid to late 1990s, it was recognized that Doppler signals could be used to visualize vasculature (Yonghua Zhao et al., 2000), thus forming an angiogram of vasculature within tissue. The development of Fourier domain OCT techniques opened the door to high-speed, high-resolution, and volumetric angiography. In 2006, Makita et al. developed techniques to perform Optical Coherence Angiography of the vasculature in the retina and choroid (Makita et al., 2006). Around the same time, moving-scatterer-sensitive OCT was developed to separate static and dynamic scattering in order to achieve more accurate Doppler velocity profiles (Ren et al., 2006). In 2007, Wang et al. further extended these techniques to perform Optical Angiography (OAG) through the intact cranium in anesthetized mice (R. K. Wang and Hurst, 2007; R. K. Wang et al., 2007).

Recent advances in imaging speeds and algorithms have led to high-resolution, large field-of-view imaging of vascular beds down to the capillary level (Srinivasan et al., 2010; Vakoc et al., 2009). A range of techniques are currently used for OCT angiography. Some techniques use the field magnitude (Mariampillai et al., 2010; Mariampillai et al., 2008), others techniques use the phase (Fingler et al., 2007; Vakoc et al., 2009), while other techniques use the complex field (An et al., 2010; Srinivasan et al., 2010; Tao et al., 2008; R. K. Wang et al., 2007), thus incorporating both magnitude and phase information.

Magnitude-based angiography techniques such as speckle variance methods, are based on $|A|$ in Eq. (1). They are insensitive to bulk phase changes, and therefore do not require bulk motion phase correction. Phase-based angiography techniques such as phase variance methods are essentially based on $\exp[j\theta]$ in Eq. (1). They require bulk phase motion correction. Complex-OCT signal based angiography techniques are based on $A=|A|\exp[j\theta]$ in Eq. (1). They also require bulk phase motion correction. Complex angiography can be viewed as high-pass filtering the complex field, which is a superposition of static and dynamic components, as shown in Eq. (2). The goal of angiography is essentially to estimate the power in the dynamic scattering component. This can be accomplished with a high-pass filtering operation, as shown in Fig. 5 and in the expression below,

$$\frac{1}{2\pi}\int_{-\pi}^{\pi} P_d(\omega)d\omega \approx \frac{1}{2\pi}\int_{-\pi}^{\pi} P(\omega)|H(\omega)|^2 d\omega \tag{19}$$

High-pass filtering the OCT signal along the slow axis achieves better sensitivity than high-pass filtering along the fast axis, enabling visualization of capillary flow (An et al., 2010; Srinivasan et al., 2010).

Angiography techniques can be understood by visualizing the electric field vector in the complex plane. In general, it is possible to distinguish two types of behavior, which are, in general present to some degree in all voxels. Firstly, axial motion leads to a linear change in the phase of the electric field vector over time (Fig. 2). The rate of phase change, or angular frequency, is used in Doppler OCT to measure particle velocity. A second type of behavior, decorrelation, is characterized by randomization of the complex field over time (Fig. 3). For point particles, decorrelation is caused by motion of the particle through the three-dimensional voxel (defined by Eq. (3) and (4)). Additionally, decorrelation can be caused by a random distribution of axial velocities, leading to a spread (uncertainty) in the angle θ over time. For red blood cells (biconcave disks with diameter of 6-8 microns and an aspect ratio of approximately 4), one would expect significant anisotropy in the scattering phase function. Therefore, decorrelation may be caused by red blood cell orientation changes as

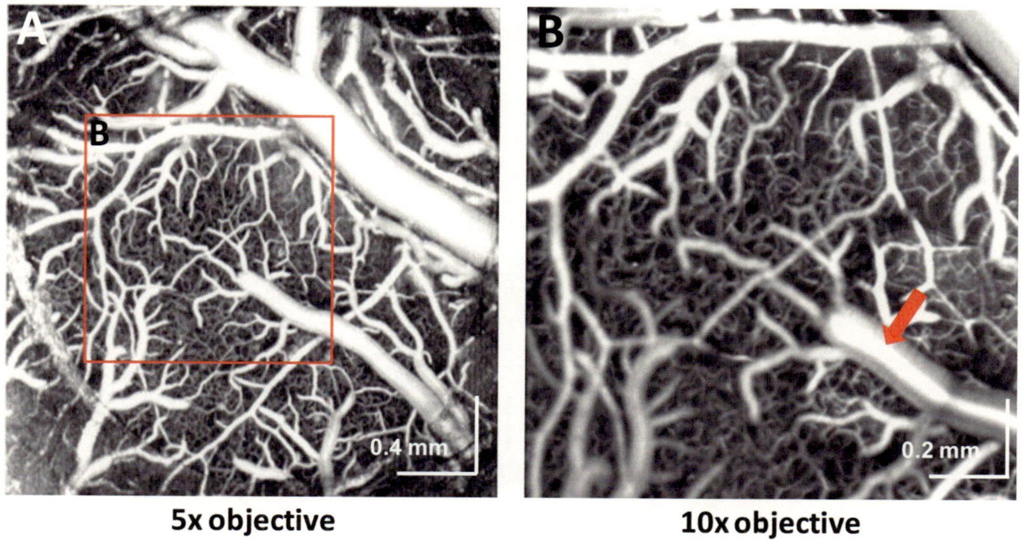

Fig. 6. OCT angiography in the rat parietal cortex through a closed cranial window. At a transverse resolution of 7 microns, the entire 3 mm window is imaged (A). At a transverse resolution of 3.5 microns, detailed microvasculature is imaged over a smaller field of view (B). The red arrow in B shows a bright "stripe" pattern along the center axis of a vein, due to the shear-induced orientation of the flat face of the red blood cells perpendicular to the probe beam.

well. In general, angiography can visualize regions with either Doppler shifting or decorrelation, since both behaviours result in power being shifted to higher frequencies (Fig. 1).

4. Absolute blood flow measurements

Blood flow is a fundamental physiological parameter. Classical methods to quantify cerebral blood flow, pioneered by Kety and colleagues (Kety, 1951), introduce a foreign, chemically inert tracer that diffuses freely across the blood brain barrier. Similar concepts are used in MRI arterial spin labeling and PET radiotracer methods to quantify perfusion.

Traditional optical imaging methods such as laser speckle and laser Doppler imaging do not provide absolute blood flow measurements. Doppler OCT has the capability to perform absolute blood flow measurements based on Doppler shifted light backscattered from moving red blood cells. Phase-resolved Doppler OCT (Yonghua Zhao et al., 2000) has become the method of choice due to its high velocity sensitivity and compatibility with Fourier domain OCT techniques. In particular, one can imagine a hypothetical three-dimensional incompressible vector field $\mathbf{v}(x,y,z)$, which gives the spatially-resolved velocity profile within vessels, and is zero outside vessels. Flow in a vessel can be interpreted as the flux of $\mathbf{v}(x,y,z)$ through any surface bisecting the vessel. Ideally, Doppler OCT measures the axial or z-projection of this three-dimensional vector field, i.e. $v_z(x,y,z)$. Therefore, flow in any vessel can be obtained from the Doppler OCT data by calculating the velocity flux through the *en*

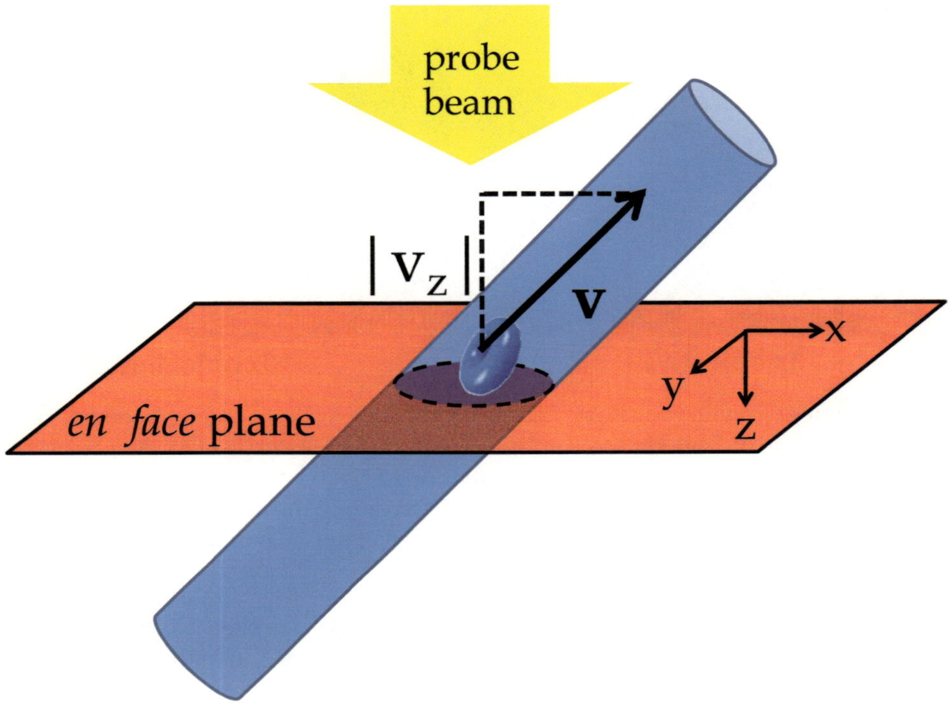

Fig. 7. Geometry for flow calculation using Doppler OCT. An ascending vessel with flow towards the incident probe beam is bisected by the *en face* plane. A red blood cell is shown, with a velocity vector given by **v**, while the magnitude of the velocity axial (z) projection is given by $|v_z|$.

face (also known as transverse or xy) plane using the following expression, (Srinivasan et al., 2010)

$$F = \iint_{ROI} v_z(x,y,z_0)dxdy \tag{20}$$

The ROI for integration is chosen to encircle the cross-section of the vessel in a particular *en face* plane, as shown in Fig. 7. Thus, by judicious choice of the surface for integration perpendicular to the measured velocity component, explicit calculation of vessel angles (Y. Wang et al., 2007) is not required to determine flow. To understand why this simple procedure works, note that Eq. (20) can be rewritten as the product of the cross-sectional area in the *en face* plane and the mean velocity axial projection.

$$F=A_{xy}\overline{v_z} \tag{21}$$

The cross-sectional area in the *en face* plane is given by

$$A_{xy}=\iint_{ROI} dxdy\,, \tag{22}$$

and the mean velocity axial projection is given by

$$\overline{v_z}=\iint_{ROI} v_z(x,y,z_0)dxdy\Big/\iint_{ROI} dxdy\,. \tag{23}$$

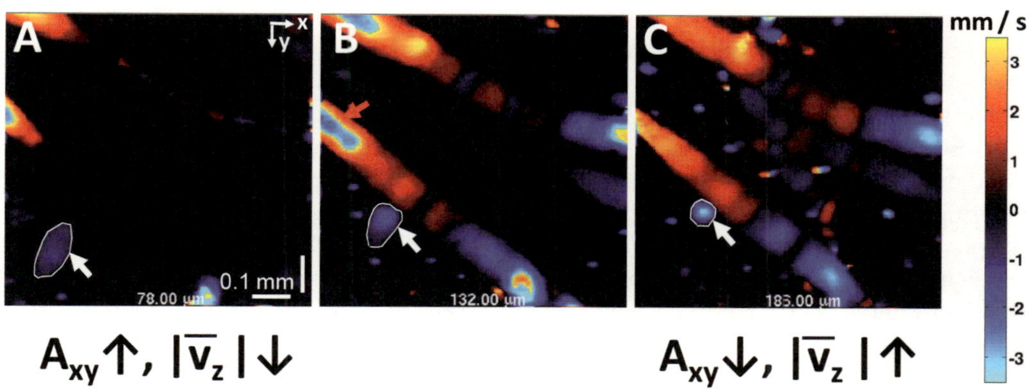

Fig. 8. Flow is conserved in a non-branching vessel. A single ascending vein at a depth (z_0) of 78 µm (A), 132 µm (B), and 186 µm (C) is shown. With increasing depth, as the vessel orientation becomes more axial, the vessel cross-sectional area (demarcated by white ROIs) in the *en face* plane decreases. At the same time, with increasing depth, the mean velocity axial projection increases in magnitude. As a result, flow, calculated as the product of these two quantities (Eq. (21)), is conserved. A region with aliasing of velocities is marked by a red arrow in B.

Keeping these equations in mind, it is instructive to view Doppler OCT images of a cortical vessel in *en face* planes at different depths, as in Fig. 8A, B, and C (z_0 = 78, 132, and 186 µm respectively). An ascending vein is demarcated by whites ROIs at each depth. Since flow in a vein drains the cortex, and by convention the +z direction points into the cortex, velocity axial projections are negative in veins. Therefore, according to Eq. (20), flow in veins is negative and flow in arteries is positive. With increasing cortical depth, the ascending vein changes from a more transverse (A) to a more axial (C) orientation. As the vein becomes more axially oriented (more parallel to the probe beam), the cross-sectional area in the *en face* plane is reduced (Eq. (22)), while the magnitude of the mean velocity axial projection is increased (Eq. (23)). Due to the fact that transverse cross-sectional area and velocity axial projection change in opposing directions, flow (as computed in Eq. (21)) is conserved. Similar methods of flow calculation, that, for instance, use an angiogram to determine the cross-sectional area in the *en face* plane more accurately, are also possible. The concept of *en face* integration to determine flow could be applied to ultrasound as well.

Using this method of flow calculation, conservation at branch points and along non-branching segments has been demonstrated (Srinivasan et al., 2011). Furthermore, Doppler OCT flow values correlated with hydrogen clearance flow values when both were measured simultaneously across multiple subjects. The technique of *en face* integration has recently been adapted to measure total retinal blood flow (Baumann et al., 2011) and glomerular blood flow (Wierwille et al., 2011).

However, there are limitations to Doppler OCT blood flow measurements. First, flow measurements are accurate only in vessels with a well-defined flow profile. Flow values are most accurate in large arteries and veins, but flow calculations necessarily fail in capillaries where the red blood cells flow in a single file. Second, the RBC velocity axial projection profile (measured by Doppler OCT) may not reflect the true flow profile, as there is an "RBC-free" zone at the periphery of the vessel lumen. Third, the presence of static scattering and dynamic scattering within voxels at the edge of vessels must be addressed by filtering or fitting techniques. Fourth, vessels must be measured at locations where they generate a Doppler shift above the detection threshold. Therefore, Doppler methods would fail where a vessel is perpendicular to the probe beam, or where velocity axial projections are not sufficiently large. Fifth, Doppler OCT relies on scattering from red blood cells, and flow measurements would therefore be inaccurate under conditions of extremely low hematocrit. Nevertheless, Doppler OCT flowmetry is non-invasive and correlates with gold standard absolute flow values across subjects (Srinivasan et al., 2011). These features make Doppler OCT an attractive technique for non-invasive longitudinal, high resolution blood flow imaging.

5. Conclusion

In conclusion, Doppler OCT and OCT angiography are complementary tools to quantitatively study vascular physiology. OCT occupies an important niche between diffuse optical imaging methods and invasive microscopic techniques. A novel technique of absolute blood flow measurement with Doppler OCT, which does not require explicit calculation of vessel angles, was recently validated in the brain (Srinivasan et al., 2011) and shown to provide flow measurements within a reasonable physiological range. This technique was recently applied in the retina (Baumann et al.) and in the kidney glomeruli (Wierwille et al., 2011). These non-invasive optical imaging technologies promise to advance longitudinal imaging of blood flow in living organ systems for basic and translational research.

6. Acknowledgment

We acknowledge support from the NIH (K99NS067050), the AHA (11IRG5440002), and the Glaucoma Research Foundation. We also acknowledge conversations with Cenk Ayata, Jonghwan Lee, Eng Lo, David Boas, Weicheng Wu, Lana Ruvinskaya, Alex Cable, James Jiang, Sava Sakadzic, Mohammed Abbas Yaseen, James Fujimoto, Iwona Gorczynska, Emiri Mandeville, and Harsha Radhakrishnan.

7. References

An, L., Qin, J., and Wang, R. K., "Ultrahigh sensitive optical microangiography for in vivo imaging of microcirculations within human skin tissue beds," Opt Express 18, 8220-8228 (2010).

Baumann, B., Potsaid, B., Kraus, M. F., Liu, J. J., Huang, D., Hornegger, J., Cable, A. E., Duker, J. S., and Fujimoto, J. G., "Total retinal blood flow measurement with ultrahigh speed swept source/Fourier domain OCT," Biomed Opt Express 2, 1539-1552 (2011).

Bjaerum, S., Torp, H., and Kirstoffersen, K., "Clutter filter design for ultrasound color flow imaging," IEEE Trans. Ultrason. Ferroelectr. Freq. Control 49, 204-216 (2002).

Chen, Z., Milner, T. E., Dave, D., and Nelson, J. S., "Optical Doppler tomographic imaging of fluid flow velocity in highly scattering media," Optics Letters 22, 64-66 (1997).

Choma, M. A., Sarunic, M. V., Yang, C. H., and Izatt, J. A., "Sensitivity advantage of swept source and Fourier domain optical coherence tomography," Optics Express 11, 2183-2189 (2003).

de Boer, J. F., Cense, B., Park, B. H., Pierce, M. C., Tearney, G. J., and Bouma, B. E., "Improved signal-to-noise ratio in spectral-domain compared with time-domain optical coherence tomography," Opt Lett 28, 2067-2069 (2003).

Denk, W., Strickler, J. H., and Webb, W. W., "2-Photon Laser Scanning Fluorescence Microscopy," Science 248, 73-76 (1990).

Dirnagl, U., Kaplan, B., Jacewicz, M., and Pulsinelli, W., "Continuous measurement of cerebral cortical blood flow by laser-Doppler flowmetry in a rat stroke model," J Cereb Blood Flow Metab 9, 589-596 (1989).

Dunn, A. K., Bolay, H., Moskowitz, M. A., and Boas, D. A., "Dynamic imaging of cerebral blood flow using laser speckle," J Cereb Blood Flow Metab 21, 195-201 (2001).

Fercher, A. F., Hitzenberger, C. K., Kamp, G., and El-Zaiat, S. Y., "Measurement of intraocular distances by backscattering spectral interferometry," Opt. Commun. 117, 43-48 (1995).

Fingler, J., Schwartz, D., Yang, C., and Fraser, S. E., "Mobility and transverse flow visualization using phase variance contrast with spectral domain optical coherence tomography," Opt Express 15, 12636-12653 (2007).

Golubovic, B., Bouma, B. E., Tearney, G. J., and Fujimoto, J. G., "Optical frequency-domain reflectometry using rapid wavelength tuning of a Cr4+:forsterite laser," Opt Lett 22, 1704-1706 (1997).

Grinvald, A., Lieke, E., Frostig, R. D., Gilbert, C. D., and Wiesel, T. N., "Functional architecture of cortex revealed by optical imaging of intrinsic signals," Nature 324, 361-364 (1986).

Hendargo, H. C., McNabb, R. P., Dhalla, A. H., Shepherd, N., and Izatt, J. A., "Doppler velocity detection limitations in spectrometer-based versus swept-source optical coherence tomography," Biomed Opt Express 2, 2175-2188 (2011).

Hillman, E. M., Boas, D. A., Dale, A. M., and Dunn, A. K., "Laminar optical tomography: demonstration of millimeter-scale depth-resolved imaging in turbid media," Opt Lett 29, 1650-1652 (2004).

Huang, D., Swanson, E. A., Lin, C. P., Schuman, J. S., Stinson, W. G., Chang, W., Hee, M. R., Flotte, T., Gregory, K., Puliafito, C. A., and Fujimoto, J. G., "Optical Coherence Tomography," Science 254, 1178-1181 (1991).

Izatt, J. A., Kulkami, M. D., Yazdanfar, S., Barton, J. K., and Welch, A. J., "In vivo bidirectional color Doppler flow imaging of picoliter blood volumes using optical coherence tomography," Optics Letters 22, 1439-1441 (1997).

Kety, S. S., "The theory and applications of the exchange of inert gas at the lungs and tissues," Pharmacol Rev 3, 1-41 (1951).

Leitgeb, R., Hitzenberger, C. K., and Fercher, A. F., "Performance of Fourier domain vs. time domain optical coherence tomography," Optics Express 11, 889-894 (2003).

Makita, S., Hong, Y., Yamanari, M., Yatagai, T., and Yasuno, Y., "Optical coherence angiography," Optics Express 14, 7821-7840 (2006).

Mariampillai, A., Leung, M. K., Jarvi, M., Standish, B. A., Lee, K., Wilson, B. C., Vitkin, A., and Yang, V. X., "Optimized speckle variance OCT imaging of microvasculature," Opt Lett 35, 1257-1259 (2010).

Mariampillai, A., Standish, B. A., Moriyama, E. H., Khurana, M., Munce, N. R., Leung, M. K., Jiang, J., Cable, A., Wilson, B. C., Vitkin, I. A., and Yang, V. X., "Speckle variance detection of microvasculature using swept-source optical coherence tomography," Opt Lett 33, 1530-1532 (2008).

Ren, H., Sun, T., MacDonald, D. J., Cobb, M. J., and Li, X., "Real-time in vivo blood-flow imaging by moving-scatterer-sensitive spectral-domain optical Doppler tomography," Opt Lett 31, 927-929 (2006).

Srinivasan, V. J., Atochin, D. N., Radhakrishnan, H., Jiang, J. Y., Ruvinskaya, S., Wu, W., Barry, S., Cable, A. E., Ayata, C., Huang, P. L., and Boas, D. A., "Optical coherence tomography for the quantitative study of cerebrovascular physiology," J Cereb Blood Flow Metab 31, 1339-1345 (2011).

Srinivasan, V. J., Jiang, J. Y., Yaseen, M. A., Radhakrishnan, H., Wu, W., Barry, S., Cable, A. E., and Boas, D. A., "Rapid volumetric angiography of cortical microvasculature with optical coherence tomography," Opt Lett 35, 43-45 (2010).

Srinivasan, V. J., Sakadzic, S., Gorczynska, I., Ruvinskaya, S., Wu, W., Fujimoto, J. G., and Boas, D. A., "Quantitative cerebral blood flow with optical coherence tomography," Opt Express 18, 2477-2494 (2010).

Swanson, E. A., Izatt, J. A., Hee, M. R., Huang, D., Lin, C. P., Schuman, J. S., Puliafito, C. A., and Fujimoto, J. G., "In vivo retinal imaging by optical coherence tomography," Opt Lett 18, 1864-1866 (1993).

Szkulmowski, M., Szkulmowska, A., Bajraszewski, T., Kowalczyk, A., and Wojtkowski, M., "Flow velocity estimation using joint Spectral and Time domain Optical Coherence Tomography," Opt Express 16, 6008-6025 (2008).

Tao, Y. K., Davis, A. M., and Izatt, J. A., "Single-pass volumetric bidirectional blood flow imaging spectral domain optical coherence tomography using a modified Hilbert transform," Opt Express 16, 12350-12361 (2008).

Vakoc, B. J., Lanning, R. M., Tyrrell, J. A., Padera, T. P., Bartlett, L. A., Stylianopoulos, T., Munn, L. L., Tearney, G. J., Fukumura, D., Jain, R. K., and Bouma, B. E., "Three-dimensional microscopy of the tumor microenvironment in vivo using optical frequency domain imaging," Nat Med 15, 1219-1223 (2009).

Vakoc, B. J., Tearney, G. J., and Bouma, B. E., "Statistical properties of phase-decorrelation in phase-resolved Doppler optical coherence tomography," IEEE Trans Med Imaging 28, 814-821 (2009).

Villringer, A. and Chance, B., "Non-invasive optical spectroscopy and imaging of human brain function," Trends in Neurosciences 20, 435-442 (1997).

Wang, R. K. and An, L., "Doppler optical micro-angiography for volumetric imaging of vascular perfusion in vivo," Opt Express 17, 8926-8940 (2009).

Wang, R. K. and Hurst, S., "Mapping of cerebro-vascular blood perfusion in mice with skin and skull intact by Optical Micro-AngioGraphy at 1.3 mu m wavelength," Optics Express 15, 11402-11412 (2007).

Wang, R. K., Jacques, S. L., Ma, Z., Hurst, S., Hanson, S. R., and Gruber, A., "Three dimensional optical angiography," Optics Express 15, 4083-4097 (2007).

Wang, Y., Bower, B. A., Izatt, J. A., Tan, O., and Huang, D., "In vivo total retinal blood flow measurement by Fourier domain Doppler optical coherence tomography," Journal of biomedical optics 12, 041215 (2007).

Weitz, D. A., Pine, D. J., Pusey, P. N., and Tough, R. J., "Nondiffusive Brownian motion studied by diffusing-wave spectroscopy," Phys Rev Lett 63, 1747-1750 (1989).

White, B. R., Pierce, M. C., Nassif, N., Cense, B., Park, B. H., Tearney, G. J., Bouma, B. E., Chen, T. C., and de Boer, J. F., "In vivo dynamic human retinal blood flow imaging using ultra-high-speed spectral domain optical Doppler tomography," Optics Express 11, 3490-3497 (2003).

Wierwille, J., Andrews, P. M., Onozato, M. L., Jiang, J., Cable, A., and Chen, Y., "In vivo, label-free, three-dimensional quantitative imaging of kidney microcirculation using Doppler optical coherence tomography," Laboratory investigation; a journal of technical methods and pathology (2011).

Wilt, B. A., Burns, L. D., Ho, E. T. W., Ghosh, K. K., Mukamel, E. A., and Schnitzer, M. J., "Advances in Light Microscopy for Neuroscience," Annual Review of Neuroscience 32, 435-506 (2009).

Yang, V. X. D., Gordon, M. L., Mok, A., Zhao, Y. H., Chen, Z. P., Cobbold, R. S. C., Wilson, B. C., and Vitkin, I. A., "Improved phase-resolved optical Doppler tomography using the Kasai velocity estimator and histogram segmentation," Opt. Commun. 208, 209-214 (2002).

Yousefi, S., Zhi, Z., and Wang, R., "Eigendecomposition-Based Clutter Filtering Technique for Optical Micro-Angiography," IEEE Trans Biomed Eng (2011).

Yun, S., Tearney, G., de Boer, J., Iftimia, N., and Bouma, B., "High-speed optical frequency-domain imaging," Opt Express 11, 2953-2963 (2003).

Zhao, Y., Chen, Z., Saxer, C., Shen, Q., Xiang, S., de Boer, J. F., and Nelson, J. S., "Doppler standard deviation imaging for clinical monitoring of in vivo human skin blood flow," Opt Lett 25, 1358-1360 (2000).

Zhao, Y., Chen, Z., Saxer, C., Xiang, S., de Boer, J. F., and Nelson, J. S., "Phase-resolved optical coherence tomography and optical Doppler tomography for imaging blood flow in human skin with fast scanning speed and high velocity sensitivity," Optics Letters 25, 114-116 (2000).

3

Phase-Resolved Doppler Optical Coherence Tomography

Gangjun Liu and Zhongping Chen
Beckman Laser Institute, University of California, Irvine.
Department of Biomedical Engineering, University of California, Irvine, USA

1. Introduction

Optical coherence tomography (OCT) is an emerging medical imaging and diagnostic technology developed by MIT in the 1990s [1]. OCT uses coherence optical gating to detect the intensity of back reflected or back scattered light from the sample. It is analogous to ultrasound tomography except that light instead of sound is used. OCT can provide a depth resolution of 1-20 μm, which is one to two orders of magnitude higher than that of conventional ultrasound. OCT is a non-contact, non invasive, fast imaging modality that provides real time, three-dimensional imaging capability. OCT has been valuable in applications in the field of medicine such as ophthalmology, cardiology, otolaryngology, pulmonology, urology, dentistry, and gastroenterology [2].

In OCT, imaging contrast originates from the inhomogeneities of sample scattering properties that are dependent on sample refractive indices. In many instances, especially in the early stages of disease, changes in sample linear scattering properties are small and difficult to measure. Additional contrast mechanisms are able to extend the capability of OCT. Doppler optical coherence tomography (DOCT) or optical Doppler tomography (ODT) is one kind of functional extension of OCT which combines the Doppler principle with OCT and provides *in-vivo* functional imaging of moving samples, flows and moving constituents in biological tissues.

The first report that measured localized flow velocity with coherence gating was demonstrated in 1991 [3]. The first two-dimensional *in vivo* ODT imaging was demonstrated in 1997 [4-6]. In early ODT systems, the Doppler frequency shift was obtained by a spectrogram method which used short time fast Fourier transformation (STFFT) or wavelet transformation [4-6]. However, spectrogram methods suffer from low sensitivity and are limited for imaging speed. Phase-resolved ODT (PRODT) was developed to overcome these limitations. This method uses the phase change between sequential A-line scans for velocity image reconstruction [7-9]. PRODT decouples spatial resolution and velocity sensitivity in flow images and increases imaging speed by more than two orders of magnitude without compromising spatial resolution and velocity sensitivity [7]. The first demonstration of PRODT was based on time domain OCT systems [7-8]. Recently, the development of Fourier domain OCT systems have greatly improved the imaging speed and sensitivity [10-12]. Fourier domain ODT systems have been demonstrated by several groups [13-17].

In this chapter, we will review the principle of ODT. Due to the high velocity sensitivity of phase-resolved method and wide use of Fourier domain systems, we will focus on the phase-resolved Doppler method with Fourier domain OCT systems. Several important issues, such as phase stability of the system, sensitivity of the PRODT method, and sample movement induced artifacts for *in-vivo* applications are discussed. In the following section, we will introduce the Doppler principle and the PRODT principle. In section 3, we will discuss the velocity sensitivity of PRODT and the ways to improve the velocity sensitivity. In section 4, we will summarize the three divisions of PRODT methods: color Doppler, Doppler variance, and power Doppler. Specifically, we will discuss the cross-correlation based algorithm for color Doppler and Doppler variance calculations. In section 5, the bulk motion induced artifact in *in-vivo* applications will be discussed. In section 6, we will introduce the recent applications of PRODT from our group. The last section is the summary and acknowledgement.

2. Theory

2.1 The Doppler principle and ODT

ODT is based on the Doppler effect, which was proposed by Austrian physicist Christian Doppler in 1842. The Doppler effect manifests as change of frequency (or wavelength) for a wave reflected or scattered from moving objects. In ODT, the light reflected or scattered from a moving sample or moving subject inside the sample, changes its frequency or wavelength. The amount of the frequency change is related to the frequency of the incident light, the velocity of the moving sample, and the angle between the incident beam direction and the moving direction of subject (or sample). Figure 1 shows a scenario where the light hits on a moving target inside a sample (for example, a red blood cell in a blood vessel).The frequency change (or shift) of the light can be obtained with the following equation:

$$\Delta f = \frac{2v \cdot \cos(\theta)}{c} f_0 = \frac{2v \cdot \cos(\theta)}{\lambda_0} \tag{1}$$

where f_0 is the central frequency of the incident light, λ_0 is the central wavelength of the incident light, v is the speed of the moving target, θ is the Doppler angle (angle between the incident light and the target moving direction), c is the light speed in vacuum.

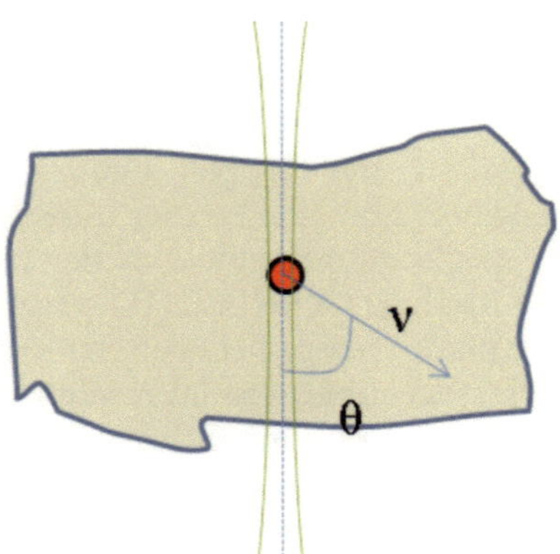

Fig. 1. Schematic of the interaction of wave and moving target inside sample .

2.2 Extraction of Doppler frequency change (shift) in ODT

In early time domain systems, the Doppler frequency shift Δf was obtained by a spectrogram method that uses the short time fast Fourier transformation (STFFT) or wavelet transformation [4-5]. In the spectrogram method, the velocity sensitivity is inversely proportional to the short-time Fourier transform window size, and the spatial resolution is proportional to the short-time Fourier transform window size [8]. Consequently, velocity sensitivity and spatial resolution are coupled. A large pixel time-window size increases velocity sensitivity while decreasing spatial resolution. In addition, the velocity sensitivity decreases with the increasing of frame rate in the spectrogram method [8]. In 2000, Zhao et al. proposed a phase-resolved method to overcome these limitations [8]. In PRODT, the Doppler frequency shift Δf is obtained by the phase change between sequential A-scans. The phase information of the fringe signal can be determined from the complex analytical signal $A_{j,z}$, where $A_{j,z}$ is the complex data at j_{th} A-scan and depth of z. The Doppler frequency shift Δf can be expressed as:

$$\begin{aligned}\Delta f &= \frac{d\phi}{2\pi \cdot dt} \\ &= \frac{\phi_{j+1,z} - \phi_{j,z}}{2\pi \cdot \Delta T} \\ &= \frac{\arg(A_{j+1,z}A_{j,z}^{*})}{2\pi \cdot \Delta T} \\ &= \frac{\tan^{-1}\left(\frac{\mathrm{Im}(A_{j+1,z})}{\mathrm{Re}(A_{j+1,z})}\right) - \tan^{-1}\left(\frac{\mathrm{Im}(A_{j,z})}{\mathrm{Re}(A_{j,z})}\right)}{2\pi \cdot \Delta T}\end{aligned} \tag{2}$$

where ΔT is the time difference between j_{th} A-scan and $(j+1)_{th}$ A-scan. In the time domain ODT system, the complex analytical signal $A_{j,z}$ is determined through analytic continuation of the measured interference fringes function by use of a Hilbert transformation. In Fourier domain ODT systems, the complex signal $A_{j,z}$ is obtained through the Fourier transformation of the acquired fringe. In this chapter, we will focus on Fourier domain PRODT systems. There are two kinds of Fourier domain ODT systems; the spectrometer-based and the swept source laser based ODT. Because the spectrometer-based ODT system shows higher phase stability and no additional phase correction is needed, we will demonstrate most of the experiments with the spectrometer-based system.

The schematic of a spectrometer-based ODT system setup demonstrated in this chapter is shown in Fig. 2. The spectrometer-based FDODT uses a super luminescent diode (SLD) light source which has a central wavelength of 890 nm and full width at half maximum (FWHM) bandwidth of 150 nm. A complementary metal–oxide–semiconductor (CMOS) based linescan camera (Sprint spL4096-70k, Basler vision technique) is used as detector. The CMOS integration time and line period are variable according to different demonstrations. The imaging process includes background signal subtraction, linear interpolation to convert data from the linear wavelength space to the linear wavenumber space, and fast Fourier transformation (FFT). The amplitude of the complex analytical signal obtained after the FFT

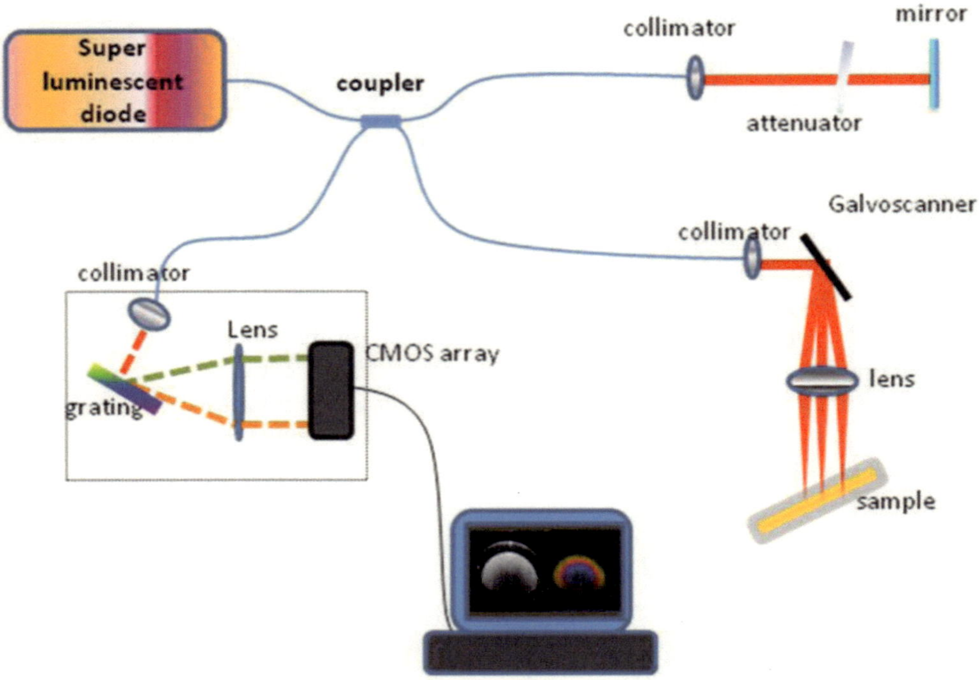

Fig. 2. Schematic of a spectrometer-based ODT system setup.

is used for OCT structure image and the PRODT images are obtained from the phase of the complex analytical signal. Figures 3(a)-(c) show the OCT images of a flow phantom. Figures 3(d), (e) and (f) show the PRODT images corresponding to Figs. 3(a), 3(b) and 3(c). The integration time was set at 47 μs and the line period was set at 50 μs. The flow phantom is made of 1% intralipid in a 500 μm diameter tube. The flow is controlled by a syringe pump. The images contain 1500 A-lines. For Fig. 3(a), 3(b) and 3(c), the angle between the tube and imaging beam was set at around 90 degrees, 85 degrees and 80 degrees, respectively, and the syringe pump speed was kept as constant. From these figures, we can verify that the Doppler frequency shift (which is proportional to the phase changes) is related to the Doppler angle. As shown in Fig. 3(a), the Doppler frequency shift is close to zero when the Doppler angle is close to 90 degrees. The Doppler frequency shift increases with the decrease of the Doppler angle (assuming the Doppler angle is between 0 degrees and 90 degrees). It should be noted that the phase is wrapped in Fig. 3(f). The velocity distribution profiles can also be determined from the PRODT images. The axial velocity distributions along white double arrow direction in Figs. 3(e) and 3(f) are shown in Fig. 4. From Eq. (1), we can also find that the Doppler frequency shift is proportional to the flow velocity if the Doppler angle is fixed. In order to verify that, we keep the angle between the incident beam and the tube constant while changing the pump speed. Figures 5 (a), (b), (c) and (d) are OCT structure images of the flow phantom pumped at, respectively, 20 μl/min, 40 μl/min, 60 μl/min, 80 μl/min. Figures 5(e), 5(f), 5(g) and 5(h) are the PRODT images of flow phantom pumped at, respectively, 20 μl/min, 40 μl/min, 60 μl/min, 80 μl/min. It should be noted that the phase is wrapped in Fig. 5(f). The increasing Doppler frequency shift with the increasing pumping speed can be clearly seen from the PRODT images.

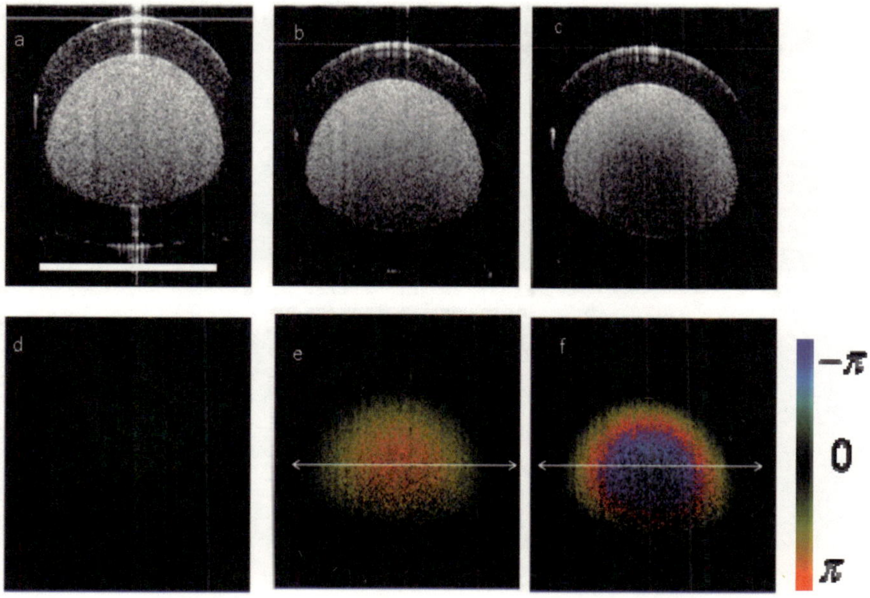

Fig. 3. (a), (b),(c) are OCT structure images of the flow phantom at a Doppler angle of around 90 degrees, 85 degrees and 80 degrees; (d), (e) and (f) are the PRODT images of the flow phantom at a Doppler angle of around 90 degrees, 85 degrees and 80 degrees. Scale bar: 500μm.

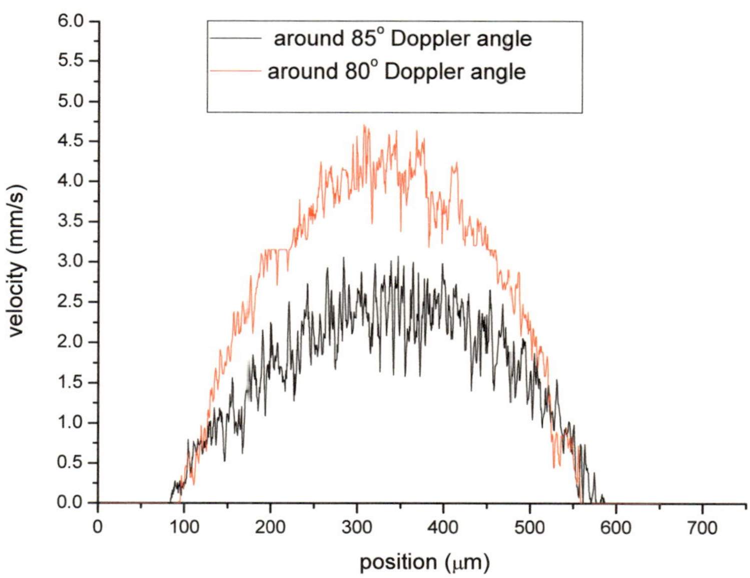

Fig. 4. Velocity profile along the double arrows in Figs. 3(e) and 3(f).

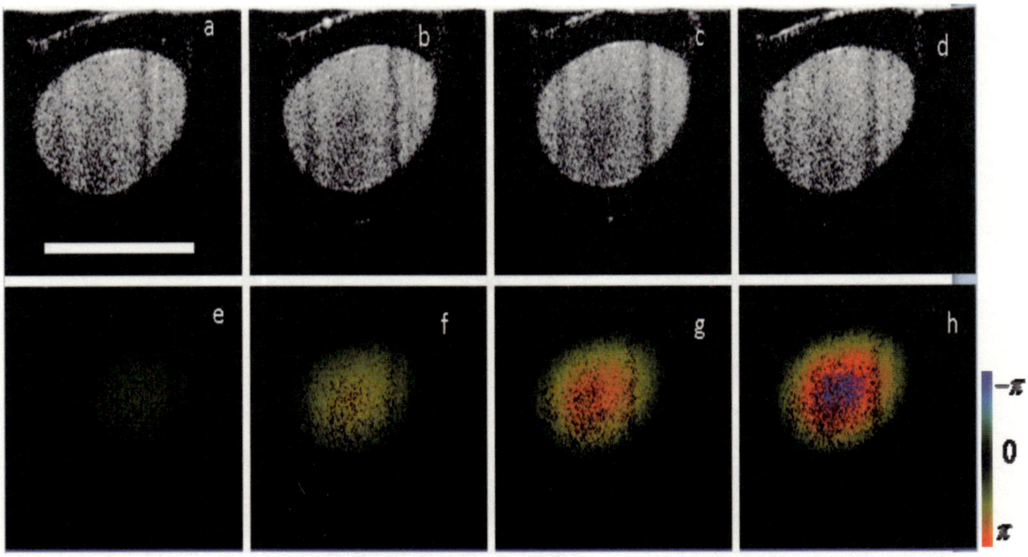

Fig. 5. (a), (b), (c) and (d) are OCT structure images of the flow phantom pumped at, respectively, 20μl/min, 40μl /min, 60μl /min, 80μl /min; (e), (f), (g) and (h) are the PRODT images of the flow phantom pumped at, respectively, 20μl /min, 40μl /min, 60μl /min, 80μl /min. Scale bar: 500μm.

3. Sensitivity of PRODT and minimum detectable Doppler shift

From Eqs. (1) and (2), the velocity of the sample can also be obtained. The minimum resolvable velocity of the system is decided by the minimum resolvable phase difference and the velocity may be expressed as:

$$v_z = \frac{\lambda_c \cdot \delta\theta}{4\pi \cdot n \cdot \Delta T} \tag{3}$$

where v_z is the velocity along the incident beam direction, λ_c is the central wavelength of the OCT system, n is the refraction index of the sample, ΔT is the time difference between adjacent A-lines, and $\delta\theta$ is the minimum resolvable phase difference. Typical phase stability for a spectrometer-based FDOCT is a few milliradians. For swept source based FDOCT, the phase stability can also reach a few milliradians to tens of milliradians range after phase correction. Assuming the A-line rate of the OCT system is 100,000 A-lines per second, the phase stability of the system is 10 milliradians and the refraction index is 1.4, the minimum velocity (along the incident beam direction) that can be resolved by an ODT system with a central wavelength of 1.3 μm is around 74 μm/s.

PRODT has been widely used for *in-vivo* imaging of blood flow in animal or human being. For these applications, the Doppler angle and blood flow velocity are usually unknown in advance. If we assume the velocity of the sample and the Doppler angle are unknown, the minimum detectable Doppler frequency shift is decided by the minimum resolvable phase difference ($d\phi$) and the time difference ΔT in Eq. (2). The minimum resolvable phase difference for an ODT system is related to the phase stability of the system that is affected by factors such as mechanical stability of the system and image SNR. The phase stability of the system can be determined by statistically analyzing the adjacent A-line phase difference of a static mirror. Figure 6(a) shows the measured phase difference of a static mirror by the spectrometer-based Fourier domain ODT system described in the previous section. The integration time was set as 22 μs and the line period was set as 25 μs, which corresponds to an A-line speed of 40,000 Hz. Figure 6(b) shows the histogram of the phase difference distribution. The phase stability is the standard deviation for the histogram of the phase difference distribution. The histogram shows a Gaussian shape-like profile with a FWHM value of 20 milliradians. In order to improve the velocity sensitivity of the PRODT system, increasing the phase stability of the system is necessary. Because there are no mechanical moving parts in the spectrometer-based Fourier domain systems, spectrometer-based Fourier domain systems usually show high phase stability. Most of the demonstrated PRODT systems use spectrometer-based Fourier domain systems.

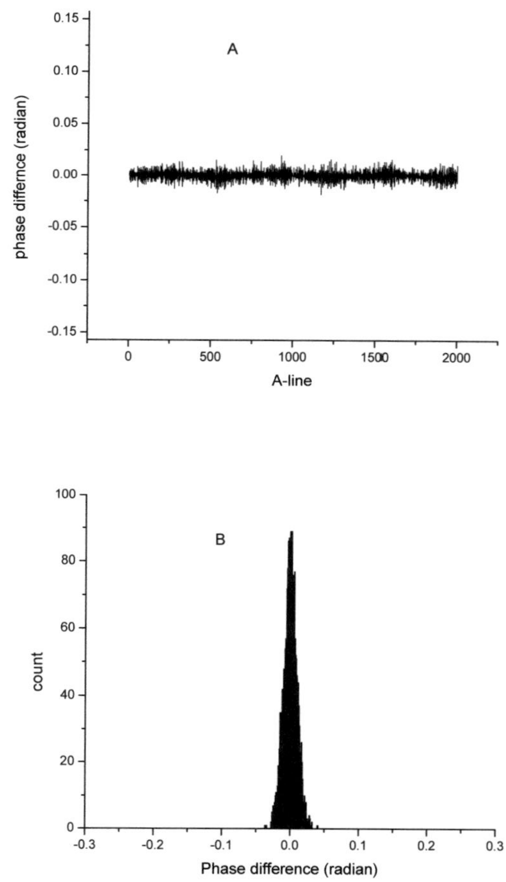

Fig. 6. Phase stability analysis of the spectrometer-based OCT system. (a) Phase differences between adjacent A-lines at the static mirror location; (b). Histogram of the phase difference distribution.

Swept source OCT (SSOCT) systems usually use tunable filters that are based on mechanically scanning of galvanometer mirrors, polygon mirrors or Fabry–Pérot (FP) filters. Due to the mechanical scanning schemes used, swept source OCT systems usually show worse phase stability than spectrometer-based OCT systems. If phase sensitive methods are used, the phase must be corrected before using the phase-resolved algorithm [16-19]. Here, we tested the phase stability of a SSOCT system. The system used a MEMS technique-based swept source laser with a central wavelength of 1310 *nm*, an FWHM spectral bandwidth of about 110 *nm*, an A-line rate of 50,000 Hz, and a total average power of 16 mW (SSOCT-1310, Axsun Technologies Inc, Billerica, MA). The system used a Mach-Zehnder type interferometer with 90% of the light in the sample arm and 10% of the light in the reference arm. A dual-balanced detection scheme was used to acquire the signal. The system works in the K-trigger mode so that no re-calibration is needed. In order to analyze the phase stability of the SSOCT system, a static mirror was used as a sample, and phase differences between adjacent A-lines at the mirror location were obtained. Figure 7(a) shows the phase difference distribution and Fig. 7(b) shows the histogram of the phase difference distribution. Although the histogram as in Fig. 7(b) shows a Gaussian-like profile with an FWHM value of 0.18 radians, there are lots of counts at the large phase difference location. This can be seen more clearly in Fig. 7(a) that shows a lot of phase jumping between adjacent A-lines. These results indicate that spectrometer-based OCT systems show much better phase stability as demonstrated in Fig. 6.

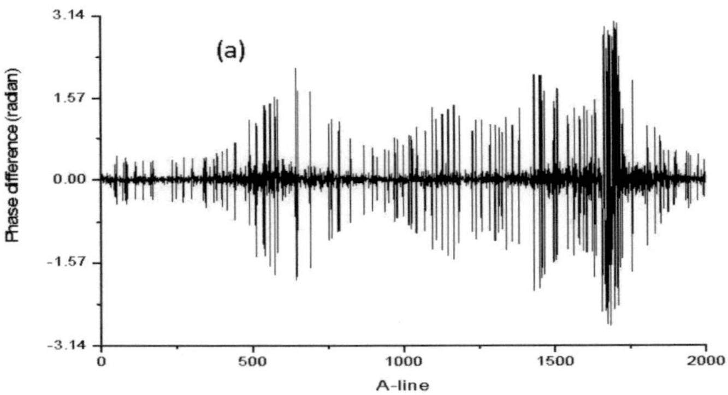

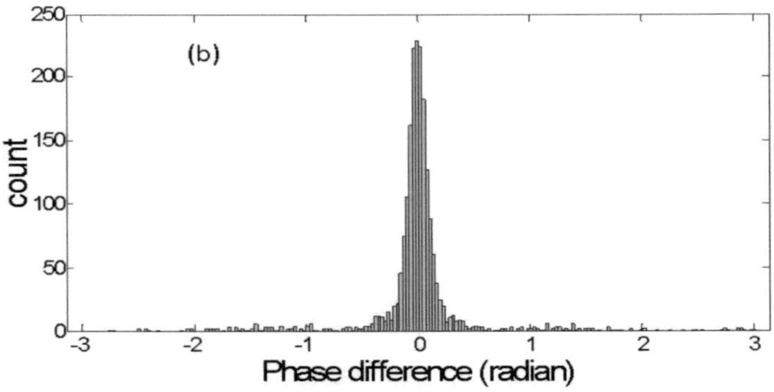

Fig. 7. Phase stability analysis of the SSOCT system. (a) Phase differences between adjacent A-lines at the static mirror location; (b) histogram of the phase difference distribution [20].

There are a number of ways to improve Doppler detection sensitivity. A static surface may be added as a reference to correct phase error and improve the phase stability. Our group has used the top surface of chick chorioallantoic membrane (CAM) as a reference to obtain the blood flow in a CAM [16]. Vakoc et al. have proposed a method to tap 1% of the sample arm light and direct it at a calibration mirror which is positioned near the maximum imaging range of the system [17]. A common-path method has been used to correct phase errors [18, 19]. Figure 8 show the effectiveness of the phase correction method [19]. The laser source is a high speed swept laser with a central wavelength of 1050 nm and a sweeping speed of 100 kHz (Axsun Technology, Billerica, MA). The laser source output is split into the reference and sample arms by a 20:80 coupler with 80% in the reference arm and 20% in the sample arm. In the reference arm, the light is further split by a 95:5 coupler. Ninety-five percent of the light in the reference is sent to cause interference with the collected back-reflection or backscattering signal from the sample. This interference signal is detected by a balanced photon detector and digitized by a high speed digitizer (ATS 9350, Alazar Technologies Inc., Pointe-Claire, QC, Canada). The remaining 5% of the light in the reference arm is sent to a non-balanced photon-detector after passing through a 1 mm thick cover slide and is then finally digitized by another channel in the digitizer [19]. The two surfaces of the cover glass will generate an inference fringe. This will produce a reference surface at a depth corresponding to the thickness of the cover glass. By subtracting a portion of the phase difference of the reference surface location from the phase difference of the sample signal, the phase error is corrected [17-19]. Figures 8(a) and 8(b) show the OCT structure image and the phase difference between successive A-lines before correction for a mirror respectively. Figure 8(c) shows the phase difference between successive A-lines after the correction. The improvement can be seen by comparing the images in Fig. 8(b) and Fig. 8(c).

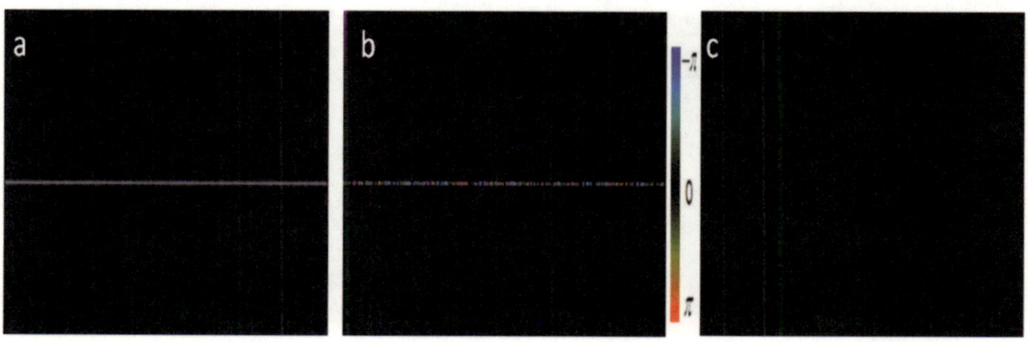

Fig. 8. (a) OCT images of a mirror; (b) adjacent A-line phase difference before correction; (c) adjacent A-line phase difference after correction [19].

Increasing the velocity sensitivity by improving the phase stability is effective. The typical phase stability of spectrometer-based ODT or SSOCT after phase correction will be a few milliradians. The biological tissue will produce adjacent A-line phase changes due to optical heterogeneity of the tissue [21, 22]. This heterogeneous index change will cause phase noise in the PRODT images. In addition, any mechanical movement from the system or environment may introduce phase noise in the PRODT images. These introduced phase noise may be larger than the phase stability of the system. Therefore, the velocity sensitivity may be determined by the phase noise instead of the system phase stability.

Another effective way to increase the velocity sensitivity is to increase the ΔT, namely decrease the A-line speed. From Eq. (3), we can find that the minimum resolvable velocity is inversely proportional to ΔT when all other parameters remain unchanged. Figure 9 shows OCT and PRODT images of a flow phantom acquired by a system with a different A-line rate. The system was the CMOS spectrometer-based FDOCT system described in previous section (Fig. 2). The flow phantom was pumped by the syringe pump at a constant speed for all of the setups. The Doppler angle was the same for all of the setups and it was fixed to be different from 90 degrees so that the Doppler frequency shift was not zero. Figures 9(a)-9(d) show the OCT images of the flow phantom. In Figures 9(a), 9(b), 9(c) and 9(d), the integration time of the CMOS camera was kept as constant (22 μs in this case) while the line periods were set as 25 μs, 50 μs, 100 μs and 200 μs, respectively. The effective A-line rates for Fig. 9(a), 9(b), 9(c) and 9(d) were, respectively, 40,000 Hz, 20,000 Hz, 10,000 Hz and 5,000 Hz. Figures 9(e), 9(f), 9(g) and 9(h) are the PRODT images of the flow phantom corresponding to the OCT images in Figs. 9 (a), 9(b), 9(c) and 9(d). The effectiveness of increasing the velocity sensitivity by reducing the A-line rates can be seen from the PRODT images in Fig. 9.

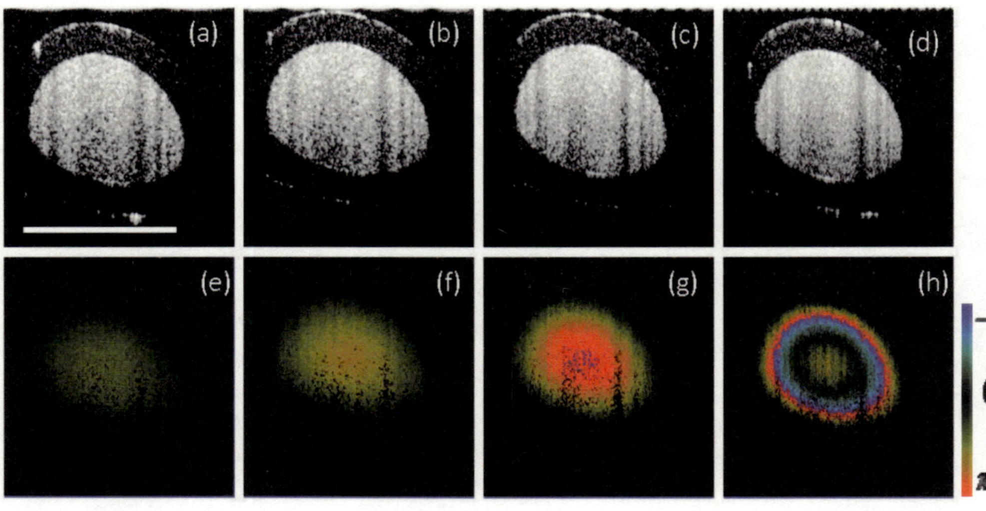

Fig. 9. (a), (b), (c) and (d) are OCT structure images of the flow phantom imaged with the line period set as, respectively, 25 μs, 50 μs, 100 μs and 200 μs; (e), (f), (g) and (h) are the PRODT images of flow phantom obtained with the detector line period set as, respectively, 25 μs, 50 μs, 100 μs and 200 μs. Scale bar: 500μm.

Although changing the A-line rate is an effective way to improve the velocity sensitivity of the PRODT system, faster A-line speed is always preferred so that the imaging time is reduced. Faster speed is especially important for real time or *in-vivo* imaging applications. Increasing the velocity sensitivity without sacrificing the A-line rate can be achieved by extending the phase-resolved algorithms to non-adjacent A-lines while still maintaining space correlation. In this way, the velocity sensitivity of the PRODT is improved while the A-lines speed is still maintained. For such cases, we can rewrite Eq. (2) as follows:

$$\Delta f = \frac{d\phi}{2\pi \cdot dt} = \frac{\phi_{m,z} - \phi_{n,z}}{2\pi \cdot \Delta T(m,n)} = \frac{\tan^{-1}\left(\frac{\text{Im}(A_{m,z})}{\text{Re}(A_{m,z})}\right) - \tan^{-1}\left(\frac{\text{Im}(A_{n,z})}{\text{Re}(A_{n,z})}\right)}{2\pi \cdot \Delta T(m,n)} \quad (4)$$

where $A_{m,z}$ is the complex data at m_{th} A-scan and depth of z, $A_{n,z}$ is the complex data at n_{th} A-scan and depth of z, and $\Delta T(m,n)$ is the time difference between m_{th} A-scan and n_{th} A-scan. When using the above algorithm, the spatial correlation between m_{th} A-scan and n_{th} A-scan should be maintained. Figure 10 shows a way to realize this scheme. Black dots in Fig. 10 show beam scanning locations in a traditional raster scanning pattern. The horizontal direction is the fast galvomirror scanning direction and the vertical direction is the slow galvomirror scanning direction. The three points (m, $m+1$ and n, indicated by the red arrows) indicate 3 locations of the OCT A-scan. Traditional phase-resolved algorithms calculate the Doppler shift with the phase difference between adjacent scanning point m and point $m+1$ at a time difference of $\Delta T(m,m+1)$. However, if the algorithm is used between points m and n, the ΔT is increased greatly because $\Delta T(m,n)$ is much larger than$\Delta T(m,m+1)$. Consequently, the minimum detectable velocity is also increased according to Eq. (3). This scheme has been adopted by several groups to image microsvascular networks [23-25]. Another method extending ΔT is to use a dual beam setup [26, 27]. Two tomograms which are slightly separated in time are obtained from the two beams that are spatially offset. The PRODT algorithm is performed between these two data sets. In this way, the $\Delta T(m,n)$ is tunable by tuning the space offset of the two beams.

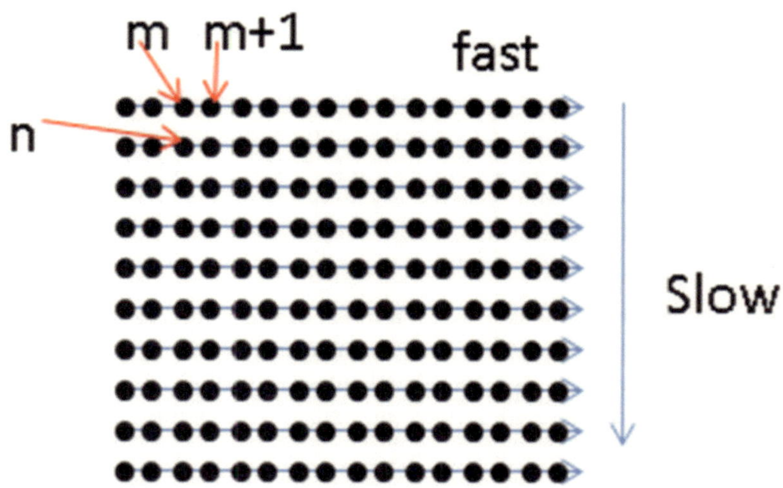

Fig. 10. Schematic of inter-frame processing scheme for PRODT.

4. Cross-correlation algorithm for PRODT, Doppler variance and power Doppler methods

ODT techniques have been widely used for flow imaging, especially blood flow in animals or human beings. Blood flow in humans or animals is complex, and the flow is pulsatile. The flow speed in a blood vessel is not a constant value and changes from the center of the blood vessel to the edge. A parabolic equation may describe the distribution of the steady blood flow along the blood vessel radius. This kind of steady flow is usually called laminar flow. Laminar flow may breakdown into a turbulent flow when the velocity becomes sufficiently high [28]. In practice, the Doppler frequency produced by a single target will produce a spectrum of Doppler frequencies or a series of frequency shifts instead of a single frequency. This spectrum broadening is attributed to several sources, such as the cone-geometrical focusing beam, Brownian motion and speckle. Brownian motion dominates the broadening of the Doppler spectrum at low flow speed, and probe-beam geometry dominates at high flow speed [29].

Depending on the Doppler frequency shift information obtained, we can display this information in a color Doppler method or a variance method. In the color Doppler imaging method, the average Doppler frequency shift is displayed as color images, and the negative and positive averaged frequency shifts are displayed in different colors [4-6,8,9], which provide quantitative information on the flow speed and flow direction. In a Doppler variance image, the variance or the standard deviation of the Doppler frequency shift is displayed [7], which can be used to quantify Brownian motion or measure transverse flow [29].

In addition, there is a power Doppler mode that displays the flow power signal by filtering out the signal form stationary tissue [30]. In Fourier domain OCT systems, the filtering process may be realized by hardware-based or software-based methods. Wang et al. developed a method called optical microangiograph (OMAG) [31-35]. In OMAG, a Doppler frequency is introduced in the lateral beam scanning direction (B-scan) so that the moving and static scattering components within the sample are separated. The Doppler frequency may be introduced by either the reference mirror mounted on A-linear piezo translation stage or by offsetting the sample arm beam from the scanning galvomirror pivot. Yuan et al. proposed a digital frequency ramping method by numerically introducing a phase shift into the original spectral interferometric signal using a Hilbert transform [36]. Tao et al. proposed single-pass flow imaging spectral domain optical coherence tomography (SPFI-OCT) with a modified Hilbert transform algorithm to separate moving and non-moving scatters [37, 38].

Instead of using the algorithm as in Eqs. (2) and (4) directly, the algorithm derived from a cross-correlation algorithm shows better performance and is usually preferred [7-9, 39, 40]. In addition, averaging can improve the signal noise ratio [7-9, 40]. Averaging could be performed in the lateral direction (temporal direction) so that the Eqs. (2) and (4) can be rewritten as [8]:

$$\bar{f} = \frac{1}{(2\pi \cdot \Delta T)} \arctan\left\{ \frac{\sum_{j=1}^{J}\left[\mathrm{Im}(A_{j+1,z})\mathrm{Re}(A_{j,z}) - \mathrm{Im}(A_{j,z})\mathrm{Re}(A_{j+1,z})\right]}{\sum_{j=1}^{J}\left[\mathrm{Re}(A_{j,z})\mathrm{Re}(A_{j+1,z}) + \mathrm{Im}(A_{j+1,z})\mathrm{Im}(A_{j,z})\right]} \right\} \tag{5}$$

where J is the number of A-lines that are averaged. Averaging could also be performed in both lateral and depth directions and Eqs. (2) and (4) become [18, 19, 20]:

$$\overline{f} = \frac{1}{(2\pi \cdot \Delta T)} \cdot \arctan\left\{ \frac{\sum_{j=1}^{J}\sum_{z=1}^{N}\left[\mathrm{Im}(A_{j+1,z})\mathrm{Re}(A_{j,z}) - \mathrm{Im}(A_{j,z})\mathrm{Re}(A_{j+1,z})\right]}{\sum_{j=1}^{J}\sum_{z=1}^{N}\left[\mathrm{Re}(A_{j,z})\mathrm{Re}(A_{j+1,z}) + \mathrm{Im}(A_{j+1,z})\mathrm{Im}(A_{j,z})\right]} \right\} \tag{6}$$

where J is the number of A-lines that are averaged, and N is the number of depth points that are averaged. The choice of J and N are dependent on application. Generally, a larger J and N will increase SNR, increase the computing time, and decrease resolution.

Doppler variance uses the variance of the Doppler frequency spectrum to map the flow. Doppler variance has the benefit of being less sensitive to the pulsatile nature of the blood flow, less sensitive to the incident angle, and may be used to obtain the transverse flow velocity [7, 29, 41, and 42]. If σ denotes the standard deviation of the Doppler spectrum, the Doppler variance σ^2 can be obtained [7]:

$$\sigma^2 = \frac{\int (f-\overline{f})^2 P(f)df}{\int P(f)df} = \overline{f^2} - \overline{f}^2 \tag{7}$$

where $\overline{f}$ is Doppler frequency and $P(f)$ is the power spectrum of the Doppler frequency shift. With the help of autocorrelation technology, the variance can be expressed as [7]:

$$\sigma^2 = \frac{1}{(2\pi \cdot \Delta T)^2}\left(1 - \frac{\left|A_{j+1,z}A_{j,z}^*\right|}{A_{j,z}A_{j,z}^*}\right) \tag{8}$$

where $A_{j,z}^*$ is the complex conjugate of $A_{j,z}$ .Similar to the color Doppler algorithms in Eqs. (5) and (6) , averaging is usually used to improve the SNR and we have:

$$\sigma^2 = \frac{1}{(2\pi \cdot \Delta T)^2}\left[1 - \frac{\left|\sum_{j=1}^{J}\left(A_{j+1,z}A_{j,z}^*\right)\right|}{\sum_{j=1}^{J}\left(A_{j,z}A_{j,z}^*\right)}\right] \tag{9}$$

$$\sigma^2 = \frac{1}{(2\pi \cdot \Delta T)^2}\left[1 - \frac{\left|\sum_{j=1}^{J}\sum_{z=1}^{N}\left(A_{j+1,z}A_{j,z}^*\right)\right|}{\sum_{j=1}^{J}\sum_{z=1}^{N}\left(A_{j,z}A_{j,z}^*\right)}\right] \tag{10}$$

where J is the number of A-lines that are averaged and N is the number of depth points that are averaged.

Figure 11 shows images of the hamster skin installed in a dorsal window chamber. The images are obtained with a charge-coupled device (CCD) spectrometer-based OCT system

[42]. Figures 11(a), 11(b), 11(c) and 11(d) show the OCT structure image, color Doppler image, Doppler variance image and power Doppler image, respectively. The color Doppler image and Doppler variance image are obtained with the Eqs. (6) and (10), respectively, with $J = 4$ and $N = 4$. The power Doppler image is obtained with a modified Hilbert method [24, 37]. From the figures, it can be found that all three methods are able to detect the blood vessels. However, the information they provide are different and this information are actually complementary. Color Doppler can give information regarding the flow direction and the speed of the flow. Doppler variance provides flow turbulence information and transverse flow velocity. Power Doppler provides the total power of the Doppler signal from the flows.

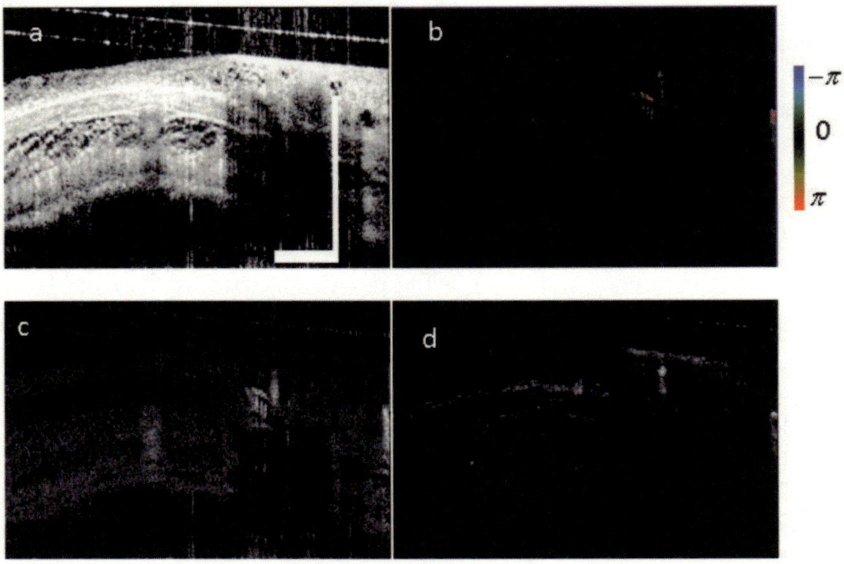

Fig. 11. OCT images of the hamster skin installed in a dorsal window chamber. (a) OCT structure image; (b) color Doppler image; (c) Doppler variance image; (d) power Doppler image. Scale bar: 500 μm.

5. Bulk-motion and *in-vivo* imaging

Because of its high spatial resolution and velocity sensitivity, Doppler OCT has been widely used for blood flow related biomedical applications [32-25, 41-48]. These applications require imaging of blood flow *in-vivo*. For *in-vivo* applications, especially awake patient imaging, axial sample movement induced by involuntary movements will introduce bulk-motion and change the Doppler frequency [9]. Both sample movement and blood flow inside the tissue will change the reflected or scattered light frequency. The Doppler frequency in the blood vessels obtained with phase-resolved method will be a linear sum of the Doppler frequency induced by the sample movement and actual blood flow [9]. Figures 12(a) and 12(b) show the *in-vivo* OCT structure and PRODT images of human retina obtained with a CCD spectrometer-base FDOCT system [41, 42, and 45]. The ODT image shows strong bulk-motion induced artifact which manifests as strong background noise, especially around the leftmost and rightmost regions in the yellow circles of Fig. 12(b). The

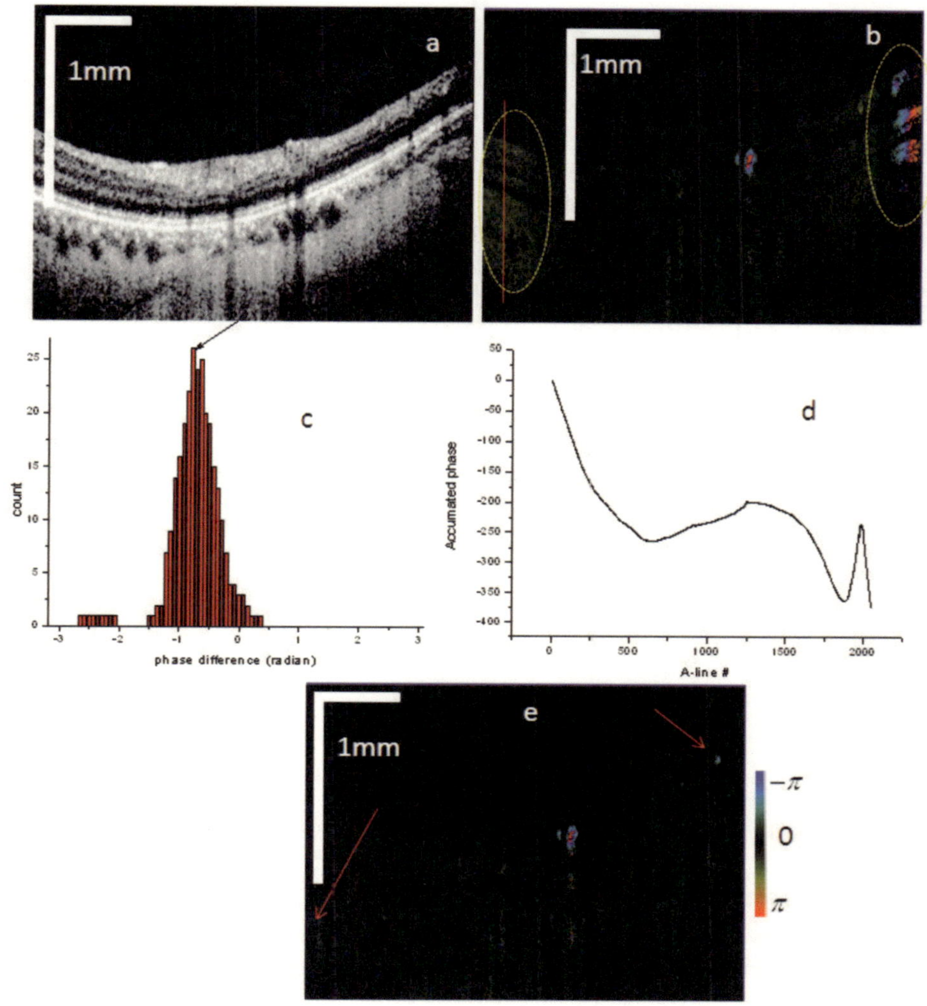

Fig. 12. Demonstration of bulk-motion correction for *in-vivo* PRODT application. (a) *In-vivo* OCT structure and (b) PRODT images without bulk-motion correction of human retina; (c) histogram of the phase difference distribution for the A-line indicated by the red vertical line in Fig.12(b); (d) accumulated bulk-motion phase of all the A-lines; (e) PRODT images with bulk-motion correction.

blood vessels in these regions are not able to be identified from the PRODT image. In order to obtain the Doppler frequency induced by the actual blood flow, the Doppler frequency induced by the sample movement must be identified and subtracted. The sample movement may be considered as a "global" effect; it will induce constant Doppler shift for the whole A-line. Most bulk-motion correction methods assume that the sample movement will induce a constant phase term for each A-line, and by subtracting this phase term, the bulk-motion induced artifacts can be corrected [9, 32, 40 and 49]. Up to now, several methods have been proposed to determine the bulk phase [9, 32, 40, 41 and

49]. Usually, the median phase or mean phase is determined from a histogram of adjacent A-line phase differences and then subtracted. Recently, averaged shift histogram-based nonparametric density estimators have shown good performance and have become popular in extracting the bulk phase [32, 41 and 49]. Figure 12(c) shows the histogram of the phase difference distribution for the A-line indicated by the red vertical line in Fig. 12(b). The location with the maximum bin count as indicated by the black arrow is taken as the bulk phase. By repeating this process for all the A-lines in the B-scan image, the bulk phases for all the A-lines are draw as Fig. 12(d). The phases in Fig. 12(d) are unwrapped and then subtracted from the phases of the corresponding A-line. Figure 12(e) shows the PRODT images after the phase-correction method has been used. The blood vessels that cannot be identified in Fig. 12 (b) are clearly visible in Fig. 12(e). The red arrows in Fig. 12(e) indicate two such vessels.

These histogram-based methods have shown success in different situations and been applied for color Doppler and OMAG [23, 32, 41 and 49]. However these methods increase the computational complexity and time. The correction may also introduce artifacts when the blood vessels are large and take most of the pixels for an A-line [35, 45]. We have shown that the Doppler variance method is not sensitive to bulk-motion and the method can be used without correcting the bulk-motion when the sample-movement-induced velocity changes gradually [42].

If ϕ_j is the bulk phase induced by sample movement at the jth A-line, when there is sample movement, we can rewrite Eq. (2) as

$$\begin{aligned}\overline{f} &= \arg(A_{j+1,z}\exp(i\phi_{j+1}A^*_{j,z}\exp(\text{-}i\phi_j))/(2\pi\cdot\Delta T)\\ &= \arg(A_{j+1,z}A^*_{j,z})/(2\pi\cdot\Delta T)+\Delta\phi_j/(2\pi\cdot\Delta T)\end{aligned} \tag{11}$$

where $\Delta\phi_j = \phi_{j+1}-\phi_j$ and $\Delta\phi_j / T$ is the Doppler frequency shift induced by the axial direction sample movement. Therefore, when there is axial sample movement, the average Doppler frequency shift detected is the linear sum of the Doppler frequency shift induced by sample movement with the Doppler frequency shift without sample movement.

However, for the Doppler variance, we can rewrite Eq. (8) as follows when there is sample movement,

$$\begin{aligned}\sigma^2 &= \frac{1}{(2\pi\cdot\Delta T)^2}\left(1-\frac{\left|A_{j+1,z}\exp(i\phi_{j+1}A^*_{j,z}\exp(\text{-}i\phi_j\right|}{A_{j,z}A^*_{j,z}}\right)\\ &= \frac{1}{T^2}\left(1-\frac{\left|A_{j+1,z}A^*_{j,z}\right|}{A_{j,z}A^*_{j,z}}\right).\end{aligned} \tag{12}$$

We can find that the Doppler variance is only a function of the amplitude of the signal and not related to the phase term of the signal. In the case where lateral averaging is used as in Eq. (9), we can rewrite it as follows when there is sample movement:

$$\sigma^2 = \frac{1}{(2\pi \cdot \Delta T)^2}\left[1 - \frac{\left|\sum_{j=1}^{J}\left(A_{j+1,z}A_{j,z}^{*}\right)\exp(i\Delta\phi_j)\right|}{\sum_{j=1}^{J}\left(\left|A_{j,z}\right|^2\right)}\right] \tag{13}$$

where $\Delta\phi_j = \phi_{j+1} - \phi_j$ and $\Delta\phi_j$ is proportional to the velocity of the axial direction sample movement. Eq. (13) can also be written as

$$\sigma^2 = \frac{1}{(2\pi \cdot \Delta T)^2}\left[1 - \frac{\left|\sum_{j=1}^{J}\left(A_{j+1,z}A_{j,z}^{*}\right)\exp(i\Delta\phi_j\text{-}i\Delta\phi_1)\right|}{\sum_{j=1}^{J}\left(\left|A_{j,z}\right|^2\right)}\right] \tag{14}$$

where $\Delta\phi_j = \phi_{j+1} - \phi_j$ and $\Delta\phi_j$ is proportional to the velocity of the axial direction sample movement. Therefore, when there is sample movement and Eq. (9) is used to calculate the Doppler variance, the value of the variance is a function of $\Delta\phi_j - \Delta\phi_1$, which is proportional to the sample-movement-induced velocity difference between the 1st A-line and the other A-lines in the averaging area. For most *in-vivo* applications, the velocity induced by sample movement changes gradually and this velocity difference in the small averaging area (usually 4-16 A-lines) is small. When both lateral and depth averaging algorithms are used as in Eq. (10), the impact of sample movement on the Doppler variance is reduced further (by N times) because ϕ_j is assumed to be constant in a single A-line.

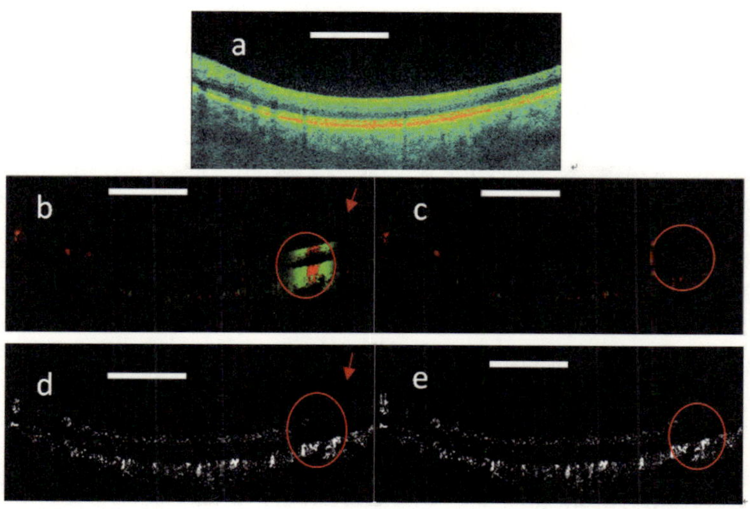

Fig. 13. (a) OCT intensity image; (b) color Doppler OCT image without bulk-motion correction; (c) color Doppler OCT image with bulk-motion correction; (d) Doppler variance OCT image without bulk-motion correction; (e) Doppler variance OCT image with bulk-motion correction. Scale bar: 1mm [42].

Figure 13 shows the OCT images of the human retinal region. The images shown have a scanning range of $5\,mm$ and include 2048 A-lines. Figure 13(a) shows the OCT structural image. Figures 13(b) and 13(c) show color Doppler images with and without bulk phase correction. Figures 13(d) and 13(e) show the Doppler variance images with and without bulk phase removal.

From Fig. 13(b), it can be seen that the color Doppler image is affected by bulk-motion. The bulk-motion increases the background signal of the color Doppler image and blood vessels cannot be identified if the bulk-motion is too strong, as shown in the region inside the red circle in Fig. 13(b). It can also be found that the bulk phase induced by bulk-motion is constant along the axial direction, which is the basis of the current bulk-motion algorithm. This also proves that the Doppler frequency induced bulk-motion can be considered as a constant variable in a single A-line. Sample movement induced motion artifacts must be corrected before applying the color Doppler algorithm. The bulk-motion-corrected image as demonstrated in Fig. 13(c) shows great improvement, and the color Doppler image demonstrates much clearer blood vessels. However, in the region where large blood vessels exist, the bulk-motion-corrected image in Fig. 13(c) shows correction artifacts as indicated by the red arrows. Although this correction artifact is not important in most imaging areas, the artifacts may cause erroneous blood vessel locations in the color Doppler image in regions with large blood vessels such as the optic disk. An improved phase-resolved algorithm has been proposed to correct this artifact [45]. Although effective, the improved algorithm increases the calculation time.

In the Doppler variance image without bulk-motion correction as shown in Fig. 13(d), the blood vessels can be seen even in the high speed sample movement region shown in the red circle. As shown in the previous section, the Doppler variance obtained with the averaged autocorrelation algorithm is affected by the sample-movement-induced velocity difference within the averaging area. We can find from Fig. 13(b) that velocity of sample movement changes gradually (please note the green to red color change in the high speed sample movement region is due to phase wrapping). The sample-movement-induced velocity change is small in the small averaging area. Because depth averaging is also used, the bulk-motion effect can be neglected here. The Doppler variance image with bulk-motion correction is also shown in Fig. 13(e) in order to verify the results. The two images [Figs. 13(d) and 13(e)] show great similarity and the high bulk-motion region as in the circle regions. However, similar to color Doppler images, histogram-based bulk-motion-correction also introduces artifacts in the final Doppler variance image as indicated by the red arrow in Fig. 13(e). The Doppler variance image [Fig. 13(d)] without bulk-motion-correction is artifact free.

6. Recent application with PRODT

Blood flow related biomedical applications with PRODT have been demonstrated for imaging ocular blood flow, mapping cortical hemodynamics for brain research, drug screening, monitoring changes in image tissue morphology and hemodynamics following pharmacological intervention and photodynamic therapy, evaluating the efficacy of laser treatment in port wine stain (PWS) patients, assessing the depth of burn wounds, imaging tumor microenvironment, and quantifying cerebral blood flow [32-25, 41-48]. There have been excellent review papers or book chapters about the advances of PRODT [2 and 50]. We will introduce the recent applications and PRODT for application beyond the flow imaging.

Recent advances of PRODT techniques have made capillary vasculature imaging possible. Our group has demonstrated fine retina microvascular networking with color Doppler, Doppler variance and OMAG techniques [41]. Figure 14(a) shows a top view of the 3-D variance reconstruction, and Fig. 14(b) shows a color-coded variance image where the retina vessels are coded with orange and the choroid ones with blue-green. Figure 14(c) gives a 3-D Doppler reconstruction of the vasculature from which one can notice the Doppler flow "artifact" in some vessels due to the Doppler angle change labeled 1 and the pulsatile nature of the blood flow labeled 2. Figures 14(d) and 14(e) show the results of 3-D OMAG. Ultrahigh sensitive PRODT techniques with inter-frame PRODT algorithm or dual beam methods have been demonstrated for several kinds of applications [23-27].

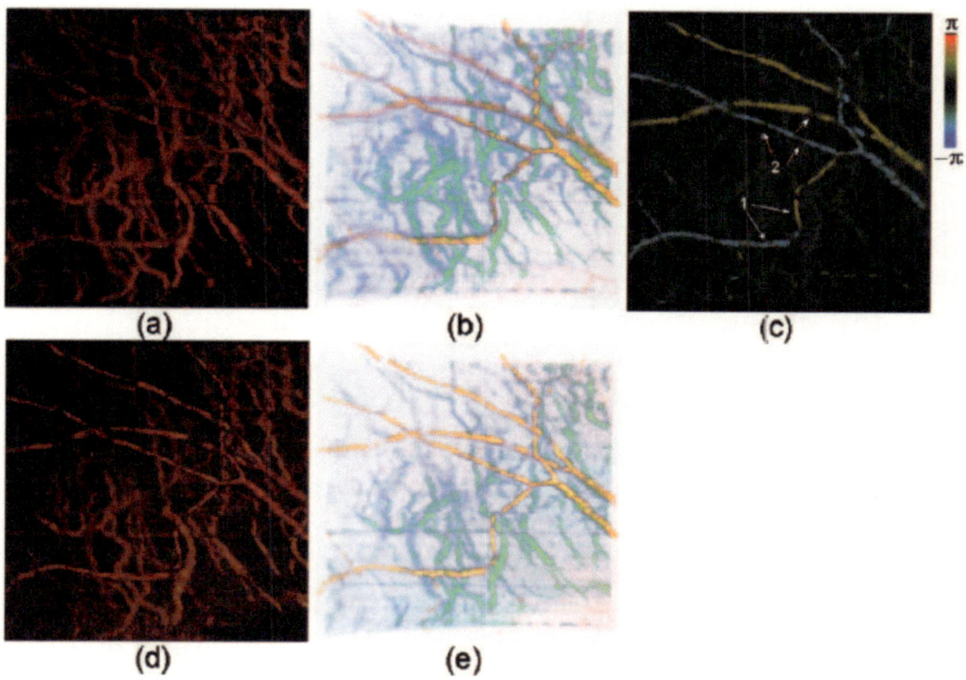

Fig. 14 Three-dimensional angiography of the human eye by different imaging modalities: (a) top view projection of 3-D variance imaging; (b) color-coded variance image; (c) 3-D ODT image; (d) and (e) show the top view and color-coded results from 3-D OMAG [41].

In addition to blood flow related applications, our group has extended the application of ODT for functional imaging of moving tissue to provide the axial direction velocity distribution in the cross-section image. Figure 15 shows the velocity distribution of a cross-sectional image obtained with the phase-resolved color Doppler method for M-Mode *ex-vivo* imaging of a vibrating swine vocal fold. The system is a swept source OCT system with A-line rate of 100,000 Hz. In Fig. 15, a quasi-periodic pattern was caused by phase wrapping, and the phase difference is wrapped between $-\pi$ and π . However, wrapped phase images also give qualitative information regarding acceleration. The absolute value of the velocity can be obtained using the following simple method.

According to Eq. (3), phase difference of $\Delta\theta = 2\pi$ corresponds to a velocity difference of $0.0525 m/s$ (here, $\lambda_c = 1.05 \mu m$, $\Delta T = 10 \mu s$). In Fig. 15, the black striations, as indicated by the white arrows, correspond to a velocity value of $n \times 0.0525 m/s$, where n is an integer. The regions with $n = 0$ are decided based upon the peak and valley location of the oscillation. The values for n in the other regions can then be decided by their relative distance to the $n = 0$ region. In Fig. 15, the maximum n is 7, and the maximum velocity is between velocities $0.3675 m/s$ and $0.42 m/s$, which correspond to n=7 and n=8 respectively. From Fig. 15, we can find that the velocity distribution in the down slope region is different from that in the up slope region. In the down slope, the velocity distribution pattern of the tissue surface is more like a sine function. The velocity changes fast at the peak and valley regions, and it changes slower at the waist region. However, in the up slope, the velocity distribution pattern cannot be seen clearly.

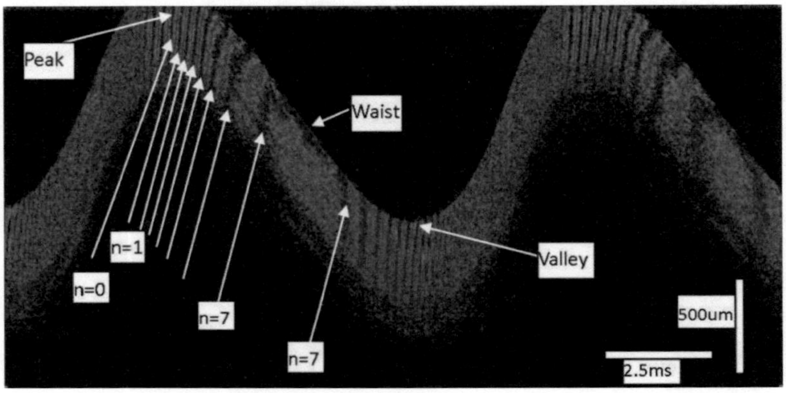

Fig. 15. Color Doppler image of the vibrating vocal fold [19].

7. Summary and conclusions

ODT has seen great improvement since its introduction a decade ago. The development of the phase-resolved method and Fourier domain method has enabled high speed and high sensitivity Doppler imaging in 3D. The sensitivity of PRODT has been improved greatly to provide capillary vascular imaging capability. The application of PRODT has extended to many aspects of biomedical imaging such as ophthalmology, otolaryngology, pulmonology, urology, dermatology and brain imaging. With the advance of OCT technology, the speed and sensitivity of ODT system will improve further, which will enable the applications of ODT technique to more fields. Finally, integration of Doppler OCT with other functional imaging modalities, such as polarization sensitive OCT, spectroscopic OCT, will enhance the potential applications of this technology further.

8. Acknowledgement

The authors thank Elaine Kato for proofreading this manuscript. We thank our former group members, Dr. Yonghua Zhao, Dr. Hongwu Ren, Dr. Lei Wang, Dr. Yimin Wang, Dr. Yi Jiang, Dr. Bin Rao, Dr. Yeh-Chan Ahn, Dr. Woonggyu Jung, Dr. Tuqiang Xie, Dr. Jianping Su, Dr. Lingfeng Yu, our current members, Dr. Jun Zhang, Ms. Wenjuan Qi, Ms. Jiechen Yin, and all those who have contributed to the Doppler OCT project at the Beckman Laser Institute and Department of Biomedical Engineering at UCI. Dr. Chen also acknowledges grant support from the National Institutes of Health (EB- 00293, NCI-91717, RR-01192, EB-00255 EB-10090, HL-103764 and HL-105215), the National Science Foundation (BES-86924), the Whitaker Foundation (WF-23281), Defense Advanced Research Program Agency (Bioflip program), Air Force Office of Scientific Research (F49620-00-1-0371, FA9550-04-0101), and the Beckman Laser Institute Endowment.

9. References

[1] D. Huang, E. A. Swanson, C. P. Lin, J. S. Schuman, W. G. Stinson, W. Chang, M. R. Hee, T. Flotte, K. Gregory, C. A. Puliafito, and J. G. Fujimoto, "Optical coherence tomography," Science 254, 1178–1181 (1991).

[2] Optical Coherence Tomography: Technology and Applications, Wolfgang Drexler (Editor), James G. Fujimoto (Editor), spinger

[3] V. Gusmeroli and M. Martnelli, "Distributed laser Doppler velocimeter," Opt. Lett. 16, 1358-1360 (1991).

[4] Z. Chen, T. E. Milner, D. Dave, and J. S. Nelson, "Optical Doppler tomographic imaging of fluid flow velocity in highly scattering media," Opt. Lett. 22, 64–66 (1997).

[5] Z. Chen, T. E. Milner, S. Srinivas, X. J. Wang, A. Malekafzali, M. J. C. van Gemert, and J. S. Nelson, "Noninvasive imaging of *in vivo* blood flow velocity using optical Doppler tomography," Opt. Lett. 22, 1119–1121 (1997).

[6] Joseph A. Izatt, Manish D. Kulkarni, Siavash Yazdanfar, Jennifer K. Barton, and Ashley J. Welch, "*In vivo* bidirectional color Doppler flow imaging of picoliter blood volumes using optical coherence tomography," Opt. Lett. 22, 1439-1441 (1997).

[7] Y. Zhao, Z. Chen, C. Saxer, S. Xiang, J. de Boer, and J. Nelson, "Doppler variance imaging for clinical monitoring of *in vivo* human skin blood flow," Opt. Lett. 25, 1358–1360 (2000).

[8] Y. Zhao, Z. Chen, C. Saxer, S. Xiang, J. de Boer, and J. Nelson, "Phase resolved optical coherence tomography and optical Doppler tomography for imaging blood flow in human skin with fast scanning speed and high velocity sensitivity," Opt. Lett. 25, 114–116 (2000).

[9] Y. Zhao, Z. Chen, Z. Ding, H. Ren, and J. S. Nelson, "Three-dimensional reconstruction of in vivo blood vessels in human skin using phase-resolved optical Doppler tomography," IEEE J. of Selected Topics in Quantum Electronics 7, 931-935 (2001).

[10] R. Leitgeb, C. K. Hitzenberger, A. F. Fercher, "Performance of fourier domain vs. Time domain optical coherence tomography," Opt. Express 11, 889-894 (2003), <a href="http://www.opticsexpress.org/abstract.cfm?URI=OPEX-11-8-889">http://www.opticsexpress.org/abstract.cfm?URI=OPEX-11-8-889</a>. [UC-eLinks]

[11] J. F. de Boer, B. Cense, B. H. Park, M. C. Pierce, G. J. Tearney, B. E. Bouma, "Signal to noise gain of spectral domain over time domain optical coherence tomography," Opt. Lett. 28, 2067-2069 (2003). [UC-eLinks]

[12] M. A. Choma, M. V. Sarunic, C. Yang,J. A. Izatt, "Sensitivity advantage of swept source and fourier domain optical coherence tomography," Opt. Express 11, 2183-2189 (2003),

[13] R.A. Leitgeb, L. Schmetterer, W. Drexler, A.F. Fercher, R.J. Zawadzki, T. Bajraszewski, Opt. Exp. 11, 3116 (2003)

[14] B.R. White, M.C. Pierce, N. Nassif, B. Cense, B.H. Park, G.J. Tearney, B.E. Bouma, T.C. Chen, J.F. de Boer, Opt. Exp. 25, 3490 (2003)

[15] L. Wang, Y. Wang, M. Bachaman, G.P. Li, Z. Chen, Opt. Commun. 242, 345 (2004)

[16] Jun Zhang and Zhongping Chen, "In vivo blood flow imaging by a swept laser source based Fourier domain optical Doppler tomography," Opt. Express 13, 7449-7457 (2005) http://www.opticsinfobase.org/abstract.cfm?URI=oe-13-19-7449

[17] B. Vakoc, S. Yun, J. de Boer, G. Tearney, and B. Bouma, "Phase-resolved optical frequency domain imaging," Opt. Express 13, 5483-5493 (2005) http://www.opticsinfobase.org/abstract.cfm?URI=oe-13-14-5483

[18] Desmond C. Adler, Robert Huber, and James G. Fujimoto, "Phase-sensitive optical coherence tomography at up to 370,000 lines per second using buffered Fourier domain mode-locked lasers," Opt. Lett. 32, 626-628 (2007) http://www.opticsinfobase.org/abstract.cfm?URI=ol-32-6-626

[19] Gangjun Liu, Marc Rubinstein, Arya Saidi, Wenjuan Qi, Allen Foulad, Brian Wong and Zhongping Chen, "Imaging vocal fold vibration with a high speed 1um swept source OCT and ODT system," *Optics Express*, 19, 11880–11889 (2011).

[20] Gangjun Liu, Lidek Chou, Wangcun Jia, Wenjuan Qi, Bernard Choi, and Zhongping Chen, "Intensity-based modified Doppler variance algorithm: application to phase instable and phase stable optical coherence tomography systems," *Optics Express*, 19, 11429–11440 (2011).

[21] Ruikang K. Wang and Zhenhe Ma, "Real-time flow imaging by removing texture pattern artifacts in spectral-domain optical Doppler tomography," Opt. Lett. 31, 3001-3003 (2006) http://www.opticsinfobase.org/abstract.cfm?URI=ol-31-20-3001

[22] Hongwu Ren, Tao Sun, Daniel J. MacDonald, Michael J. Cobb, and Xingde Li, "Real-time in vivo blood-flow imaging by moving-scatterer-sensitive spectral-domain optical Doppler tomography," Opt. Lett. 31, 927-929 (2006) http://www.opticsinfobase.org/abstract.cfm?URI=ol-31-7-927

[23] J. Fingler, R. J. Zawadzki, J. S. Werner, D.Schwartz, and S. E. Fraser, "Volumetric microvascular imaging of human retina using optical coherence tomography with a novel motion contrast technique," Opt. Express 17, 22190-22200 (2009). http://www.opticsinfobase.org/abstract.cfm?URI=oe-17-24-22190

[24] L. An, J. Qin, and R. K. Wang, "Ultrahigh sensitive optical microangiography for in vivo imaging of microcirculations within human skin tissue beds," Optics Express 18, 8220-8228 (2010).

[25] Yeongri Jung, Zhongwei Zhi and Ruikang K. Wang, "Three-dimensional optical imaging of microvascular networks within intact lymph node *in vivo*", J. Biomed. Opt. 15, 050501

[26] S. Zotter, M. Pircher, T. Torzicky, M. Bonesi, E. Götzinger, R. A. Leitgeb, and C. K. Hitzenberger, "Visualization of microvasculature by dual-beam phase-resolved Doppler optical coherence tomography," Opt. Express 19, 1217-1227 (2011). http://www.opticsinfobase.org/abstract.cfm?URI=oe-19-2-1217

[27] S. Makita, F. Jaillon, M. Yamanari, M. Miura, and Y. Yasuno, "Comprehensive in vivo micro-vascular imaging of the human eye by dual-beam-scan Doppler optical coherence angiography," Opt. Express 19, 1271-1283 (2011). http://www.opticsinfobase.org/abstract.cfm?URI=oe-19-2-1271

[28] David H. Evans, W. Norman McDicken, Doppler Ultrasound: Physics, Instrumental, and Clinical Applications, 2nd Edition (John Wiley Sons, 2000)

[29] H. Ren, K. M. Brecke, Z. Ding, Y. Zhao, J. S. Nelson, and Z. Chen, "Imaging and quantifying transverse flow velocity with the Doppler bandwidth in a phase-resolved functional optical coherence tomography," Opt. Lett. 27, 409-411 (2002). http://www.opticsinfobase.org/abstract.cfm?URI=ol-27-6-409

[30] H. Ren, Y. Wang, J. S. Nelson, and Z. Chen, "Power optical Doppler tomography imaging of blood vessel in human skin and M-mode Doppler imaging of blood flow in chick chrioallantoic membrane," in Coherence Domain Optical Methods and Optical Coherence Tomography in Biomedicine VII, V. V. Tuchin, J. A. Izatt, and J. G. Fujimoto, eds., Proc. SPIE 4956, 225-231 (2003).

[31] R. K.Wang, S. L. Jacques, Z. Ma, S. Hurst, S. R. Hanson, and A. Gruber, "Three dimensional optical angiography," Optics Express, vol. 15, no. 7, pp. 4083–4097, 2007.

[32] R. K. Wang and S. Hurst, "Mapping of cerebro-vascularblood perfusion in mice with skin and skull intact by Optical Micro-AngioGraphy at 1.3 μm wavelength," Optics Express, vol. 15, no. 18, pp. 11402–11412, 2007.

[33] L. An and R. K. Wang, "In vivo volumetric imaging of vascular perfusion within human retina and chcroids with optical micro-angiography," Optics Express, vol. 16, no. 15, pp. 11438–11452, 2008.

[34] R. K. Wang and L. An, "Doppler optical micro-angiography for volumetric imaging of vascular perfusion in vivo," Optics Express, vol. 17, no. 11, pp. 8926–8940, 2009.

[35] L. An, H. M. Subhash, D. J. Wilson, and R. K. Wang, "High resolution wide-field imaging of retinal and choroidal blood perfusion with optical micro-angiography," Journal of Biomedical Optics, vol. 15, no. 2, 2010.

[36] Z. Yuan, Z. C. Luo,H. G. Ren, C.W. Du, and Y. Pan, "A digital frequency ramping method for enhancing Doppler flow imaging in Fourier-domain optical coherence tomography," *Optics Express*, vol. 17, no. 5, pp. 3951–3963, 2009.

[37] Yuankai K. Tao, Anjul M. Davis, and Joseph A. Izatt, "Single-pass volumetric bidirectional blood flow imaging spectral domain optical coherence tomography using a modified Hilbert transform," Opt. Express 16, 12350-12361 (2008) http://www.opticsinfobase.org/abstract.cfm?URI=oe-16-16-12350

[38] Yuankai K. Tao, Kristen M. Kennedy, and Joseph A. Izatt, " Velocity-resolved 3D retinal microvessel imaging using single-pass flow imaging spectral domain optical coherence tomography," Opt. Express 17, 4177-4188 (2009) . http://www.opticsinfobase.org/abstract.cfm?uri=oe-17-5-4177

[39] C. Kasai, K. Namekawa, A. Koyano, R. Omoto, "Real-Time Two-Dimensional Blood Flow Imaging Using an Autocorrelation Technique," IEEE Trans. Sonics Ultrason, SU-32(3), 458-464(1985).

[40] V. X. Yang, M. L. Gordon, A. Mok, Y. Zhao, Z. Chen, R. S. Cobbold, B. C. Wilson, and I. A. Vitkin, "Improved phase-resolved optical Doppler tomography using Kasai velocity estimator and histogram segmentation," Opt. Commun. 208, 209-214 (2002)

[41] Lingfeng Yu and Zhongping Chen, "Doppler variance imaging for three-dimensional retina and choroid angiography," J. Biomed. Opt. 15, 016029 (2010)

[42] Gangjun Liu, Wenjuan Qi, Lingfeng Yu, and Zhongping Chen, "Real-time bulk-motion-correction free Doppler variance optical coherence tomography for choroidal capillary vasculature imaging," Opt. Express 19, 3657-3666 (2011) http://www.opticsinfobase.org/abstract.cfm?URI=oe-19-4-3657

[43] Z. Chen, Y. Zhao, S. M. Srivivas, J. S. Nelson, N. Prakash, and R. D. Frostig, "Optical Doppler Tomography," IEEE J. Select. Topics Quantum Electro. 5, 1134 (1999).

[44] Z. Chen, T. E. Milner, S. Srinivas, A. Malekafzali, X. Wang, M. J. C. Van Gemert, J. S. Nelson, "Characterization of Blood Flow Dynamics and Tissue Structure Using Optical Doppler Tomography," Photochemistry and Photobiology 67, 56-60 (1998).

[45] Bin Rao, Lingfeng Yu, Huihua Kenny Chiang, Leandro C. Zacharias, Ronald M. Kurtz, Baruch D. Kuppermann and Zhongping Chen,"Imaging pulsatile retinal blood flow in human eye", JBO Letters, 040505(2008).

[46] J. Nelson, K. Kelly, Y. Zhao, and Z. Chen, "Imaging blood flow in human port wine stain in situ and in real time using optical Doppler tomography", Archives of Dermatology, 137, 741-4 (2001).

[47] Vakoc BJ, Lanning RM, Tyrrell JA, Padera TP, Bartlett LA, Stylianopoulos T, Munn LL, Tearney GJ, Fukumura D, Jain RK, Bouma BE. Three-dimensional microscopy of the tumor microenvironment in vivo using optical frequency domain imaging. Nat Med. 2009 Oct;15(10):1219-23.

[48] Vivek J. Srinivasan, Sava Sakadžić, Iwona Gorczynska, Svetlana Ruvinskaya, Weicheng Wu, James G. Fujimoto, and David A. Boas, "Quantitative cerebral blood flow with Optical Coherence Tomography," Opt. Express 18, 2477-2494 (2010) http://www.opticsinfobase.org/abstract.cfm?URI=oe-18-3-2477

[49] Shuichi Makita, Youngjoo Hong, Masahiro Yamanari, Toyohiko Yatagai, and Yoshiaki Yasuno, "Optical coherence angiography," Opt. Express 14, 7821(2006). http://www.opticsinfobase.org/abstract.cfm?URI=oe-14-17-7821

[50] HrebeshM. Subhash, "Biophotonics Modalities for High-Resolution Imaging of Microcirculatory Tissue Beds Using Endogenous Contrast: A Review on Present Scenario and Prospects", International Journal of Optics, Article ID 293684 (2011).

4

3-D Ultrahigh Resolution Optical Coherence Tomography with Adaptive Optics for Ophthalmic Imaging

Guohua Shi*, Jing Lu, Xiqi Li and Yudong Zhang
Institute of Optics and Electronics,
Chinese Academy of Sciences,
Shuangliu, Chengdu,
P R China

1. Introduction

By use of broad bandwidth light source, the potential of OCT is demonstrated to perform noninvasive optical biopsy of the human retina (D. Huang, et al, 1991). OCT is based on low coherence interferometry (R. C. Youngquist, et al, 1987), in which the pattern of interference between the reference and object beams is used to determine the amount of light reflected back from a certain point within the volume of the sample under study. The broad bandwidth source is used for illumination, so the two beams only produce an interference pattern when their optical paths difference is less than the coherence length of the source. This means that the bandwidth of the source determines the axial resolution of the OCT system. Therefore, by using ultra-broad bandwidth light source (such as Ti: Al2O3 laser, laser generated from a photo crystal fiber, ultra-broadband SLD), the cross section image as biopsy is achieved successfully(A. Unterhuber, et al, 2003, Yimin Wang, et al, 2003, D.S. Adler, et al, 2004).

The transverse resolution in ophthalmic OCT is determined by beam-focusing conditions on the retina (Bratt E. Bouma, et al, 2002). The smaller achievable spot size means the higher transverse resolution. For an ideal eye, a large diameter beam would produce a small theoretical spot size. However, in practice, for large pupil diameters, mono-chromatic aberrations of the human eye blur the retinal images. Although the axial resolution of ophthalmic OCT has been improved dramatically, the transverse resolution is still limited to 15-20 μm in retinal ultra high resolution OCT (UHR OCT) tomograms because of the small pupil diameter used.

Adaptive optics (AO) can correct the aberration in real time. By using adaptive optics, the optical resolution of retina camera is significantly increased by correcting the ocular aberrations across a large pupil. Combined OCT with AO, 3-D ultrahigh resolution is achieved. The increase of transverse resolution permits the observation of human retinal structures at the cellular level in vivo.

* Corresponding Author

2. Resolution of OCT

Unlike conventional microscopy, the axial and transverse optical resolutions of OCT are independent, because of its unique mechanism. Either Time Domain OCT or Fourier Domain OCT, the axial resolution for OCT imaging is determined by the coherence length of the illumination source (R. Leitgeb, et al, 2003). Therefore, the shorter the coherence length, the higher the axial resolution is. Thus, the axial resolution is inversely proportional to the bandwidth of light source. Assumes a Gaussian spectral illumination source, the axial resolution Δz is

$$\Delta z = \frac{2\ln 2}{\pi}(\frac{\lambda_0^2}{\Delta\lambda}). \tag{1}$$

Where λ_0 is the center wavelength of the illumination source and $\Delta\lambda$ is the 3dB bandwidth of tits spectrum. Equation (1) reveals that to increase axial resolution the broad band spectral sources is required. By use of ultra-broad bandwidth light sources, the ultrahigh axial resolution optical coherence tomography can be achieved.

While the axial resolution in OCT is governed by the source coherence length, OCT's transverse resolution is the same as optical microscopy, and is determined by the focusing properties of the illumination beam which is limited by diffraction and aberrations of optical system (Born. M and Wolf. E, 1980). Ideally, the transverse resolution is

$$\Delta x \approx 1.22\lambda_0(\frac{f}{d}). \tag{2}$$

Where f is the focal length of objective and d is its effective aperture. Theory, by using high NA objective to focus a small spot size, the high transverse resolution can be achieved. In practice, when the case of a fixed numerical aperture, the optical system aberration determine the focus size.

The transverse resolution in ophthalmic UHR OCT is constrained by the pupil size of eye, which determines smallest achievable spot size on the retina. However, in practice, human eyes is not a perfect optical system for large pupil diameter, it has wave front aberrations which deteriorate the transverse resolution of OCT (Junzhong Liang, et al, 1993). Although the axial resolution of ophthalmic OCT has been improved dramatically, the transverse resolution is still limited to 15-20 μm in retinal UHR OCT tomograms because of the small pupil diameter used (H.C. Howland, et al, 1977).

3. Wave front aberrations of human eye

3.1 Zernike mode aberrations

We can use the wave front aberration to describe the transverse imaging properties of ophthalmic imaging optical system perfectly. It is defined as the optical path difference (OPD) between the perfect spherical wave front and the actual wave front for every point over the eye's pupil. The ideal eye focuses a perfect spot (Airy disk) on retina. Actually, the existence of eye's wave front aberration blur the focused spot on retina significantly (J. Liang, et al, 1997).

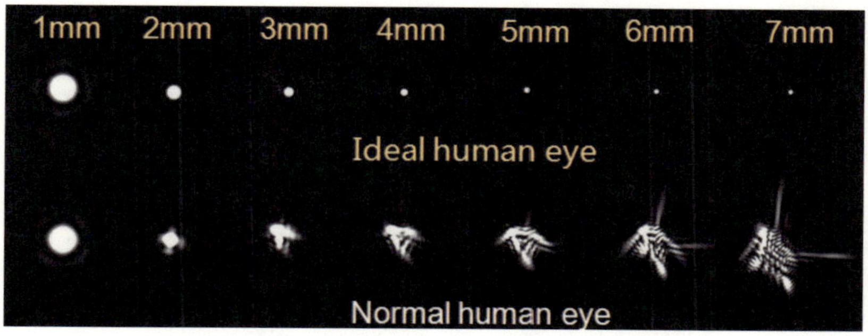

Fig. 1. The ideal and reality PSF change with pupil size.

Fig 1 shows the ideal and reality PSF that change with pupil size. In theory, with the increase of pupil size, the ideal PSF will rapidly become smaller because of the diffraction effects. It's mean the improvement of transverse resolution. In fact, for a normal human eye (without refractive disease) the reality PSF will became smaller at first, and will achieve the minimum when the pupil size is 3mm. Because the smaller pupil size means the smaller wave front aberration. Then, with the increase of pupil size, the wave front aberrations increased dramatically, so the reality PSF become rapidly expanding.

Fortunately, most of normal human eyes just have the 3mm pupil size. But for ophthalmic imaging, transverse resolution of 3mm pupil size is not enough. Therefore, the key issue is how to correct the wave front aberration which is introduced by the large pupil. The wave front aberration may be mathematically represented and broken down into its constituent aberrations (such as defocus, astigmatism, coma, spherical aberration, etc.) using a Zernike decomposition.

$$\varphi(\vec{r}) = \sum_{k=1}^{N} a_k Z_k(\vec{r}) \tag{3}$$

Where $\varphi(\vec{r})$ is the wave front phase. $Z_k(\vec{r})$ and a_k is the Zernike mode and its corresponding coefficient. Zernike polynomials are set of orthogonal polynomials on a circular domain. It is defined as

$$Z_k = \begin{cases} \left.\begin{array}{l} \sqrt{2(n+1)}R_n^m(\rho)\cos(m\theta)......k = odd \\ \sqrt{2(n+1)}R_n^m(\rho)\sin(m\theta)......k = even \end{array}\right\} ......m \neq 0 \\ \sqrt{n+1}R_n^m(\rho)..m = 0 \end{cases} \tag{4}$$

Where $R_n^m(\rho)$ is

$$R_n^m(\rho) = \sum_{s=0}^{(n-m)/2} \frac{(-1)^s (n-s)!}{s!\left(\frac{n+m}{2}-s\right)!\left(\frac{n-m}{2}-s\right)!}\rho^{n-2s} \tag{5}$$

Where m and n is angular frequency and the radial frequency separately. They are constant integers and satisfy

$$m \leq n, n - |m| = even; \tag{6}$$

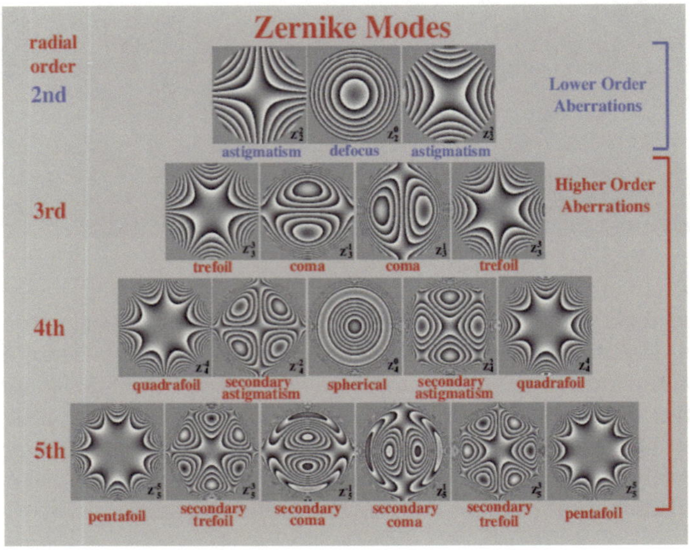

Fig. 2. The Zernike modes wave front aberrations

Fig. 2 and 3 shows the Zernike modes wave front aberrations and its corresponding point spread function (PSF). Glasses and contact lenses have been used to correct the lower order aberrations (defocus and astigmatism) of eye. However, it has been well known that the human eye also suffers from the higher order aberrations, in addition to typical defocus and astigmatic errors. Moreover the higher order aberrations different from each subject, and change over time. So it is impossible to solve higher order aberrations by optical design.

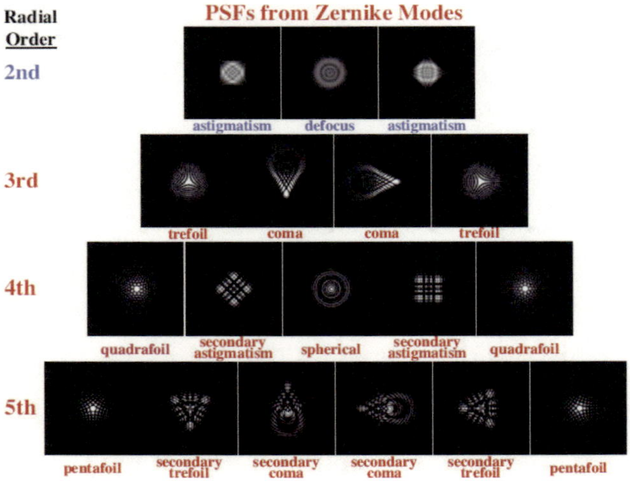

(a) (b)

Fig. 3. The PSF of each Zernike modes wave front aberration.

3.2 Hartmann-Shack wave front sensor

In order to correct the wave front aberrations of the eye, we must measure the aberrations at first. In reality, every refracting ocular surface generates aberrations, and they contribute differently to the overall quality of the retinal image. The monochromatic aberration of the complete eye, considered as one single imaging system, can be measured using a large variety of wave front sensing techniques. However, from 1994, with the development of human eye Hartmann-Shack wave front sensor, the researchers of the human eye wave front aberration have a more in-depth understanding, recognizing that the human eye aberrations in addition to defocus, astigmatism, but also there are other more complex higher-order aberrations (J. Liang, et al, 1994, Ning Ling, et al, 2001, Heidi Hofer, et al, 2001).

Figure 4 shows the measuring principle of Hartmann-Shack wave front sensor (Ning Ling, et al 2001). The Hartmann-Shack wave front sensor is consist of a micro-lens array and a CCD camera. The incident wave front is divided into several sub-apertures by micro lens array, then image by CCD camera.

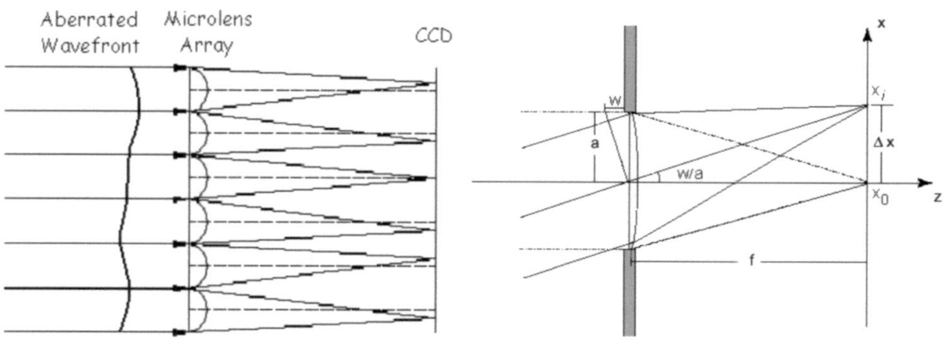

(a) (b)

Fig. 4. (a) The schematic diagram of Hartmann-Shack wave front sensor; (b) Focal spot displacement caused by the incident wave front tilt

If the incident wave front is ideal plane wave front, set the centroids of sub-apertures focal spots as reference position (x0, y0). When the incident wave front have aberrations, then the centroids of sub-apertures focal spots (xi, yi) will deviate from reference position. The offsets of X and Y direction are proportional to the X and Y directions average slope of the wave front. Wave front slope (in wavelength/sub-aperture unit) can be expressed as

$$g_{xi} = \frac{x_i - x_o}{\lambda f} = \frac{\iint \frac{\partial \varphi(x,y)}{\partial x} ds}{\iint ds}, \quad g_{yi} = \frac{y_i - y_o}{\lambda f} = \frac{\iint \frac{\partial \varphi(x,y)}{\partial y} ds}{\iint ds} \tag{7}$$

Where φ(x, y) is the phase of incident wave front, f is the focal length of micro lens array, and λ is the wavelength of incident light.

After obtain the sub-aperture wave front slope, the wave front reconstruction algorithm can calculate the phase distribution function φ(x, y). There are many kinds of wave-front reconstruction algorithm that can be used in different applications. In order to measure higher-order aberrations for the human eye, Zernike wave front reconstruction mode method is more appropriate.

Through the derivative of Zernike polynomials and within each sub-aperture averaging, the average slope of the sub-aperture can be established the relationship with the Zernike mode coefficients.

$$\begin{cases} g_{x_m} = \sum_{n=1}^{N} a_n \left. \frac{\iint_{\sigma_m} \frac{\partial Z_n(x,y)}{\partial x} dxdy}{\iint_{\sigma_m} dxdy} \right|_m \\ g_{y_m} = \sum_{n=1}^{N} a_n \left. \frac{\iint_{\sigma_m} \frac{\partial Z_n(x,y)}{\partial y} dxdy}{\iint_{\sigma_m} dxdy} \right|_m \end{cases}, \tag{8}$$

Where σ_m is the corresponding integral area of the detected aperture M on the unit circle. Write the all the sub-aperture's slope and the Zernike mode coefficient in vector form.

$$\begin{aligned} \vec{g} &= \left(g_{x_1}, g_{y_1}, g_{x_2}, g_{y_2}, \ldots\ldots, g_{x_M}, g_{y_M}\right)^T \\ \vec{a} &= \left(a_1, a_1, \ldots\ldots a_N\right)^T \end{aligned} \tag{9}$$

Where $\vec{g}$ is slope vector and $\vec{a}$ is Zernike mode coefficient vector. Then the Eq. (8) can be written

$$\vec{g} = D\vec{a} \tag{10}$$

Where D represents the relationship matrix of slope vector $\vec{g}$ and Zernike mode coefficient vector $\vec{a}$. So the generalized inverse of D is the wave front reconstruction matrix of Zernike wave-front reconstruction mode method. Thus, the Zernike mode coefficient vector $\vec{a}$ can be obtain by

$$\vec{a} = [(D^T D)^{-1} D^T] \cdot \vec{g} = D^+ \cdot \vec{g}$$

Using Zernike mode coefficient vector $\vec{a}$, we can calculate the phase distribution function φ(x, y), get the Zernike wave front aberrations, calculate the PSF of whole optical system.

Fig. 5 is the results of a volunteer measured by H-S sensor in our lab (Ning Ling, et al 2001). H-S sensor can not only achieve the wave front measurement of eye, but aslo can get the system PSF, MTF, encircled energy. And it measures in real time, thus can measure the wave front aberrations changes with time. International Organization for Standardization have recommended Zernike polynomial to describe wave front aberrations of human eye. So H-S sensor has become the most important techniques of optometry research.

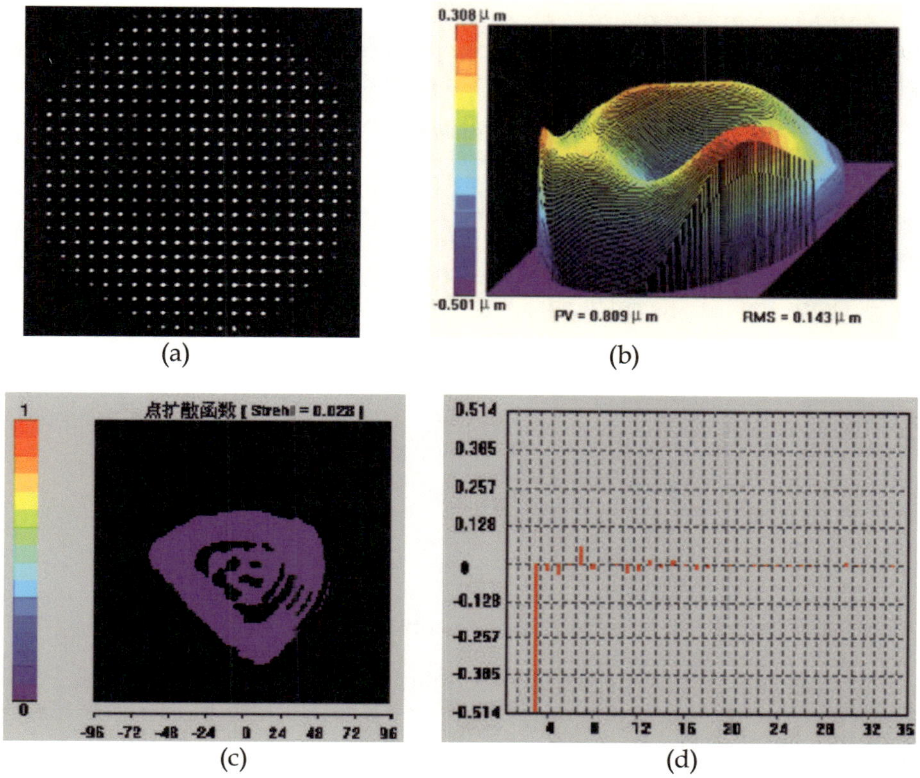

Fig. 5. (a) is the spot array of a volunteer obtained by H-S sensor; (b) is the wave front reconstructed by Zernike wave-front reconstruction mode method; (c) is the PSF of volunteer eye; (d) is the first 35 order Zernike coefficient

4. Principle of adaptive optics

4.1 Wave front corrector

When the wave front aberrations of the eye are measured precisely and in real time, it is possible to correct them by using a wave front correcting device that compensates the eye's aberrations. This is a direct application of Adaptive Optics (AO) on the eye imaging. In the ideal case, the AO system produces retinal images with perfect transverse resolution.

Adaptive optics was first used in large astronomical telescopes (Fried D L, 1997), which includes wave front sensor, wave front corrector and control system. Fig. 6 is the typical adaptive optics system. The basic principle of adaptive optics is phase conjugation (R.K.Tyson, 1991). The electric field of an incident light can be expressed as

$$E_1 = |E| e^{i\varphi} \tag{12}$$

Where the φ is the phase of incident light and it is affected by external disturbance, such as temperature variation, atmospheric turbulence, eye aberrations and so on. The function of adaptive optics system is to produce phase that is the conjugate of the incident light. Thus, the phase error (wave front aberration) is compensated, and the incident light became an ideal plane wave. This lead to a diffraction limit resolution image.

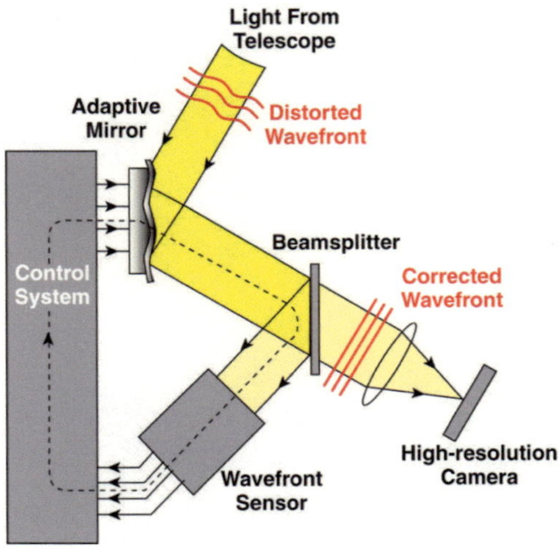

Fig. 6. Schematic diagram of a typical adaptive optics system.

Wave front corrector is the core component in adaptive optics system. It determines the performance, size and cost of the adaptive optics. The wave front corrector changes its surface by driving the actuators push or pull the thin mirror. This produces an opposite wave front phase which is measured by wave front sensor to correct the aberrations of optical system. Different types of wave front corrector have been used to correct eye's aberrations, such as liquid crystal spatial light modulators (E.J. Fernandez, et al, 2005), micro-mechanical deformable mirror (Y. Zhang, et al, 2006), bimorph deformable mirror (Robert J. Zawadzki, et al 2005) and deformable mirrors (Yudong Zhang, et al 2001). Their pictures are shown in Fig. 7.

Type	No. of the actuators	Stroke	Size	Cost
liquid crystal spatial light modulator	800×600	One wavelength	21 x 26 mm	lower
micro-mechanical deformable mirror	12×12	3μm	4mm×4mm	lower
bimorph deformable mirror	35	32μm	10mm	expensive
deformable mirror	37	4μm	Ø40mm	Most expensive

Table 1. Comparison of four wave front corrector.

Table 1 is the comparison of four types of wave front corrector. Liquid crystal spatial light modulator has the minimum stroke, which is just one wavelength, and it has the lowest optical power efficiency. Micro-mechanical deformable mirror is low cost and small size, but its stroke (3-6μm) is not enough for correcting large aberrations. Though deformable mirror is the wild used wave front corrector, but its bulky size and expensive cost restricts its application for retinal imaging. Synthetically, the bimorph deformable mirror is the cost-effective wave front corrector.

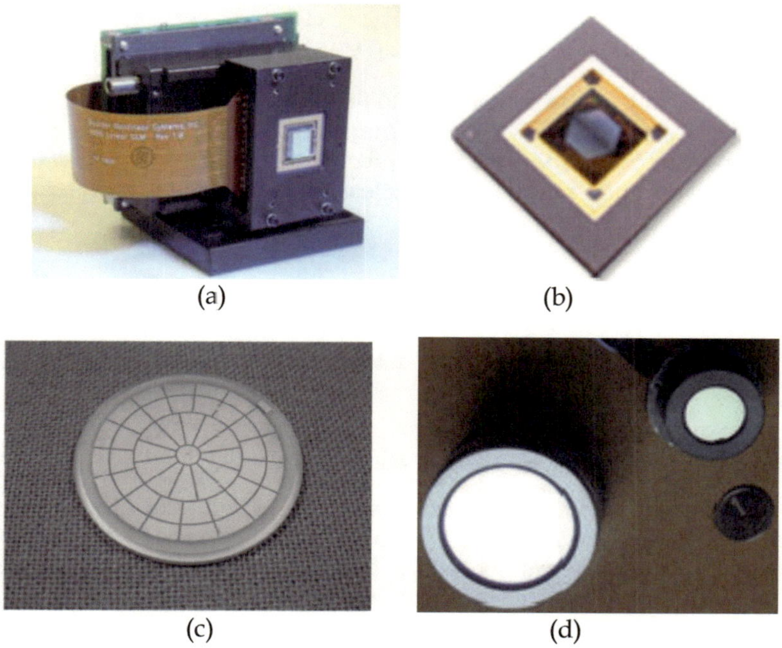

Fig. 7. Pictures of four wave front corrector. (a) liquid crystal spatial light modulator; (b) micro-mechanical deformable mirror; (c) bimorph deformable mirror; (d) deformable mirror.

4.2 Direct slope method for adaptive optics

Except liquid crystal spatial light modulator, the other wave front correctors correct aberrations by applying voltage to actuators to change surface shape of the thin mirror. Thereby, the control algorithm is important because it is the vital link between the wave front sensor and the wave front corrector in an adaptive optics system. According to Eq. (11) can reconstruct incident wave front. But calculating each actuator's drive voltage from the reconstructed wave front require complex decoupling algorithm, which is a complex process. Direct slope method is the most widely applied control algorithm (Wenhan Jiang, Huagui Li, 1990). It uses the wave front slope as control variables instead of wave front phase. So it is particularly suitable for the AO system that include H-S wave front sensor.

Assuming an ideal optical system, the sub-aperture of H-S sensor detects the slop generated by wave front corrector. So the slop of x and y direction in the i th sub- aperture is

$$\begin{aligned} G_{xi} &= \sum_{j=1}^{n} V_j R_{xij} \\ G_{yi} &= \sum_{j=1}^{n} V_j R_{yij} \end{aligned} \qquad i=1,2,3,4\cdots\cdots n \tag{13}$$

Where R_{xij} and R_{yij} are the slop of x and y direction in the i-th sub-aperture when the j-th actuator applied unit drive voltage alone. V_j is the drive voltage of the j-th actuator. n is the number of actuator. Therefore, Eq. (13) can be expressed as

$$G = DV \tag{14}$$

D is called influence function slope matrix and its elements are R_{xij} and R_{yij}. It is determined by adaptive optics system itself, and can be measured by adaptive optics system itself too. Wave front slop vector G is measured by wave front sensor, which is defined as Eq. (9) shows. V is the drive voltage matrix. So, using least square method, V is

$$V = D^{+}G \tag{15}$$

Where D^{+} is the generalized inverse matrix of D, and called as control matrix. When the AO system is working, the H-S sensor measures the slop of incident wave front. Then according to Eq. (15), we can get the drive voltage and control the wave front corrector to correct the wave front aberration.

5. Adaptive optics optical coherence tomography

University of Rochester take the lead in the use of adaptive optics for ophthalmic imaging (D. T. Miller et al, 1996, J. Liang, et al, 1997). They combined the AO with fundus camera. By using AO to correct the aberration caused by large pupil size (6 mm), the transverse resolution of fundus camera achieved 2μm, and imaged three cone classes in the living human eye successfully (Austin. Roorda & DavidR.Williams, 1999). But the axial resolution of AO- Camera is lower, so the AO-CSLO (Adaptive Optics Confocal Scanning Laser Ophthalmoscope) and AO-OCT (Adaptive Optics Optical Coherence Tomography) have been invented one after the other (A.Roorda, et al, 2002, D. T. Miller, et al, 2003).

Fig. 8 shows the 3-D PSF comparison of AO-Camera, AO-CSLO and AO-OCT. The width and height of the scale bar represent the axial and transverse resolution separately. So it is clear that AO-OCT have the smallest 3-D PSF. Thus, AO-OCT is the highest resolution for ophthalmic imaging in vivo so far. Since 2003, many research groups carried out the study of AO-OCT, and realized the 3-D imaging of different kinds of human retinal cell in vivo.

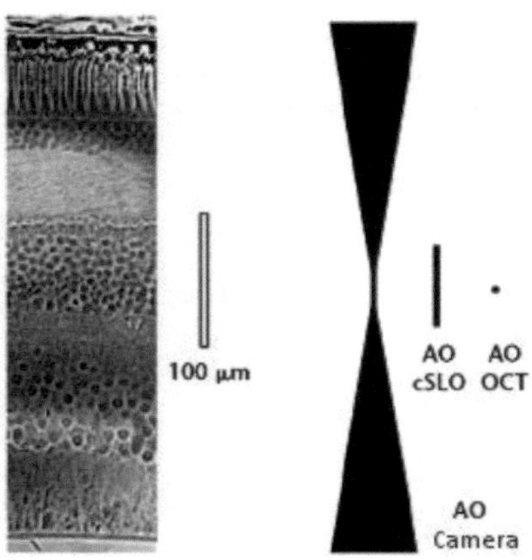

Fig. 8. The 3-D PSF comparison of ophthalmic imaging techniques.

5.1 Adaptive optics combined with time domain OCT

In 2003, D. T. Miller et al. have been first tried to combine an enface coherence gated camera with AO for enface OCT imaging with axial resolution (2μm) and high transverse resolution, and obtained the images of in vitro bovine retina (D. T. Miller, et al, 2003). In 2004, B. Hermann merged the ultrahigh-resolution time domain optical coherence tomography (UHROCT) with adaptive optics (AO), resulting in high axial resolution (3um) and improved transverse resolution (5-10 um) is demonstrated for the first time in human retinal imaging in vivo (B. Hermann, et al, 2003).

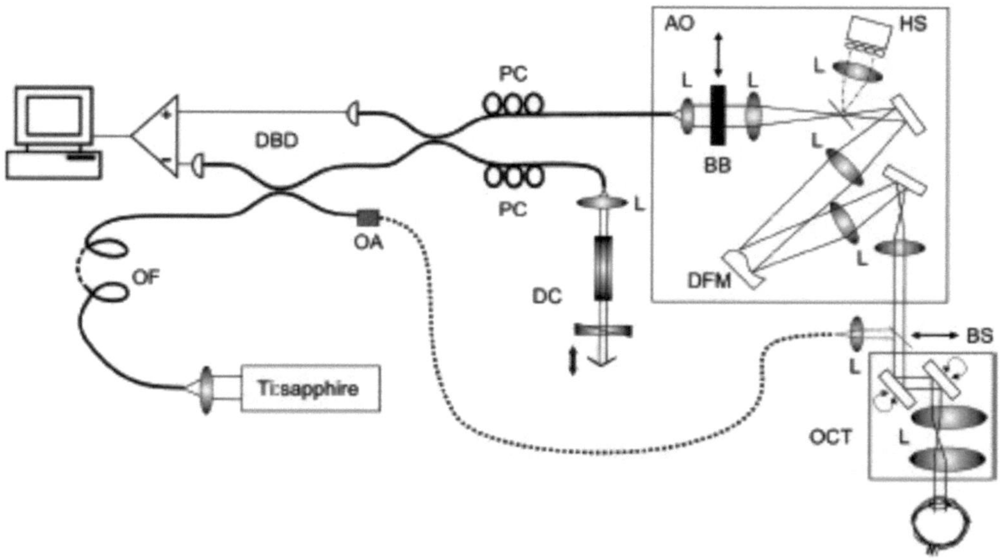

Fig. 9. The AO-OCT system which is developed by B. Hermann, et al, in 2003. DBD, dual balanced detection; PCs, polarization controllers; OA, optical attenuator; OF, 100 m of optical fiber; DC, dispersion compensation; L's, achromatic doublet lenses; BB, removable beam blocker; DFM, deformable mirror; BS, removable beam splitter.

Fig.9 is the schematic diagram of B. Hermann's AO-OCT system. A closed-loop AO system, based on a real time Hartmann-Shack wave front sensor operating at 30Hz and a 37-actuator membrane deformable mirror, is interfaced to an UHR OCT system, based on a commercial OCT instrument, employing a compact Ti: sapphire laser which's center wavelength is 800 nm with 130 nm bandwidth. The AO system was designed to conjugate the exit pupil of the eye on to the deformable mirror, in to the H-S sensor. The diameter of the measurement beam entering the eye was increased from 1mm to 3.68mm. When the correction was achieved, the system was switched to the UHR OCT imaging mode by removal of the beam blocker and the beam splitter.

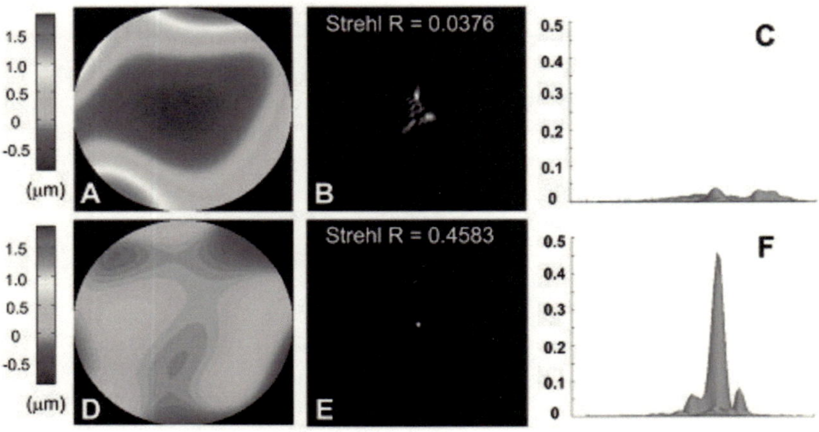

Fig. 10. Wave front for the A, uncorrected and D, corrected case and the associated PSFs for the B, C, uncorrected and E, F, corrected cases are indicated.

After corrected the eye aberration by AO, the residual of uncorrected wave front aberration is 0.1um (see Figs. 10A and 10D)., and the Strehl ratio improvements of a factor of more than 10 (Figs. 10B and 10E) were achieved, resulting in a significantly improved PSF profile (Figs. 10C and 10F). Fig. 11 illustrates the significantly effect of aberration correction in AO UHR OCT image.

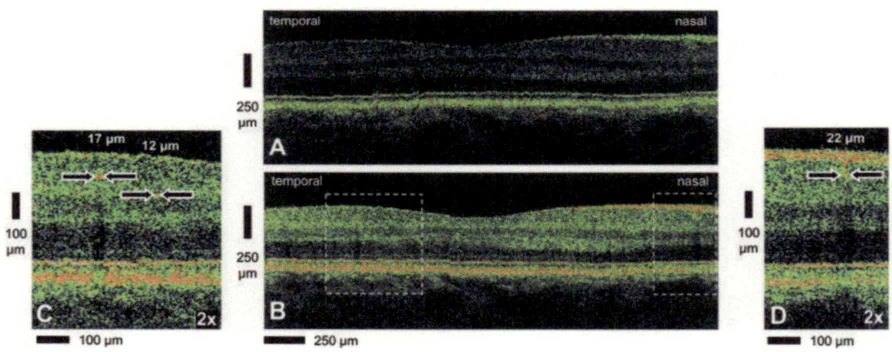

Fig. 11. In vivo AO UHR OCT tomograms of a normal human eye in the foveal region for the A, uncorrected as well as B, corrected case (600 A-scans over a line of 2.8 mm, transverse sampling rate of ~5μm). B, SNR improvement of up to 9 dB as well as 5-10μm transverse in addition to 3μm axial resolution could be achieved by wave-front corrections introduced by a 3.68 mm diameter beam. C, D, Small features within the ganglion cell layer, as well as inner plexiform layer, that might correspond to vessels with 12-22μm diameter are clearly visualized in twofold enlargements.

Guohua Shi et al have used AO to correct the aberration of a 6mm pupil size to improve the transverse resolution furthermore (Shi Guohua, et al, 2007 and 2008). But the earlier AO-OCT system combined AO with TD-OCT, so the imaging speed is slow. As the reference shows the fastest A-scan rate of TD-OCT is 8KHz (A.M. Rollins, 1998). Therefore, although using AO to correct the aberration of a 6mm pupil size, the AO-TDOCT can't achieve the 3-D image mosaic of retinal tomography image, because of the human eyes jitter. Thus, the AO-TDOCT system can't provide the high resolution C-scan OCT image of retinal cell. In addition, the wave front sensor is very sensitive to the back-reflections from the lenses of the optical system. So the optical system must use off-center illumination geometry, and this increases the difficulty of optical adjustment.

5.2 Adaptive optics combined with spectral domain OCT

The combination of AO and TD-OCT, a resolution approaching a few microns in three dimensions is possible. With the development of Fourier Domain OCT the imaging speed and signal-to-noise ratio have a greatly improved (R. Leitgeb, et al, 2003, J.F. de Boer, et al, 2003). This provides a technical approach to overcome the retinal jitter to achieve en-face OCT image of retinal cells. In 2005, AO has been combined with free space parallel SD-OCT and fiber based SD-OCT (R. Zawadzki, et al, 2005, Y. Zhang, et al, 2005). These instruments have been reported to achieve lateral and axial resolutions up to 3μm and 2-3μm in the eye, respectively. The instruments, however, were tailored for specific experiments that did not emphasize volumetric imaging of single cells.

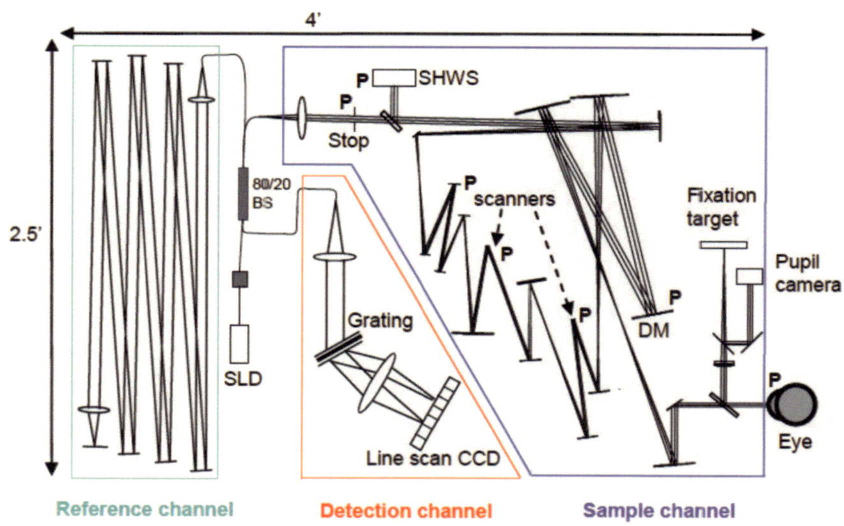

Fig. 12. Layout of the AO- SDOCT retina camera. The camera consists of three channels: (1) sample channel, (2) reference channel, and (3) detection channel. The AO system is integrated into the sample channel. BS, DM, and P refer to the fiber beam splitter, AOptix deformable mirror, and planes that are conjugate to the pupil of the eye, respectively.

In 2006, Yan Zhang established an AO-SDOCT (adaptive optics spectral domain optical coherence tomography) system for high-speed volumetric imaging of cone photoreceptors (Yan Zhang, et al, 2006). In order to overcome retinal jitter, the SDOCT components based on a fast line scan camera which's A-scan rate is 75KHz, and a shorter distance of raster scans (38 A-scans per B-scan). Thus, retinal motion artifacts were minimized by quickly acquiring small volume images of the retina with and without AO compensation. Fig. 12 is the layout of its system. A SLD (λ_0= 842 nm, $\Delta\lambda$ = 50 nm) illuminates the retina. In the sample arm, it uses reflective optics to minimize the back-reflections of the optical system. The pupil of the eye conjugated to the wave front corrector (an AOptix deformable mirror has 37 actuators with a maximum stroke of 32μm for defocus correction), the X-Y scanner and the 20×20 lenslet array of the H-S sensor. The closed-loop rate of AO components is 12 Hz.

The result of correcting aberration shows as Fig. 13(a). AO compensation clearly reduces the magnitude of the aberrations and increases the Strehl ratio at the SLD wavelength of 842nm from 7% to 35%. As an alternative image quality metric, Fig. 13(b) shows a root mean square (RMS) trace of the measured wave aberrations for the same subject before and during AO dynamic correction. By correcting the wave front aberration of 6.6mm human eye pupil size, the transverse resolution is 3μm.

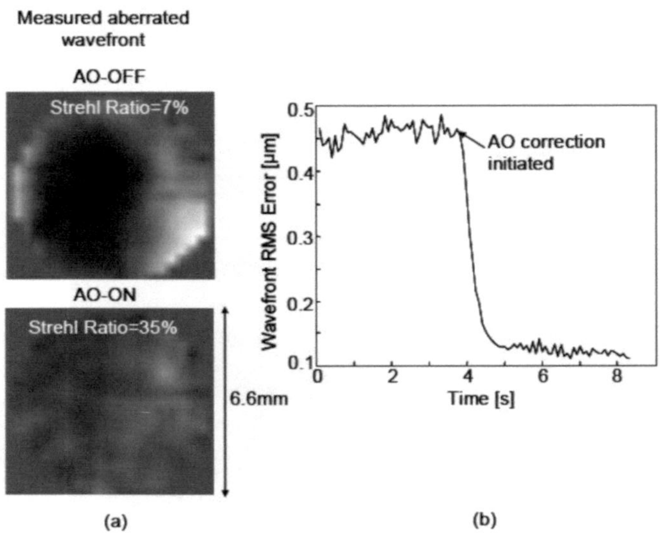

Fig. 13 (a) Residual of wave front aberrations across a 6.6 mm pupil in one subject as measured by the H-S sensor before and after AO compensation. Wave front phase is represented by a gray-scale image with black and white tones depicting minimum (-1.0μm) and maximum (1.19μm) phase, respectively. (b) An RMS trace of the residual wave aberrations is shown for one subject before and during dynamic AO correction.

Figure 14 shows C-scan image in vivo at the posterior tips of the OS with and without AO working. The volume images is a small patches of 2° retinal eccentricity retina which is 38×285×1100μm (width × length × depth) with a sampling density of 1×1×2.2μm duration of 150ms. The Fig.14 demonstrated that the AO-SDOCT was necessary for observing individual cone photoreceptor cells and led to a significant increase in the SNR (about 7-8dB) in C-scan images.

In recent years, there has been a variety of AO-SDOCT device. David Merino et al use adaptive optics to enhance simultaneous en-face optical coherence tomography and scanning laser ophthalmoscopy (David Merino, et al, 2006). RobertJ. Zawadzki et al

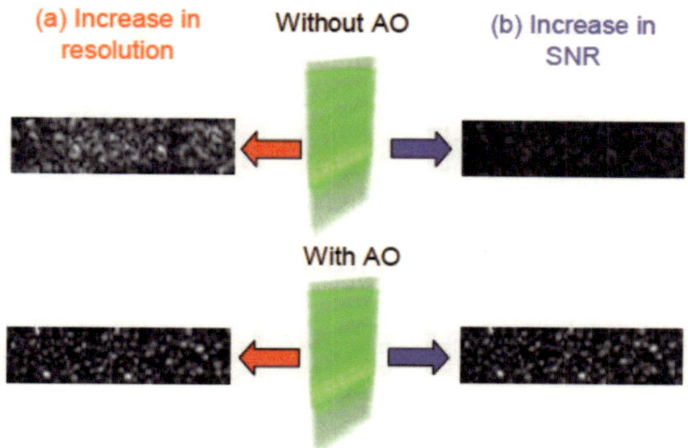

Fig. 14. (a) C-scan images at the posterior tips of the OS show an increase in transverseresolution with AO. The two images are normalized to their own gray scale so as to permit better visualization of the cone photoreceptor structure. (b) The same C-scan images in (a), but adjusted to the same gray scale.

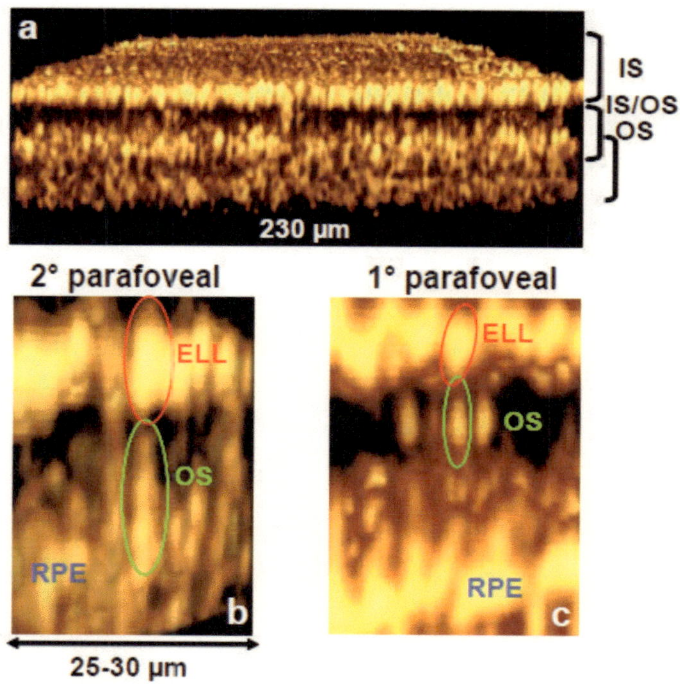

Fig. 15. In vivo cellular resolution retinal imaging at ~2.25 deg eccentricity: (a). Three dimensional morphology of photoreceptor ellipsoids, together with the outer segments is visualized. Two different volumes showing the detailed micro-structural architecture of single photoreceptors at two eccentricities: ~2.25 and ~1.12 deg (b, c).

employed two deformable mirror to enhance the correcting capability of aberration for AO-OCT system (RobertJ. Zawadzki, et al 2007). Barry Cense et al combined polarization-sensitive optical coherence tomography with adaptive optics to research birefringent of nerve fiber laye (Barry Cense, et al, 2009). The 3-D image of retinal photoreceptor has been achieved in vivo which is shown in Fig. 15 (Enrique J. Fernández, et al, 2008). In Fig. 15(a), the 3-D structure of the ellipsoids, together with the OS, was recognizable. This opens the door to study the possible connection between pathologies associated to the loss or alteration of photoreceptor elements, including the internal process of renewing photoactive discs. With development of AO-OCT technology, more and more retinal cells will be achieved 3-D imaging in vivo, and will provide a powerful imaging tool for establish the relationships between the disease with retinal image at 3-D cellular level.

6. Conclusion

This chapter provides a technical overview of the AO-OCT for ophthalmic imaging. The overview includes a detailed description of Zernike modes wave front aberration, Hartmann-Shack wave front sensor, the fundamental of adaptive optics technology, and the development process of AO-OCT technology. OCT provides the high axial resolution, and AO the complementary high transverse resolution. Combined AO with OCT, will achieve 3-D ultrahigh resolution, and it have realized 2-D and 3-D image of signal photoreceptor. The AO-OCT musters a potentially powerful imaging tool whose 3-D resolution and sensitivity in the eye can substantially surpass those of any current retinal imaging modality. However, most of the AO system is not only expensive but also larger diameter devices, resulting in AO-OCT system have a big size. Although the invention of MEMS deformable mirror reduces the size of AO-OCT system, its small stroke limits its ability of aberration correction. Therefore, in the future to invent a smaller aperture, larger stroke and cheaper wave front sensor is the critical issue.

7. Acknowledgment

This research was supported by the National Science Foundation of China (Grant No. 61108082), the Knowledge Innovation Program of the Chinese Academy of Sciences (Grant No.KGCX2-Y11-920)

8. References

A. Unterhuber, B. Povazˇ ay, B. Hermann, et al. (2003). Compact, low-cost Ti: Al2O3 laser for in vivo ultrahigh-resolution optical coherence tomography. *Optics Letters.*, Vol. 28, No.11, pp 905-907.

A.M. Rollins, M.D. Kulkarni, S. Yazdanfar, et al. (1998). In vivo video rate optical coherence tomography. *Optics Express.*, Vol. 3, No. 6, pp 219–229.

A.Roorda, F. Romero-Borja, W. Donnelly Iii, H. Queener, T. J. Hebert, and M. C. W. Campbell. (2002). Adaptive optics scanning laser ophthalmoscopy. *Opt. Express.*, Vol. 10, pp 405–412

Austin. Roorda & DavidR.Williams. (1999). The arrangement of the three cone classes in the living human eye. *NATURE.*, Vol. 397

B. Hermann, E. J. Fernández, A. Unterhuber, H. Sattmann, A. F. Fercher, W. Drexler, P. M. Prieto, and P. Artal. (2004). Adaptive optics ultrahigh resolution optical coherence tomography. *Opt. Lett.*, Vol. 29, pp 2142-2144

Barry Cense, Weihua Gao1, Jeffrey M. Brown, et al. (2009). Retinal imaging with polarization-sensitive optical coherence tomography and adaptive optics. *Opt. Express.*, Vol. 17, No. 24

Born. M and Wolf. E, (1980), Principles of Optics 7th edn , Publishing hourse of electronics industry, ISBN 7-121-01256-1, Beijin, China

Brett E. Bouma, Guillermo J. Tearney. (2002), Handbook of optical coherence tomography, Marcel Dekker, Inc. ISBN 0-8247-0558-0, Newyork, USA

D. Huang, E. A. Swanson, C. P. Lin, et al. (1991). Optical coherence tomography. *Science.*, Vol. 254, No. 5035, pp 1178-1181.

D. S. Adler, T.H. Ko, A.K. Konorev, et al. (2004). Broadband light source based on quantμm-well superlμminescent diodes for high-resolution optical coherence tomography. *Quantμm Electronics.*, Vol. 34, No. 10, pp 915-918.

D. T. Miller, D. R. Williams, G. M. Morris, and J. Liang. (1996). Images of cone photoreceptors in the living human eye. *Vision Res.*, Vol. 36, pp 1067–1079

D. T. Miller, J. Qu, R. S. Jonnal, and K. E. Thorn. (2003). Coherence Gating and Adaptive Optics in the Eye. *Proceedings of SPIE.*, Vol. 4956, pp 65-72

David Merino and Chris Dainty et al. (2006). Adaptive optics enhanced simultaneous en-face optical coherence tomography and scanning laser ophthalmoscopy. *Optics Express.*, Vol. 14, pp 3345-3353

E.J. Fernandez, B. Povazˇ ay, B. Hermann, et al. (2005). Three-dimensional adaptive optics ultrahigh-resolution optical coherence tomography using a liquid crystal spatial light modulator. *Vision Research.*, Vol. 45, No. 28, pp 3432-3444.

Enrique J. Fernández, Boris Hermann, Boris Považay, et al. (2008). Ultrahigh resolution optical coherence tomography and pancorrection for cellular imaging of the living hμman retina. *Opt. Express.*, Vol. 16, No. 15

Enrique J. Fernández, Boris Hermann, Boris Považay, et al. (2008). Ultrahigh resolution optical coherence tomography and pancorrection for cellular imaging of the living hμman retina, *Opt. Express.*, Vol. 16, No. 15

F. Lexer. (1999). Dynamic coherence focus OCT with depth-indenpent transversal resolution. *Journal of Modern Optics.*, Vol. 46, No. 3, pp 541-553.

Fried D L. (1977). Topical issue on adaptive optics. *Opt.Soc. Am.*,1977, Vol. 67, No. 3.

Guohua Shi, Yun Dai, Ling Wang, et al. (2008). Adaptive optics optical coherence tomography for retina imaging. *Chinese Optics Letters.*, Vol. 6, No. 6, pp 424-425

H.C. Howland. (1977). A subjective method for the measurement of monochromatic aberrations of the eye. *Journal of the Optical Society of America A.*, Vol. 67, No. 11, pp 1508–1518.

Heidi Hofer, Pablo Artal, Ben Singer, Juan Luis Aragón, and David R. Williams. (2001). Dynamics of the eye's wave aberration. *JOSA A.*, Vol. 18, No. 3, pp. 497-506

J. Liang, B. Grimm, S. Goelz, and J. F. Bille. (1994). Objective measurement of wave aberrations of the human eye with use of a Hartmann–Shack wave-front sensor. *J. Opt. Soc. Am. A.* Vol. 11, pp 1949–1957

J. Liang, D. R. Williams and D. T. Miller. (1997). Supernormal vision and high resolution retinal imaging through adaptive optics. *Journal of Optical Society of America A.*, Vol. 14, pp 2884-2892

J. Liang, D. R. Williams, and D. T. Miller. (1997). Supernormal vision and high-resolution retinal imaging through adaptive optics. *Opt. Soc. Am. A.*, Vol.14, pp 2884–2892

J.F. de Boer, B. Cense, B.H. Park, et al. (2003). Improved signal-to-noise ratio in spectral-domain compared with time-domain optical coherence tomography. *Optics Letters.*, Vol. 28, No. 21, pp 2067-2069

Junzhong Liang, Gerald Westheimer. (1993). Method for measuring visual resolution at the retinal level. *Opt. Soc. Am. A.*, Vol. 10, No. 8, pp 1691～1696

Ning Ling, Xuejun Rao, Zheping Yang, Cheng Wang. (2001). Wave front sensor for measurement of vivid hμman eye. *The 3rd International workshop on adaptive optics for industry and medicine.*, pp.85-90

R. C. Youngquist, S. Carr, and D. E. N. Davies. (1987). Optical coherence-domain reflectometry: a new optical evaluation technique. *Opt. Lett.* , Vol. 12, pp 158-160.

R. Leitgeb, C.K. Hitzenberger, A.F. Fercher. (2003). Performance of Fourier domain vs. time domain optical coherence tomography. *Optics Express.*, Vol. 11, No. 8, pp 889-894.

R. Zawadzki, S. Jones, S. Olivier, M. Zhao, B. Bower, J. Izatt, S. Choi, S. Laut, and J. Werner. (2005). Adaptive optics optical coherence tomography for high-resolution and high-speed 3-D retinal in vivo imaging. *Opt. Express.*, Vol. 13, pp 8532-8546

R.K.Tyson. (1991). Principles of adaptive optics. Academic PressInc, SanDiego,

Robert J. Zawadzki, Steven M. Jones, Scot S. Olivier, et al. (2005). Adaptive-optics optical coherence tomography for high-resolution and high-speed 3-D retinal in vivo imaging. *OPTICS EXPRESS.*, Vol. 13, No. 21

RobertJ. Zawadzki, StaceyS. Choi, Steven M. Jones, et al. (2007). Adaptive optics–optical coherence tomography: optimizing visualization of microscopic retinal structures in three dimensions. *J.Opt.Soc.Am.A.*, Vol. 24, No. 5

Shi Guohua, Ding Zhihua, Dai Yun, Rao Xunjun, Zhang Yudong. (2007). Adaptive optics optical coherence tomography. *Proceedings of SPIE.*, Vol. 6534, No. 1

Wenhan Jiang, Huagui Li. (1990). Hartmann-Shack wavefront sensing and wavefront control algorithm, *Proc.of SPIE.*, Vol. 1271, No. 82

Y. Zhang, J. Rha, R. S. Jonnal, and D. T. Miller. (2005). Adaptive optics spectral optical coherence tomography for imaging the living retina. *Opt. Express.*, Vol. 13, pp 4792-4811

Y. Zhang, S. Poonja, and A. Roorda. (2006). MEMS-based adaptive optics scanning laser ophthalmoscopy. *Opt. Lett,*. Vol. 31, pp 1268–1270

Yan Zhang, Barry Cense, Jungtae Rha, et al. (2006). High-speed volμmetric imaging of cone photoreceptors with adaptive optics spectral-domain optical coherence tomography. *Opt. Express.*, Vol. 14, No. 10, pp 4380-4394

Yimin Wang, Yonghua Zhao, Hongu Ren, et al. (2003). Ultrahigh resolution optical coherence tomography using continuμm generation from a photo crystal fiber. Coherence Domain Optical Methods and Optical Coherence Tomography in Biomedicine, *Proceedings of SPIE.*, Vol. 4956

Yudong Zhang, Ning Ling, Xuejun Rao, Xingyang Li, Cheng Wang, Xuean Ma, Wenhan Jiang. (2001). A small adaptive opticl system on table for hμman retinal imaging. *The 3rd International workshop on adaptive optics for industry and medicine.*, pp 97～104

5

Quasi–Nondiffractive Beams for OCT–Visualization: Theoretical and Experimental Investigations

Larisa Kramoreva, Elena Petrova and Julia Razhko
Gomel State Medical University, Gomel State Technical University, Republican Research Center for Radiation Medicine and Human Ecology, Gomel, Belarus

1. Introduction

Optical coherence tomography (OCT) is a method for imaging the internal structure of biological tissue *in vivo* with micron resolution. OCT has been recognized as an extremely promising tool for the diagnosis of pathological changes in biological tissue (Chauhan et al., 2001; Fercher et al., 2003). The coherence–domain range in OCT is performed by using a Michelson interferometer. By measuring singly back scattered light as a function of depth, OCT has the potential to image the structure of tissue with a high resolution and sensitivity. It is of importance for a diagnostics of structures inside a cornea, a cornea edema, for a quantitative imaging of the optic disc in glaucoma, for an evaluation of retinal thickness, etc. in ophthalmology. The high axial resolution of OCT is realized by the use of a broadband light source whereas the lateral resolution is determined by the numerical aperture (NA) of the focusing lens. Although a high NA of a conventional focusing lens in the sample arm of the imaging optical system enables high lateral resolution imaging, but low axial resolution. A low NA is required to achieve a large depth of focus, but in this case we deal with the low lateral resolution. The improvement of the axial–lateral resolution is a very important problem in imaging OCT-systems. Furthermore, a restriction of an imaging method is closely connected with a problem of tissue light–scattering: it leads to the decreasing in the focal depth of a probing beam and an image involves a "noisy"–speckle field superimposed on imaged structures as a result of scattering by a volume medium.

The impairment of optical mediums transparency, for example corneal caligo, opacity of vitreous body, cataract, causes the significant light scattering in the sample arm of OCT. In the case, when different pathologies in the macular area or in the optic nerve area occur the OCT–method doesn't give us a possibility to determine the reason of partial or complete sight loss. Fig. 1 demonstrates the non–informative OCT–image of retina for a patient with the cataract diagnosis (Fig. 1, a). After the surgical removal of opaque lens the retinal detachment was detected by the OCT–retest (Fig. 1, b). Before the surgical removal of the lens the retinal detachment was not detected by other methods, even the method of direct opthtalmoscopy. Fig. 1, c, d shows the OCT– image of the optic nerve area in a normal state (Fig. 1, c) and when we deal with the destruction in the vitreous body (Fig. 1, d). Thus clinical investigations (Fig. 1, a-d) indicate the impossibility of correct image registration under the condition of strong tissue scattering (Kramoreva & Rozhko, 2010).

A scattering problem in OCT has been solved by numerical analysis of OCT-images. A possibility to estimate scattering properties of tissue layers by the dependence of OCT signal on a probing depth was demonstrated in several publications (Andersen et al, 2004; Schmitt & Knuttel, 1993; Turchin et al., 2003). In the majority of papers, the theoretical models of OCT signal that are employed in reconstruction algorithms use two optical parameters to describe the scattering medium: the total scattering coefficient and the backscattering coefficient (Schmitt & Knuttel, 1993; Turchin et al., 2003) or the total scattering coefficient and mean cosine of scattering angle. In other case the reconstruction algorithm allows one to estimate three scattering parameters, namely, the total scattering coefficient, the backscattering probability, and the variance of the small-angle scattering phase function. The reconstruction procedure for scattering parameters in a multilayer medium has a poor accuracy with the decrease in the thickness of a single layer (Andersen et al, 2004).

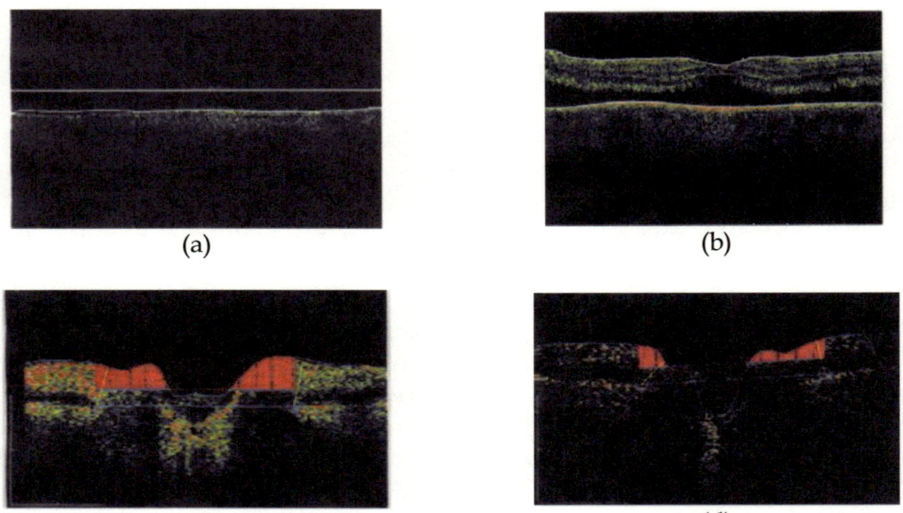

(a) (b)

(c) (d)

Fig. 1. The OCT - images of the macular area before (a) and after (b) the surgical removal of the opaque lens and the OCT - images of the optic nerve area in a normal state (c) and with the destruction in the vitreous body (d).

Therefore it is very important to improve the reconstruction algorithm of the OCT-signal. However, the contemporary design of optical elements is capable to improve the system resolution and image quality even before the final stage of computer processing.

From the viewpoint of foresaid the growing interest to various types of quasi-nondiffractive light beams (for example, a Bessel beam) is caused by the availability of unique properties: the large focal length of the beam, the suppressed diffraction divergence of the central part of the beam inside the focal length, the reconstruction of the transversal structure of the beam at the shielding of its central zone and a submicron structure of the axial maximum (for a nonparaxial and evanescent Bessel beam). These properties are promising for practical applications requiring the laser beam with a large focal depth, including the interferometry of cylindrical objects (Belyi, et al., 2005; Dresel, et al., 1995), the coherent microscopy (Leitgeh et al, 2006),the optical manipulation of microparticles (Arlt, et al., 2001; Garces-Chavez et al., 2002), etc. Together with advantages referred above Bessel beams have several drawbacks due to the feature of shaping units (Kramoreva & Rozhko, 2010). It reduces Bessel beam's efficiency in OCT–optical schemes. On the one hand, the development of new methods of the Bessel beam's generation with improved properties of the beam is a shortcut to an upgrading of the OCT–image problem.

On the other hand the electro–magnetic radiation absorption and the influence of tissue optical activity and scattering are the main optical effects under the condition of tissue probing.

Therefore, the knowledge about the objective laws of reflection and refraction for the probing radiation at the medium boundary is a necessary condition for high-quality diagnostics, for example, in the field of the polarizing sensitive tomography.

2. Generation of broadband Bessel-like beams: theory and experiment

The quasi-nondiffractive beam with the transverse intensity profile approximately corresponding to the zero-order Bessel function may be experimentally realized in the manner, which provides the annular-field generation in the far-field zone of the optical scheme. Traditionally simple ways of generation of the zero-order Bessel beam include the use of the annular ring mask placed at the front focal plane of the lens; the use of the refractive linear and logarithmic axicons illuminated by the collimated laser beam or the computer–generated axicon–type hologram (McGloin & Dholakia, 2005). However, for a probing Bessel beam, such disadvantages as the low energy-conversion efficiency, the nonuniform axial intensity (the residual sharp oscillation around the average intensity) within a focal length of a beam or the nonuniform of the central–core width of focal segment of the beam (Burval, 2004), can lead to a degradation of the image quality in different optical schemes including OCT.

In this section we consider the method of the creation of diffraction-free beams including the use of optical elements with a strong spherical aberration. Such features as the long beam focal length, the effective suppression of axial intensity oscillations, and the ability to form the beam with the given number of rings and the cone angle are the significant advantages of diffraction-free beams formed using optical elements with a strong spherical aberration over traditional Bessel beams formed by the axicons.

2.1 Investigation of two-element scheme axicon–lens with the high numerical aperture: experimental setup and results

The scheme of an experimental set-up is shown in Fig. 2. Gaussian beam from the He-Ne laser 1 (λ= 0.63 μm) is expanded by the collimator 2 up to the diameter of 2 cm. The linear axicon 3 has the apex angle α = 186 deg. The thick plane-convex high-NA-lens 4, having the form of a half-ball with curvature radius 9.5 mm and refractive index 1.5, is placed behind the axicon in the area of the existence of the Bessel beam. CCD-matrix 6 serves for the registration of 2D structure of the output field.

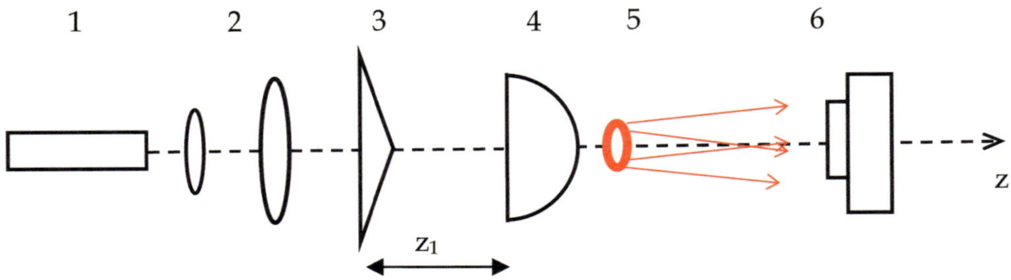

Fig. 2. Experimental setup for the generation of the Bessel-like beam light beam: 1- He-Ne laser; 2-the collimator; 3- the axicon; 4 - the lens with strong spherical aberration; 5 - the annular field in a focal plane; 6- CCD - matrix.

The high-NA-lens 4 focused the Bessel beam into the extended annular field by the external diameter in 0.9 mm. Such annular field serves as a source of a Bessel-like beam generation with the z-dependent cone angle. Fig. 3 demonstrates the transformation of the extended annular field into the Bessel-like beam with z-dependent cone angle γ for different distances z along the focal region of the high-NA-lens (the paraxial focal distance of high-NA-lens is f=1.9 cm). The ratio of external diameter to internal one for annular field is r=2.25 at the starting scanning position in z=1.5cm (Fig. 3, a). The ratio r decreases to 1.2 with the growth of z (Fig. 3, c) and at the distance z=2.3 cm the annular field transforms into the light cloud with the spiral-like structure (Fig. 3, d).

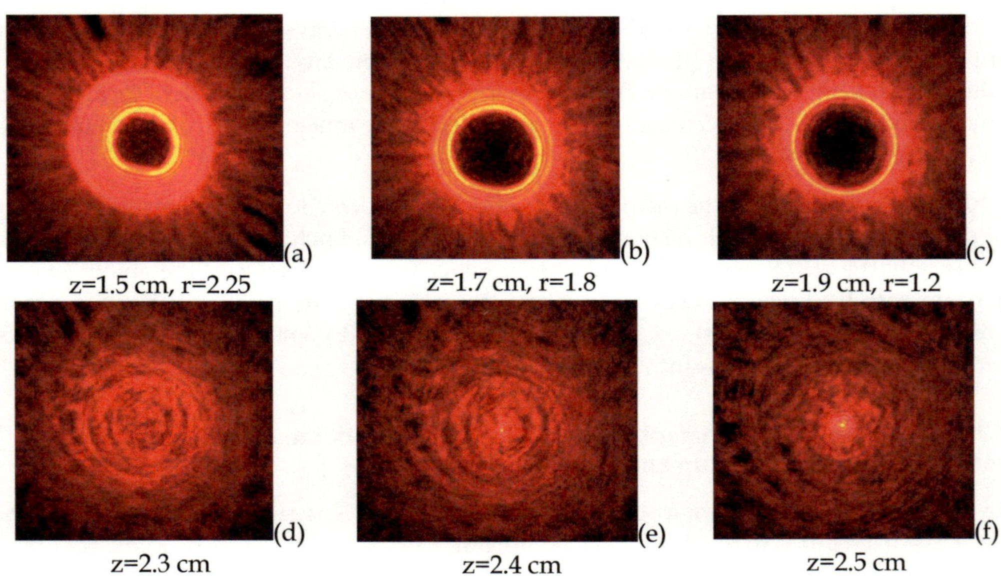

Fig. 3. Evolution of the Bessel-like beam from the extended annular field in two element scheme axicon–high NA-lens, z_1=10 cm.

Origination of the Bessel-like beam with the z-dependent cone angle was captured in Figs. 3, e, d. During the evolution of the Bessel-like beam the external diameter of the annular field remains constant (0.9 mm), but the diapason of variation in the internal diameter is changing from 0.4 mm to 0.8 mm.

The results of measurement of the output beam intensity on the distance z_1 between the axicon and the lens, when a motion of the lens along the optical axis occurs are shown in Figs. 4; 5.

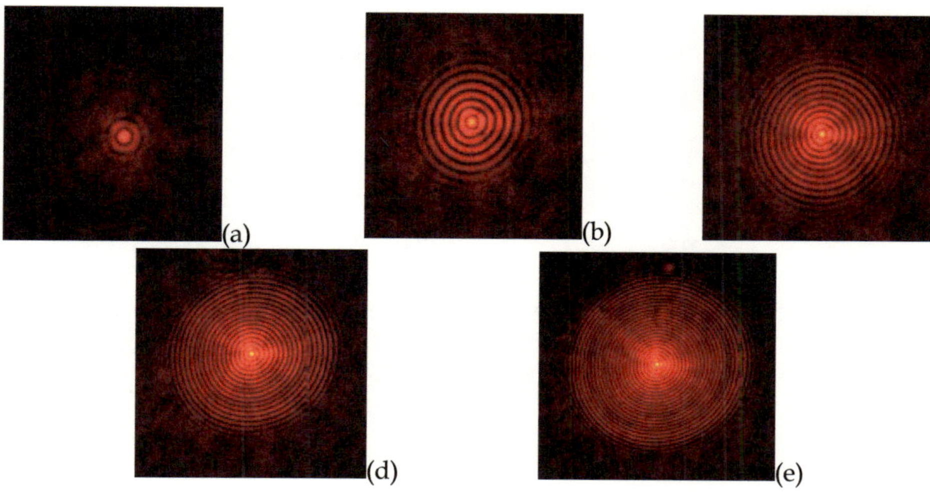

Fig. 4. Photos of the transverse section of the beam at the distance of z_1= 3.5 cm (a); 5.5 cm (b); 6.5 cm (c); 9.5 cm (d); 11.5 cm (e). The distance between the axicon and the CCD-matrix is equal to 64cmhotos of the transverse section of the beam at the distance of z_1= 3.5 cm (a); 5.5 cm (b); 6.5 cm (c); 9.5 cm (d); 11.5 cm (e). The distance between the axicon and the CCD-matrix is equal to 64cm.

On condition of small z_1 the central part of the field is seen to obtain the Bessel-like structure with a small number of rings (Fig. 4, a). With the growth of z_1 the number of rings N increases (Figs. 4; 5, a). A small change of z_1 leads to the essential increase of N and the diameter of the beam (Figs. 4; 5, b). Moreover the boundary between annular field and background is not sharp, but smoothed. It should be noted the growth of the diameter depends linearly on z_1, but the number of rings depends nonlinearly. As a result, the average cone angle of the beam increases, however the speed of this growth decreases (Fig. 5, c). It is an interesting fact that the axial intensity increases with the growth of the number of beam rings (with increasing of z_1) inside the half-focal length of the Bessel beam (after the axicon the focal length of the Bessel beam is ~32 cm) (Fig. 5, d).

Fig. 6 shows the dependence of the diameter of the annular maximum with the serial number N=10 on the distance z. The diameter is seen to increase linearly with z therefore the cone angle changes inversely to z.

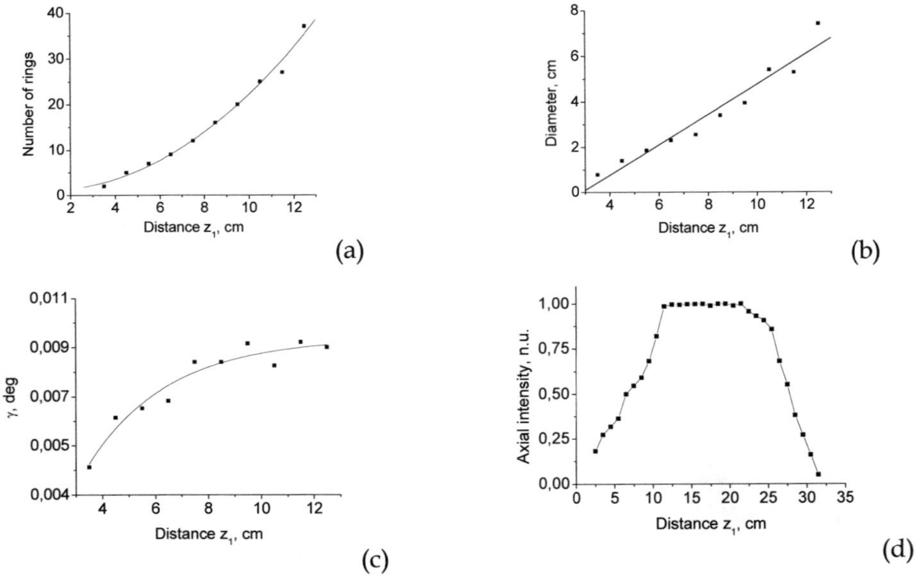

Fig. 5. Dependence on the distance of the number of rings N (a), the diameter of the beam (b), the average cone angle γ (c) and the on-axis intensity (d). Note that in the process of measurements the distance between the axicon and CCD-matrix is unaltered.

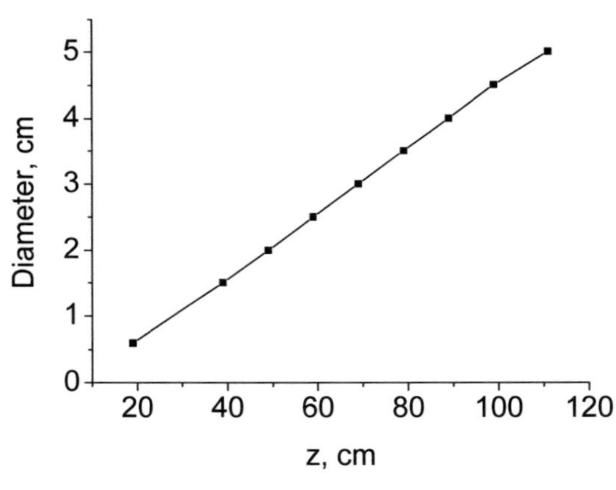

Fig. 6. Change in the Bessel-like beam size D along the longitudinal coordinate z (number of rings N = 10).

2.2 Analysis using Huygens–Fresnel diffraction integral

A quantitative calculation of the scheme with the high-NA lens needs in the application of the vector theory of diffraction. Within the framework of this chapter we will limit ourselves by a scalar approximation (Jaroszewicz & Morales, 1998). Output field amplitude $a(\rho, z)$ for the system of thin lens–axicon–high-NA-lens (Fig. 7) describes by the formula:

$$a(\rho,z)=-\frac{k^2}{zz_1}\int\exp\left[-\frac{\rho_2^2}{w^2(z_0)}+ik\frac{\rho_2^2}{2R(z_0)}-ik\gamma\rho_2+ik\frac{\rho_2^2+\rho_1^2}{2z_1}\right]J_0\left(\frac{k\rho_2\rho_1}{z_1}\right)\rho_2\,d\rho_2\times$$

$$\int\exp\left[-ik\frac{\rho_1^2}{2f^2}-ik\beta\rho_1^4-ik\gamma\rho_2-ik\frac{\rho^2+\rho_1^2}{2z}\right]J_0\left(\frac{k\rho\rho_1}{z_1}\right)\rho_2\,d\rho_2 \qquad (1)$$

where k is a wave number, ρ, ρ_1, ρ_2 are radial coordinates for planes R, L2, A (Fig. 7), $w(z_0) = w_0\,[1+\lambda^2 z_0^2/\pi^2 w_0^4]$ is the radius of area of the focused Gaussian beam as the function on the longitudinal coordinate z_0, w_0 is a minimal radius of beam, J_0 is the Bessel function of zero order (m=0), f_2 is the focal length of the high-NA-lens L2, $R(z_0)$ is a radius of wave front curvature for the Gaussian beam at the axicon, λ is a wavelength, γ is the cone angle of the axicon, β is an aberrant coefficient for the lens L2.

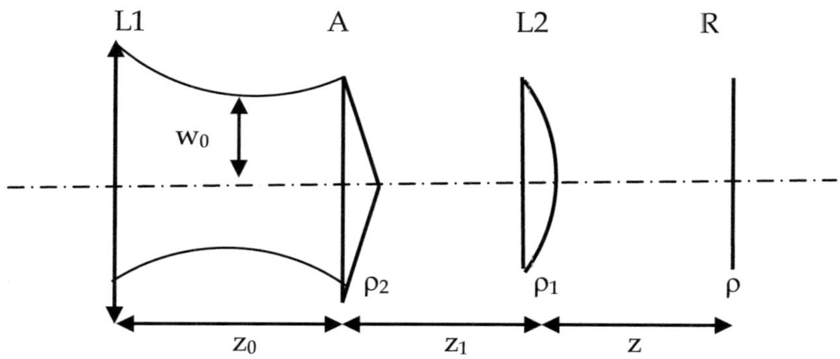

Fig. 7. Optical scheme for the evaluation of diffraction integral.

Results of the calculation for the output field are shown in Fig. 8. The calculation was made for the case when distance between the axicon and the output plane preserves unchangeable (equal to 64 cm), but the distance z_1 between the axicon and the lens changes. It is seen that a strong dependence of the structure of field on z_1 takes place due to spherical aberrations. In the case when z_1.is lower or equal to the paraxial focal length (1.5 cm), the field is a wide ring with the internal radius tending to zero when z_1.increases (Fig. 8, a, b). Sharp change of the field type from wide ring into the beam with intensive axial maximum and oscillated periphery takes place, when z_1 exceeds a little larger the focal length. Fig.8, c, d shows a small modulation depth of the multi-ring field. With further increase of z_1 the modulation depth increases in near-axial region.

Thus, the model of spherical lens satisfied the description of properties of the generated light beam (for example, the dependence of the ring number on distance z_1). It is necessary to notice that this model is not strict because it does not take into account such effects as the dependence of the transmission coefficient of spherical surface on the incident angle.

The conclusion can be made that two-element optical scheme composed of the axicon and the high-NA-lens allows one to create compact a generator of z-dependent Bessel–like beams, where the ring number can be changed due to the shift of lens along the optical axis.

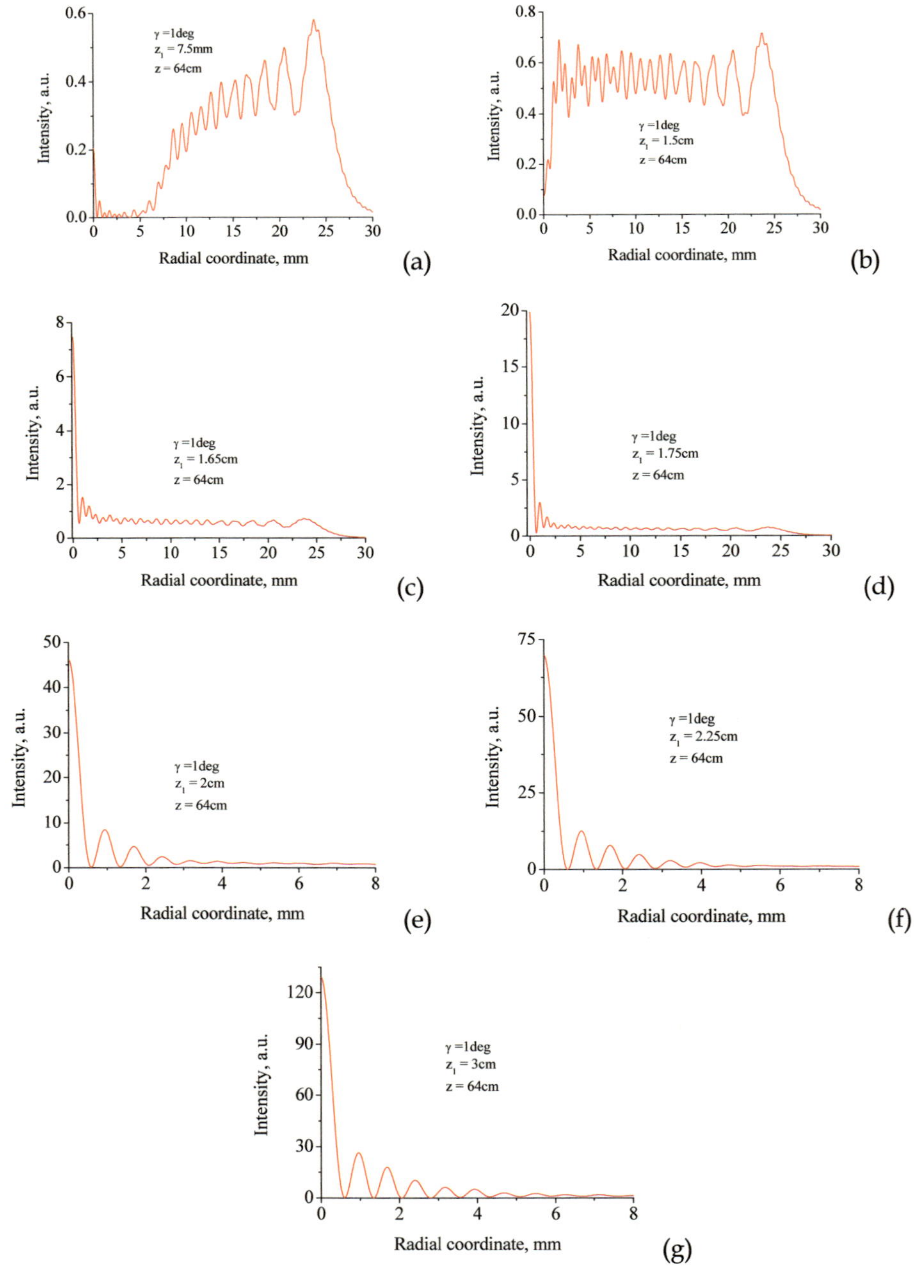

Fig. 8. The influence of the distance between the axicon and the high-NA-lens on the structure of the far- field.

2.3 Scheme with Fourier–transformation of the annular field: formation of the beam with uniform axial intensity and propagation features

The investigation of the far field is the aim of further analysis of the optical scheme with the axicon and the high- NA lens. In the scheme in Fig. 2 the Fourier-transforming lens was used additionally. The front focal plane of this lens was placed in the focal area of high-NA lens (Fig. 9). The focal distance of second lens was equal to 60 cm.

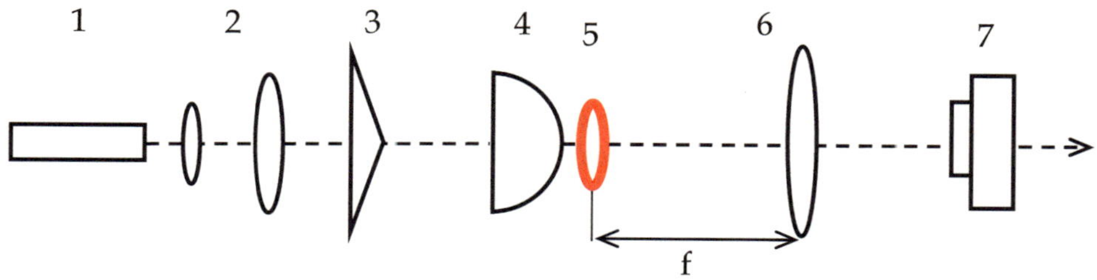

Fig. 9. Experimental setup for the generation of the quasi-Bessel light beam: 1– the He-Ne laser; 2– the collimator; 3– the axicon; 4 – the lens with strong spherical aberration; 5 – the annular field; 6 – the Fourier transforming lens; 7 – CCD – matrix

The field in the back focal plane of the lens and at the further distance had the Bessel type multi–ring structure. This can be easily explained with the use of the thin lens instead of high- NA lens 4. In this case the output field will be a Fourier-transformation of a thin annular beam formed in focal plane after the thin lens. Such a field is known to be the Bessel beam with high accuracy. When the high-NA-lens is used, the thin ring is not formed due to the spherical aberration which influences later on the field in far zone. The Fourier-transformation of the annular field with the large width leads to the formation of some superposition of Bessel beams with different the cone angles and relative phases. The superposition of Bessel beams exhibit new properties, which are not typical for partial Bessel beams. The use of different Bessel beam's superpositions opens the possibility for field synthesis with the given transverse and longitudinal structure. Furthermore, such Bessel–like beam is characterized by a large length of the area, where the axial intensity closes to uniform (within the limit of 13 m the variation of axial intensity amounted to ~ 4% (see Fig. 10)).

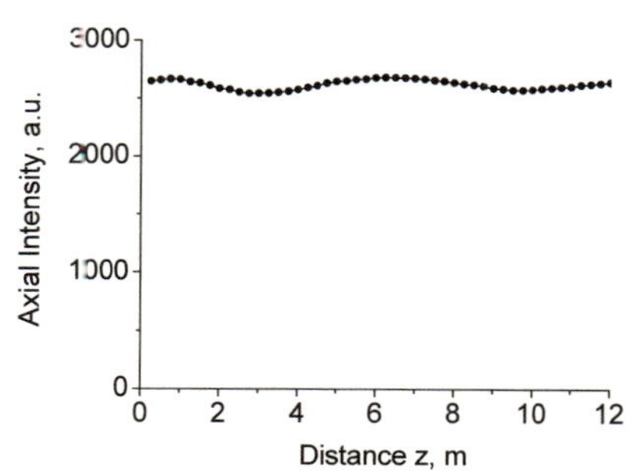

Fig. 10. Axial intensity as a function of longitudinal distance z after the Fourier-transforming lens.

This result points out that the annular fields with the large ratio of ring width to average diameter can generate a wideband on angular spectrum Bessel beam with the uniform long-distance focal area.

2.4 Investigation of properties of broadband Bessel–like beams

Two types of objects can be identified among a large variety of light-scattering objects. There are foreign inclusions with distinct boundaries and cloudy media. A matted surface and solutions of suspensions respectively are two-dimensional and three-dimensional analogs of the first type of the medium; a milky scatterer and milky emulsions are analogs of cloudy media. It was shown experimentally (Belyi et al., 2006) that a beam profile reconstruction occurs upon a passage of the Bessel beam through scattering media (solutions of suspensions, emulsions, and matted surfaces). The influence of scattering media on the structure of broadband Bessel-like beams has also been investigated.

Fig. 11 demonstrates the radial distribution of the intensity for the Gaussian beam and broadband Bessel-like beam at their propagation without the matted diffuser (curve 1) and with the matted diffuser (curve 2) along the optical axis of the scheme.

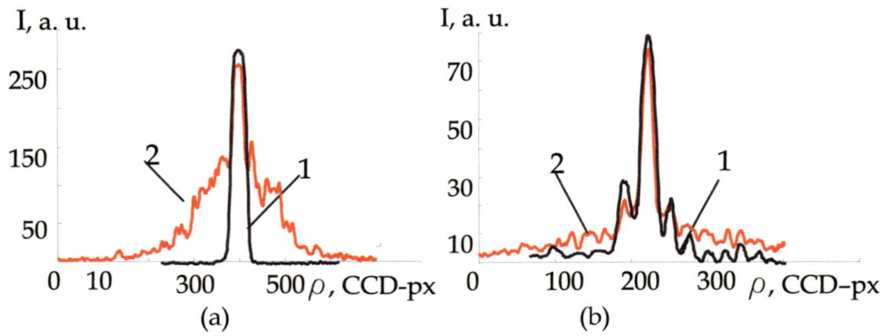

Fig. 11. Radial distribution of intensity: (a) for the Gaussian beam - the curve 1 corresponds to the Gaussian beam profile without the diffuser and the curve 2 is the result of the Gaussian beam passage through the diffuser; (b) the Bessel-like beam - the curve 1 corresponds to the Bessel-like beam profile without the diffuser and the curve 2 is the result of the Bessel-like beam passage through the diffuser

The matted diffuser as the scattering medium was located at the distance of 20 cm after the lens 4 (in the Fig. 2). The width of the Gaussian beam and the width of the central maximum of the Bessel-like beam were chosen out to be approximately identical and about 450-460 μm. The registration plane was located at the distance of 10 cm after the matted diffuser in both of cases. For the Gaussian beam an appearance of a considerable speckle - noise leads to the distortion of the overall picture of the intensity profile. In case of the Bessel-like beam propagation through the light-scattering medium the structure of the central maximum and the rings remain insignificant against speckle-noise (Kramoreva & Rozhko, 2010).

In another case a "regeneration" phenomena of the Bessel-like beam is investigated, when a metal ball with the diameter of 2 mm was chosen as an obstacle for the Bessel-like beam. The ball has been placed at the distance of 34 cm from the high-NA-lens 4 (in the Fig. 2) in the center of the Bessel–like beam and has overlapped the central and partially the first annular maxima. The registration of the transverse distribution of the intensity has been made at several distances from the ball. In Fig. 12, a, b the 2D distribution of intensity is shown for two distances from the obstacle (lower side of the beam is not shown, i.e. it has been covered by the support for the ball).

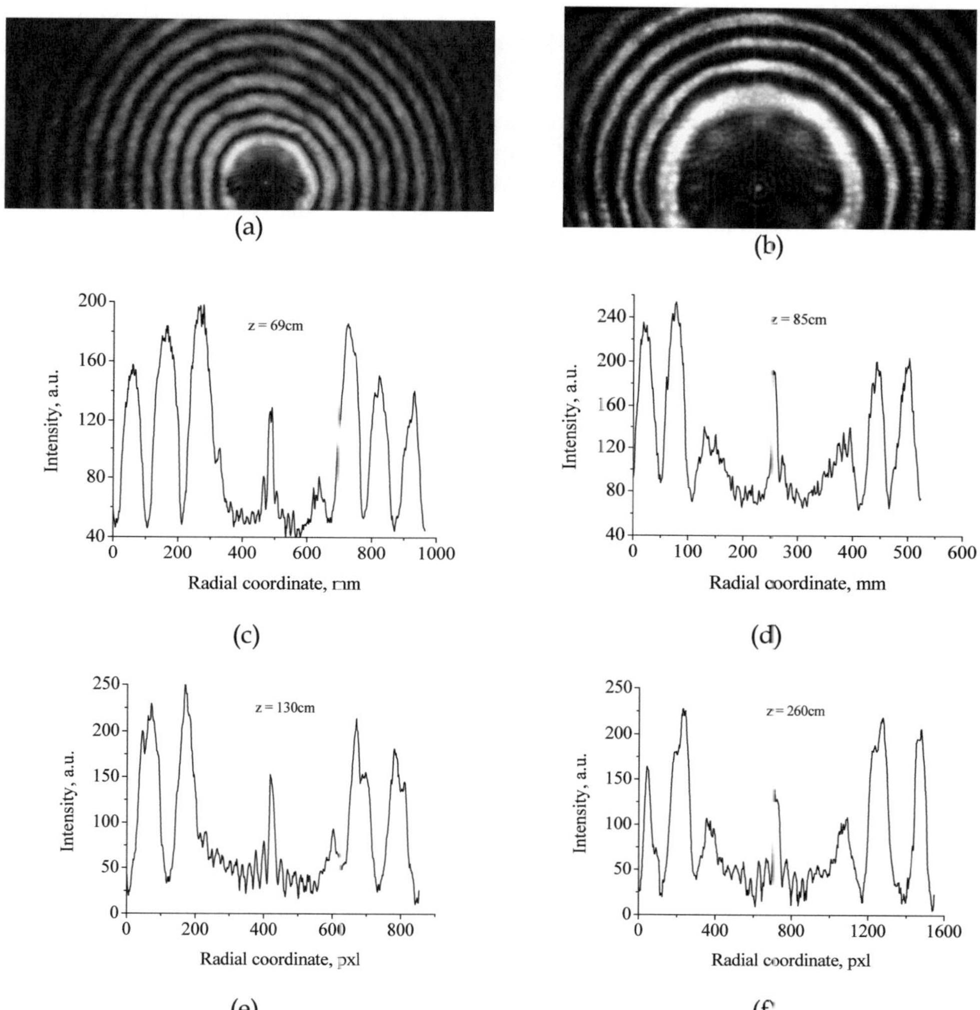

Fig. 12. Photos of transverse intensity distribution of z- dependent Bessel-like beam at distances 69 cm (a) and 260 cm (b) from the ball. 1D intensity distribution of central part of the beam at various distances z (c-f).

Macroscopic dip of the intensity in the center of the beam is the consequence of screening the field by the ball. In the shadow area the multi-ring field which coincides in its sight with Bessel one can be observed. The 1D-cuts of intensity of the shadow field for various z are shown in Fig. 12, c-f.

In this section we present the experimental investigation and the numerical simulation of spatial and angular properties of the light field irradiated by the annular source formed in the scheme composed the axicon and the lens with the strong spherical aberration. The cone angle of such beam decreases smoothly when the beam propagates along the optical axis. The number of rings of the beam depends on the distance between the axicon and the lens. As a result, the pointed scheme is promising for the creation of compact sources of the z-dependent Bessel beam. Using the additional Fourier-transforming lens, the generated field presents itself the Bessel beam with wide angular spectrum. The axial intensity of the beam is characterized by high uniformity at large distance.

The shadow field generated by the beam during the screening of the central zone by the circular obstacle has been investigated. The shadow field is shown to have conical nature, which can be identified on its annular spatial spectrum. The fact that the shadow field appearing at the presence of the obstacle with the ideal edge has azimuthally-symmetrical amplitude-phase distribution is of important practical application. Consequently, the presence of any edge defects will influence on the structure of the shadow field. This opens the possibility to create the method of optical diagnostics of the quality of micro-reliefs. Moreover, the minimal presence of a speckle – noises under the condition of light-scattering is promising for quality improving the tissue structures visualization in the systems of OCT.

In conclusion it is necessary to pay attention to the peculiar type of Bessel light fields, which are formed in conditions of total internal reflection. They are called evanescent light beams. The improved lateral resolution of optical systems using the evanescent Bessel beams as a probe radiation is a rather real possibility.

2.5 Evanescent Bessel beam: theory and simulation analysis

It is known that resolution depends on the diameter of a probing light beam: the less the diameter of the beam, the higher the resolution of the system. Therefore, the growing interest to nonparaxial and evanescent Bessel lights is caused by the availability of submicron structure of the axial maximum, different polarization properties and energy characteristics (Grosjean et al., 2003; Novitsky et al., 2008 as cited in Kurilkina et al., 2010; Rushin & Leizer, 1999; Zhan, 2006).

According to so-called "evanescent field" phenomenon, the appearance of an evanescent field is associated with light internally reflection phenomena when the Gaussian light beam travels from the first optical medium n_1 into the second optical medium with a refraction index n_2 so that $n_2 < n_1$ (for example, for a cornea $n_1=1.38$ and an aqueous humor $n_2=1.336$ or for a lens $n_1=1.413$ and a vitreous humor $n_2=1.336$). In general an evanescent mode is the wave–guide propagation mode which is known per se and therefore needs not be more specifically described. It is notable that the amplitude of a wave in this mode diminishes rapidly along the direction of its propagation, but the phase does not change. The evanescent Bessel beam has the following features: significantly reduced diameter comparing to the emitted beam; a central lobe is significantly smaller in size than the wavelength of radiation in the medium where the evanescent Bessel beam is generated (a second medium n_2); and a retained tight focus profile along the direction of beam propagation within the desired distance. This desired distance is relatively large for near-field applications (up to several wavelengths), and can be even more increased by using the third medium interposed between the first and the second media, provided that the refraction index of the second medium is less than the refraction index of each of the first and the third media.

If the propagation direction of circular polarized evanescent Bessel beam is a perpendicular to a boundary of two isotropic media (under a condition of total internal reflection ($n_1 > n_2$)) the representation of transversal component of electric vector for circular polarized evanescent Bessel beam in the optical less dense medium n_2 is (Goncharenko et al., 2001):

$$E_{\perp}^{\pm} = \mp i \sin(\gamma_2)\left[e_+ J_{m-1}(q\rho)\exp(-i(\varphi \mp \alpha)) + e_- J_{m+1}(q\rho)\exp(i(\varphi \mp \alpha))\right]\exp(-\chi z + im\varphi) \quad (2)$$

Here ρ, φ, z are the cylindrical coordinates, $J_m(q\rho)$ is the m-order Bessel function, $k_0 = 2\pi/\lambda$, γ_2 – the cone angle of the Bessel beam in the second medium n_2, $q = \sqrt{(k_0 n_2)^2 + \chi^2}$ - the transversal component of the wave vector, $\sin(\gamma_2) = q/k_0 n_2$, $\tan(\alpha) = \chi/k_0 n_2$, $k_z = i\chi$ is z-projection of the wave vector, $e_{\pm} = (e_1 \pm ie_2)/\sqrt{2}$ are unit circular vectors, e_1, e_2 are unit-vectors of the right (+) and the left (-) circular polarization. In common case, according to Eq. 2 the evanescent Bessel beam is a superposition of two circular-polarized Bessel beams with a different space structure. If m = 0, the transversal component of the electric vector is:

$$E_{\perp}^{\pm} = \mp\sqrt{2}\sin(\gamma_2) J_1(q\rho)[e_1 \sin(\varphi - \alpha) - e_2 \cos(\varphi - \alpha)]\exp(-\chi z) \quad (3)$$

As seen from Eq. 3 in the optical less dense medium n_2 the polarization of the evanescent Bessel beam m=0 becomes linear one.

Azimuthal, radial and z- components of an energy flow of the evanescent Bessel beam are (Goncharenko et al., 2001):

$$S_\rho = \frac{4\chi q^3}{k_0^4}\frac{m}{q\rho} J_m^2(q\rho)\exp(-2\chi z), \quad S_\varphi = \frac{2(\varepsilon_1 + \varepsilon_2)k_0}{n_1 q}\frac{m}{q\rho} J_m^2(q\rho)\exp(-2\chi z) \quad (4)$$

$$S_z = \left[J_{m-1}^2(q\rho) - J_{m+1}^2(q\rho)\right]\exp(-2\chi z),$$

where $n_{1,2} = \sqrt{\varepsilon_{1,2}}$.

According to Eq. 4 for the evanescent Bessel beam m=0 only the longitudinal z-component of the energy flow occurs in an energy balance, for the evanescent Bessel beam of high order all three components of energy flow are nonzero one.

The important feature of the evanescent Bessel beam is the ability of a spatial localization of its energy. For n_1=2.3, γ_1=40 deg., the diameter of the central lobe for the beam within the range of a evanescent field existence is: $d(\gamma) \approx 4.8\frac{\lambda}{2\pi n_1 \sin(\gamma_1)} \approx 0.5\lambda$.

The penetration depth of the beam inside the medium depends on the cone angle of the evanescent Bessel beam. The growth in the cone angle leads to the penetration depth decrease as an exponential damping (Fig. 13, a). Fig. 13, b demonstrates a "virtual" jump of energy of the beam into the optically less dense medium.

So, the theoretical analysis demonstrates the ability of the evanescent Bessel beam to realize the localization of light field in a subwavelength space region; the evanescent Bessel beam has a significantly reduced diameter and small number of rings in comparison to initial Bessel beam. The narrow central maximum of evanescent Bessel beam is a nondiffractive one within the range of the evanescent field's existence in comparison to the evanescent Gaussian field. According to the given consideration the evanescent Bessel beam has a promising perspective for application in optical near–field microscopy and OCT.

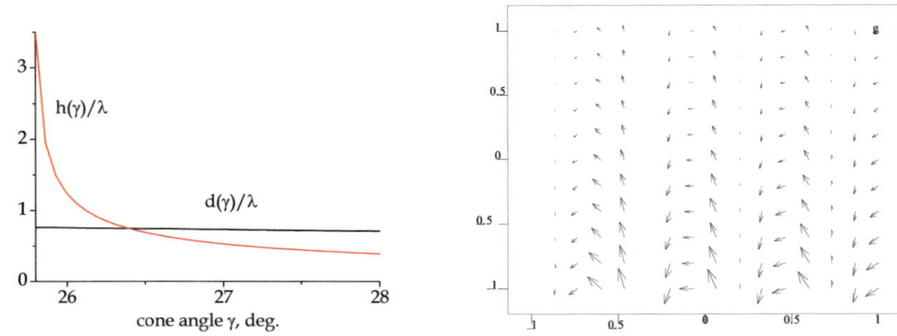

(a) (b)

Fig. 13. Evanescent Bessel beam behavior: the dependence of the penetration depth h and the central lobe diameter d on the cone angle γ (a); a vector field of the evanescent beam (b).

3. Influence of absorption and optical activity on spatial properties of the quasi-nondiffractive beam

For the optimization of probing condition by the quasi-nondiffractive beam availability of absorption and optical activity in tissues are to be taken into account.

Several publications concern the analysis of nondiffracting beams interaction with an optically active or absorbing medium. The displaying properties of the Bessel beams behavior at their propagation in an optically active media is investigated to a greater extent than for the absorbing media. So, the analysis of Bessel beam behavior propagation along one of the optical axes in biaxial crystals is presented by Kazak et al., 1999. Berry & Jeffray, 2006 have analyzed the image of a conical refraction in terms of singular optics focusing their attention on the fact that the Bessel vortex beams in biaxial crystals are the beams with eigen polarization. Fadeeva & Volyar, 2010 revealed the abnormal zone, where a diffraction-free beam can propagates through a purely chiral crystal as if they do in an isotropic medium. According to the proposed theory even a purely chiral crystal without linear birefringence can generates optical vortices in an initially vortex-free Bessel beam. Spatial features and the polarization pattern of non-paraxial Bessel beams were investigated by Petrova, 2000 in natural optically active media. It is shown that the value of the Bessel beam cone angle influences on the behavior of specific plane-of-polarization rotation.

The problems of Bessel beam interaction with the absorbing media are investigated in a modest way. As regard the interaction of the Bessel beam with the absorbing medium,

Zamboni-Rached, 2006 has developed a method for the simulation of longitudinal intensity pattern of propagating beams in absorbing media. As a particular case, the diffraction-attenuation resistant beams were obtained so that the beams are capable of maintaining both, the size and the intensity of their central spots for long distances compared to ordinary beams. The referred method for absorbing media was developed from appropriate superposition of ideal zero-order Bessel beams. Such beams maintain their resistance to diffraction and absorption even when they are generated by the finite apertures (Zamboni-Rached et al, 2010). At present the behavior of energy flows under a condition of the Bessel beam interaction with absorbing media is studied poorly. However the knowledge about a distribution of energy flows are important to understand the subtle effect of energy swapping inside the beam. Under a condition of interaction of the Bessel beam with the absorbing cylinder a problem is solved partially by Khilo et al., 2005. An analysis of TE- and TH-polarized input field both, the reflection and energy coefficients allows one to evaluate the laser energy loss in an absorbing cylinder and the heat distribution in the cross section.

In this section some features of the interaction of the Bessel beam with a semi-infinite media with absorption and optical activity are presented.

3.1 Bessel beam and absorbing medium: theory and simulation analysis

When incident Bessel beam passes from the transparent isotropic medium with the refraction index n_0 into the semi-infinite isotropic absorption medium n, the refractive index $n = n' + i n''$ and the longitudinal component of wave vector $\tilde{k}_z = k_{z1} + i k_{z2}$ are complex values. Solutions of Maxwell's equations for TE-, TH-polarized Bessel beam within absorption medium are (Khilo et al., 2005; Petrova & Kramoreva, 2010):

$$E_\rho^{TH} = -\frac{i\tilde{k}_z}{2}\left(J_{m+1}(q\rho) - J_{m-1}(q\rho)\right), \quad E_\varphi^{TH} = -\frac{\tilde{k}_z}{2}\left(J_{m+1}(q\rho) + J_{m-1}(q\rho)\right),$$
$$E_z^{TH} = qJ_m(q\rho)$$
$$E_\rho^{TE} = \frac{ik_0}{2}\left(J_{m+1}(q\rho) + J_{m-1}(q\rho)\right), \quad E_\varphi^{TE} = \frac{k_0}{2}\left(J_{m+1}(q\rho) - J_{m-1}(q\rho)\right),$$
$$E_z^{TE} = 0. \tag{5}$$

Where q is a radial wave number, $q = k_0 n \sin(\gamma)$, γ is the cone angle of the Bessel beam in an absorbing medium. All amplitudes in Eq. 5 involve a common phase factor $\exp[i\tilde{k}_z z + im\varphi]$. For TH- polarized Bessel beam longitudinal (z), radial (ρ), and azimuth (φ) components of Pointing vector and heat flow are

$$S_z = \frac{c}{8\pi} k_0 \left(k_z'\varepsilon' + k_z''\varepsilon''\right)\left\{J_{m-1}^2(q\rho) + J_{m+1}^2(q\rho)\right\}\exp[-2k_z'' z]$$

$$S_\rho = \frac{c}{8\pi} k_0 q\varepsilon'' J_m(q\rho)\left\{J_{m-1}(q\rho) - J_{m+1}(q\rho)\right\}\exp[-2k_z'' z] \tag{6}$$

$$S_{\varphi} = \frac{c}{8\pi} k_0 \varepsilon' \frac{m}{\rho} J_m^2(q\rho)\exp[-2k_z'' z]$$

$$Q(q\rho) = \frac{\omega}{4\pi} \varepsilon'(\omega)\left| E(q\rho)\right|^2 \exp[-2k_z'' z], \quad (7)$$

where $E(q\rho)E^*(q\rho) = |k|^2\left(J_{m-1}^2(q\rho) + J_{m+1}^2(q\rho)\right) + 2q^2 J_m^2(q\rho)$

Eqs. 6, 7 and Fig. 14 show that the radial energy flow of the Bessel beam and the availability of heat evolution/absorption areas inside the beam cross-section occur due to absorption.

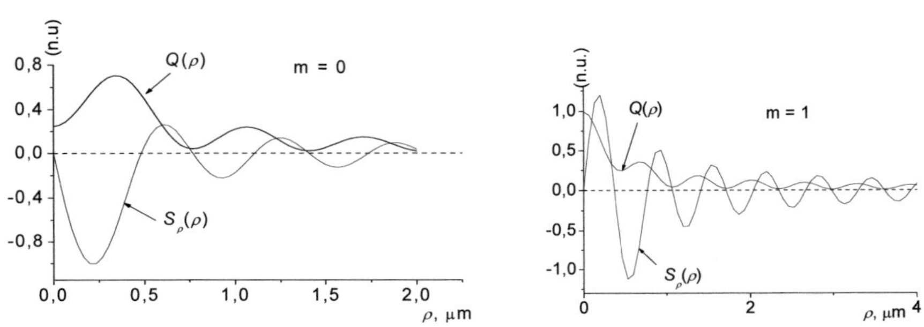

(a) (b)

Fig. 14. Dependence of the radial energy flow and heat flow on the radial coordinate for the Bessel beam with m = 0 (a) and m=1 (b).

Here zero-values of radial energy flow coincide with the minimum or maximum of the heat evolution area in the cross section of the Bessel beam. This property can be useful for the thermal action on tissues in therapeutic area. The heat evolution is a maximal in the region of minimal radial energy flow values. The propagation direction of the radial energy flow S_ρ depends on the order of the Bessel beam. For the Bessel beam with an order m=0 the radial energy flow is directed to the beam axis (Fig.15, a). When we deal with the high order (m=1) Bessel beam, the azimuthal component of energy flow appears and the radial energy flow moves away from the beam axis (Fig. 15, a).

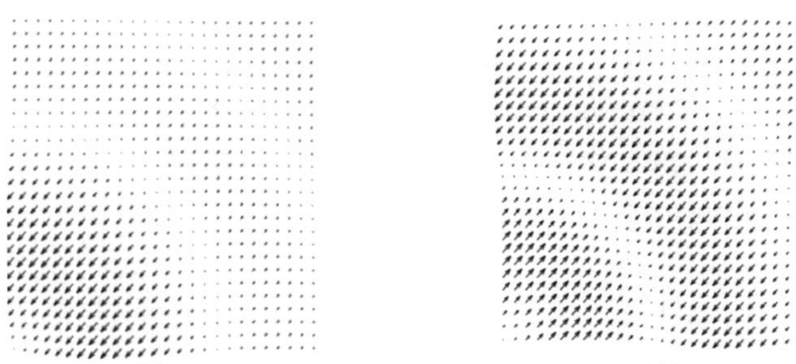

(a) (b)

Fig. 15. Vector field of the radial energy flow for the Bessel beam of different order: m=0 (a), m=1 (b).

Another feature of the beam behavior is that the initiation of azimuthal component of energy flows only for the high-order Bessel beam propagating through an absorbing medium. The change in the azimuthal and radial energy flow direction occurs for different higher m-order of the Bessel function. Fig. 16 shows the oscillation phase shifts in $\pi/2$ and the extension of near-axis minimum with the growth in m. Numerical simulations demonstrate the growth of oscillation frequency in the energy flow under the condition when the cone angle increases (Fig. 17).

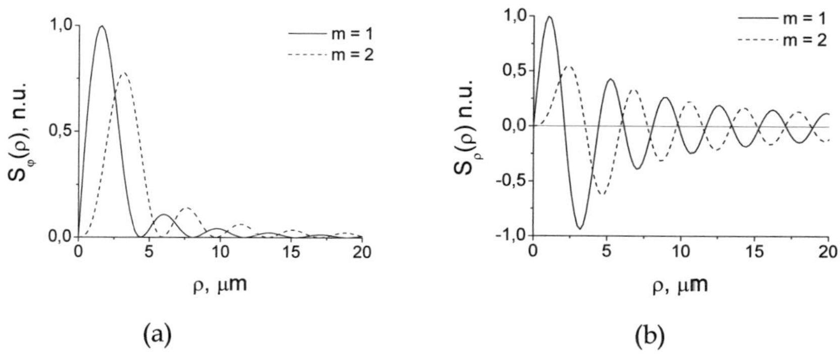

Fig. 16. Energy flow against m –order Bessel beam in an absorbing medium.

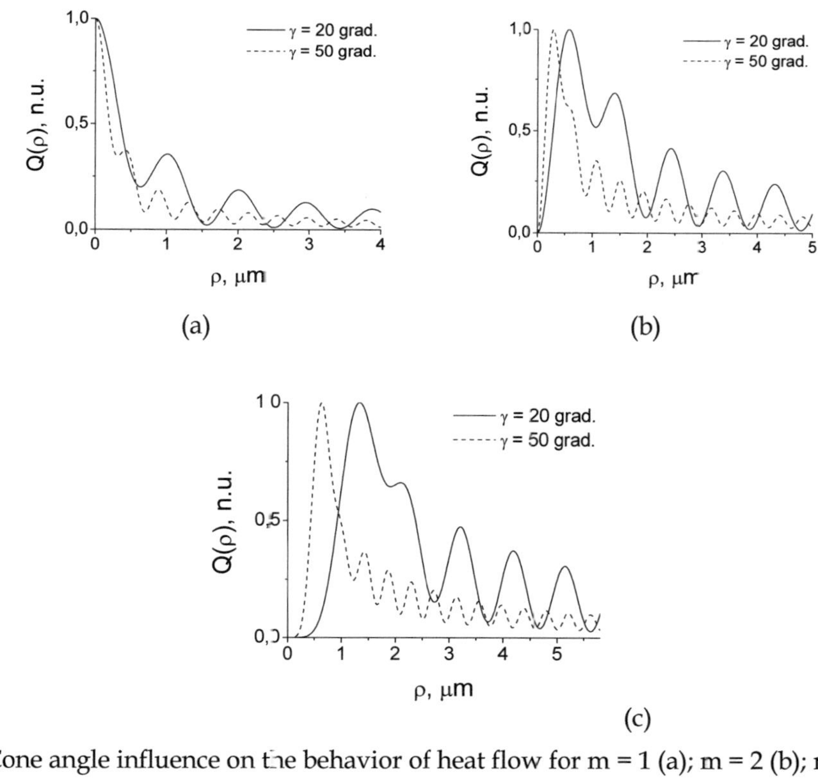

Fig. 17. Cone angle influence on the behavior of heat flow for m = 1 (a); m = 2 (b); m = 4 (c).

In this case the smoothing of $Q(\rho)$ oscillations is the feature for the given function and it is the effect of radial flow contribution in the energy balance of the Bessel beam.

3.2 Bessel beam and optically active medium: theoretical analysis

When TH-polarized Bessel beam travels from the non-absorbing medium n_1 to semi-infinite optically active medium the boundary condition describes by the expression:

$$E_{\tau i}^{TH} + E_{\tau r}^{TH} + E_{\tau r}^{TE} = E_{\tau t}, \quad H_{\tau i}^{TH} + H_{\tau r}^{TH} + H_{\tau r}^{TE} = H_{\tau t}, \tag{8}$$

This formula describes the normal incidence of the beam to the boundary of mediums.

In an optically active medium the refracted field is a circular-polarized Bessel beam with transverse and longitudinal components (Petrova, 2000):

$$\begin{gathered}
E_{\rho}^{\pm} = \pm i\left(\frac{m}{q\rho} J_m(q\rho) \pm \cos(\gamma_{\pm}) J'_m(q\rho)\right), \\
E_{\varphi}^{\pm} = -\left(\cos(\gamma_{\pm})\frac{m}{q\rho} J_m(q\rho) \pm J'_m(q\rho)\right), \quad E_z^{\pm} = \sin(\gamma_{\pm}) J_m(q\rho), \\
H_{\rho}^{\pm} = \sqrt{\varepsilon}\left(\frac{m}{q\rho} J_m(q\rho) \pm \cos(\gamma_{\pm}) J'_m(q\rho)\right), \\
H_{\varphi}^{\pm} = \pm i\sqrt{\varepsilon}\left(\cos(\gamma_{\pm})\frac{m}{q\rho} J_m(q\rho) \pm J'_m(q\rho)\right), \\
H_z^{\pm} = \mp i\sqrt{\varepsilon}\sin(\gamma_{\pm}) J_m(q\rho).
\end{gathered} \tag{9}$$

Where $\gamma_{\pm}$ is the cone angle of the Bessel beam in the optically active medium, $\cos(\gamma_{\pm}) = \cos(\gamma_0)[1 \pm (\alpha/\sqrt{\varepsilon})\tan^2(\gamma_0)]$, γ_0 is the cone angle of Bessel beam without taking into account a gyrotropic parameter α.

The relationship between the electric vector E and the magnetic vector B is: $B = \mp i n_{\pm} E$, where $n_{\pm} = \sqrt{\varepsilon} \pm \alpha$. The transverse component of the electric vector for m = 0 is described by formula: $E_{\perp}(q\rho) = -\frac{i\cos(\gamma_{\pm})}{\sqrt{2}}(e_{\rho} + i\tau_{\pm} e_{\varphi}) J_1(q\rho)$, where e_{ρ}, e_{φ} are unit-vectors for radial and azimuthal directions, $\tau_{\pm} = 1/\cos(\gamma_{\pm})$ is an ellipticity parameter. In paraxial approximation for the circular polarized Bessel beam the transverse component of electric vector is: $E_{\perp}(q\rho) - i[(e_1 \pm i e_2)/2] J_1(q\rho)\exp(\mp i\varphi)$, where e_1, e_2 are unit-vectors of the right (+) and the left (–) circular polarization.

In this case, coefficients of reflection r_{TH}^{TH}, r_{TE}^{TH} and refraction $t_{\pm}^{TH}$ (±) are

$$r_{TH}^{TH} = \frac{\sqrt{\varepsilon_2}\cos(\gamma_i) - n_1\cos(\gamma_0)}{\sqrt{\varepsilon_2}\cos(\gamma_i) + n_1\cos(\gamma_0)},$$

$$r_{TE}^{TH} = \frac{2\alpha n_1\cos(\gamma_i)\cos(\gamma_0)\tan^2(\gamma_0)}{(n_1\cos(\gamma_0) + \sqrt{\varepsilon_2}\cos(\gamma_i))(n_1\cos(\gamma_i) + \sqrt{\varepsilon_2}\cos(\gamma_0))}, \quad (10)$$

$$t_{\pm}^{TH} = \frac{n_1\cos(\gamma_i)(n_1\cos(\gamma_i) + \sqrt{\varepsilon_2}\cos(\gamma_{\mp}))}{(n_1\cos(\gamma_0) + \sqrt{\varepsilon_2}\cos(\gamma_i))(n_1\cos(\gamma_i) + \sqrt{\varepsilon_2}\cos(\gamma_0))}.$$

The upper index denotes the incident TH-polarized Bessel beam, the lower index – the reflected TH- or TE-polarized beam and also the refracted (±) circular-polarized beam. Therefore, the reflected field contains two mutually orthogonal polarized modes. The gyrotropic parameter α can be found by the measurement of the reflected field intensity.

According to Eq. 10 (±) circular-polarized Bessel beams propagate in an optically active medium with different phase velocities and refractive coefficients. The transversal component of electric field $E_{\perp}^{TH}$ with using of a rotation matrix $\hat{U}(\beta z)$ can be represents as following expression:

$$E_{\perp}^{TH}(\alpha) = t^{(1)}\left[-\frac{m}{q\rho}J_m(q\rho)\cos(\gamma_2)\hat{U}(\varphi_1(z))\begin{pmatrix}0\\1\end{pmatrix} + iJ'_m(q\rho)\cos(\gamma_2)\hat{U}(\varphi_1(z))\begin{pmatrix}1\\0\end{pmatrix}\right] -$$
$$-\alpha C_1\left[i\frac{m}{q\rho}J_m(q\rho)\begin{pmatrix}1 & 0\\0 & -C_2\end{pmatrix}\hat{U}(\beta z)\begin{pmatrix}1\\0\end{pmatrix} + J'_m(q\rho)\begin{pmatrix}C_2 & 0\\0 & -1\end{pmatrix}\hat{U}(\beta z)\begin{pmatrix}0\\1\end{pmatrix}\right], \quad (11)$$

where:

$$C_1 = \frac{2\,n_1\cos(\gamma_i)\cos(\gamma_0)\tan^2(\gamma_0)}{(n_1\cos(\gamma_0) + \sqrt{\varepsilon_2}\cos(\gamma_i))(n_1\cos(\gamma_i) + \sqrt{\varepsilon_2}\cos(\gamma_0))}, \qquad C_2 = \frac{n_1\cos(\gamma_i)}{\sqrt{\varepsilon_2}},$$

$\beta = k_0\alpha/\cos(\gamma_0)$ is the specific plane-of-polarization rotation,

$$\varphi_1(z) = \tan^{-1}\left[\frac{\tan(\beta z)}{\cos(\gamma_0)}\right],$$

$$\cos(\gamma_2) = \sqrt{\sin^2(\beta z) + \cos^2(\beta z)\cos^2(\gamma_0)}, \qquad \hat{U}(\beta z) = \begin{pmatrix}\cos(\beta z) & \sin(\beta z)\\ -\sin(\beta z) & \cos(\beta z)\end{pmatrix}$$

$$t^{(1)} = \frac{2n_1\cos(\gamma_i)}{n_1\cos(\gamma_0) + \sqrt{\varepsilon_2}\cos(\gamma_i)}$$

Eq. 11 is the invariant expression to sign reversal as $\cos(\gamma_0) \to -\cos(\gamma_0)$. Practically, it means the invariance of polarization modes to the change in the propagation direction of incident Bessel beam.

For the demonstration of TH→TE transformation phenomena we rewrite Eq. 11 as:

$$E_{\perp} = t_{+}^{(1)}\left[E_{\perp}^{+}\exp(i\beta z) + \tau\, E_{\perp}^{-}\exp(-i\beta z)\right]\exp[i(k_z z + m\varphi] \quad (12)$$

where $E_{\perp}^{\pm} = E_{\rho}^{\pm} e_{\rho} + E_{\varphi}^{\pm} e_{\varphi}$, $\tau = t_{-}^{TH} / t_{+}^{TH}$.

For paraxial approximation, when $\tau \to 1$, therefore

$$E_{\perp} = i\sqrt{2}\, t_{+}^{TH} \exp[ik_z z]\left[\cos(\beta z) E_{\perp i}^{TH} + i \sin(\beta z) E_{\perp i}^{TE}\right]. \quad (13)$$

Here $E_{\perp i}^{TH,TE}$ are transversal components of incident TH-, TE-polarized beam. Output field is the superposition of TH-and TE-Bessel beams and the amplitude ratio for beams depends on distance z in an optically active medium complies with the simple harmonic law. When $\beta z = (2d + 1)\pi/2$, and an integer number $d = 0$, we deal with the converting TH-polarization of the Bessel beam into the beam with TE-polarization. Estimation of an oscillation period is $z = \pi/2\beta \sim 3$mm, when $\alpha = 5\times10^{-5}$, and $\lambda = 0.63$ μm.

Thus, the incidence of linear-polarized quasi-nondiffractive light beam on the boundary with semi-infinity optically active media leads to the appearance of two mutually orthogonal linear-polarized modes in the reflected field. The gyrotropic parameter can be found by the measurement of the reflected field intensity for nonparaxial beams.

So, when the paraxial circular-polarized quasi-nondiffractive beam propagates in semi-infinity optical active medium the refracted field is the superposition of TH-and TE-Bessel beams and the amplitude ratio for beams depends on longitudinal distance z in the optically active medium by the simple harmonic law and TH↔TE mode transformation phenomenon occurs for this case.

In common theoretical analysis allows one to recognize clearly the interaction features of the quasi-nondiffractive beam with semi-infinity absorbing and optically active media. However, the representation of bio-tissue as a bi- or multi-layer combination of the studied above media is a necessary condition for more correct simulation and optimization of probing condition by optical scanning systems.

4. Future research

Our further researches concern on a modernization of the interference technique based on axicon optics. The comparative analysis of the OCT images for different types of probe beams is the focus of our investigations.

The use of the axicon optics in the time–domain OCT was first investigated by Ding et al., 2002. Ding et al. reported on the incorporation of an axicon lens into the sample arm of the interferometer. Using the axicon lens with a top angle of 160 degrees, the researchers maintained lateral resolution of 10 mm or better over a focusing depth of at least 6 mm. The focusing spot has the intensity that is approximately constant over a greater depth range than when a conventional lens is used. Recently, using the spectral–domain OCT, Leitgeb et al., 2006 proposed a non-dual path imaging scheme for imaging of biological samples. It is known, that conical lenses are used for shaping of Bessel beam field distribution in a range of the focal length, whereas they create a ring shape in the far field. The authors used the advantage of the ring–shaped intensity distribution generated by the axicon in the far field: when this field is focused into the back focal plane of the microscope objective, the intensity distribution at the sample position after the objective is a Bessel field with an extended focal range. Leitgeb et al. demonstrated 1.5 μm resolution across a 200 μm depth of focus. Lee & Rolland, 2008 reported on the feasibility of using a custom-made micro-optic axicon to create a Bessel beam for the illumination and imaging of biological samples using the spectral-domain OCT. The effectiveness of implementing axicon micro-optics has been demonstrated by imaging a biological sample of an African frog tadpole at various positions of the axial distance. The Bessel beam images show invariant resolution and signal-to-noise ratio over at least of 4 mm focal range, while the Gaussian beam images are already out of focus at the axial distance of 1 mm.

We project to conduct the investigations on a base of the Twyman-Green interferometer. The basic configuration of such interferometer is illustrated in Fig.18.

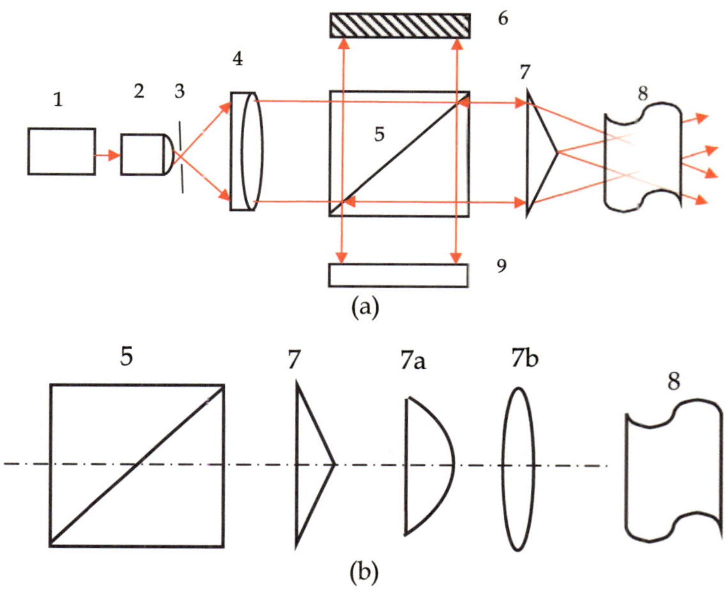

Fig. 18. The optical scheme of the Twyman-Green interferometer with the Bessel beam (a) and the sample arm of the Twyman-Green interferometer with the Bessel - like beam (b):1 - the coherent light, 2 - the microscope objective, 3 - the spatial filter, 4 - the collimator, 5 - the beam splitter, 6 - the reference mirror, 7 - the axicon, 7a - the high NA lens, 7b - the Fourier lens, 8 - the object under test, 9 - CCD. Optical elements 7-7a-7b serves for the generation of the Bessel-like light beam with the uniform axial intensity

The setup consists of a light source 1, a microscope objective 2, a spatial filter 3, a collimator 4, a beam splitter 5, a reference mirror 6, the axicon 7, an object under test 8, and CCD 9.

The light from the source is expanded and collimated by a telescopic system that usually includes the microscope objective 2 and the collimator 4. To obtain a clean wavefront, without diffraction rings on the field the optical components must be as clean as possible. For an even cleaner beam a spatial filter (pinhole) 3 may be used at the focal plane of the microscope objective. The quality of the wavefront that is produced by this telescope, does not need to be extremely high, because its deformations will appear on both interfering wavefronts and not produce any deviations of an interference pattern.

The sample arm of the interferometer involves the axicon for the Bessel beam shaping in the first case (Fig.18, a) and the system of axicon–high NA lens–Fourier lens (7–7a–7b see in Fig.18, b) for the Bessel–like beam shaping with the uniform axial intensity in the second case. The advantage of the given scheme is compactness and a high stability against vibrations.

5. Conclusion

The investigations on improving the quality of OCT-images are currently being pursued in many leading research centers. The methods for solving the problem of improving the axial and lateral resolution of OCT optical schemes and the quality of OCT-images have been resulted from the extensive studies on the optics of Bessel and conical light beams. The idea consists of the necessity to use quasi-nondiffractive Bessel beams and their superpositions as a probe radiation. Such an approach is completely justified owing to the spatial features of Bessel and conical beams, which by their nature are interference fields due to many planar waves. The wave vectors of these waves cover a conical surface causing the formation of a stable interference pattern in the area of the beam focal length. The properties which make Bessel and conical light beams promising in various biomedical sectors are: the suppressed diffraction divergence of the beam pre-axial region, the high lateral resolution in combination with a long focal length, and the reconstruction effect that enables the interaction condition of coherent radiation with an ensemble of microparticles situated in the direction of beam propagation to be significantly smoothed. However, the main drawback of quasi-nondiffractive Bessel beams is the dependence of the axial beam intensity on the axial coordinate. This degrades the energy efficiency of the probe system in various optical systems (in particular, optical tomography systems), which use quasi-nondiffractive Bessel beams.

The development of new methods for forming quasi-diffraction-free beams, including using optical elements with strong spherical aberration, will enable a long focal length of a conical beam and help to achieve the uniform axial intensity.

The theoretical analysis demonstrates the ability of evanescent Bessel beam to localize light field in a sub-wavelength space region. A narrow central maximum of evanescent Bessel beam is a nondiffractive one inside the area of its existence in comparison with the evanescent Gaussian field. In this consideration the use of the evanescent Bessel beam is a promising perspective for improvement of lateral resolution in OCT-system.

New methods of quasi-nondiffractive light beam shaping and the knowledge about the features of interaction of quasi-nondiffractive light beam with different multilayer media allow one to optimize the probing conditions by quasi-nondiffractive light beam. It can be confidently stated that the use of quasi-diffraction-free beams as the probe radiation for increasing simultaneously the lateral and the axial resolution of the OCT optical systems opened a new era for improving the optical tomography.

6. Acknowledgment

Authors would like to thank Vladimir Belyi and Nikolai Khilo (B.I. Stepanov Institute of Physics of the National Academy of Science, Minsk, Belarus) for their support of research, for many productive discussions on the subject and for valuable comments and help during the preparation of this material.

7. References

Andersen, P. E.; Thrane, L.; Yura, H. T.; Tycho, A.; Jorgensen, T. M.; Frosz, M. H. (2004). Advanced modeling of optical coherence tomography systems, *Phys. Med. Biol.*, Vol.49, No. 7, pp. 1307–1327

Arlt, J.; Garces-Chavez, V.; Sibbett, W.; Dholakia, K. (2001). Optical micromanipulation using a Bessel light beam, *Opt. Comm.*, Vol. 197, pp.239-245

Belyi, V.; Kroening, M.; Kazak, N.; Khilo, N.; Mashchenko, A.; Ropot, P. (2005). Bessel beam based optical profilometry, *Proceeding of SPIE 2005 Europe International Symposium Optical Systems Design*, Vol. 5964, pp.59640L1–59640L12, Jena, Germany, Sept. 12–16, 2005

Belyi, V.; Kazak, N.; Khilo, N.; Kramoreva L.; Mashchenko, A.; Ropot, P.; Yushkevich, V. (2006). Influence of scattering media on regular structure and speckle of quasi-nondiffractive Bessel light beams. *Proceeding of SPIE 2006 International Conference Speckle06: Speckles, From Grains to Flowers,* Vol.6341, pp. 6341O-1–6341O-6, Nimes, France, Sept. 13–15, 2006

Berry, M. V.& Jeffray, M.R. (2006). Chiral conical diffraction, *J. Opt. A: Pure Appl. Opt.*, Vol.8, pp.363–372

Burval, A. (2004). Axicon imaging by scalar diffraction theory, In: Stockholm. [Electronic resource], 27.07.2009, Available from http:// kth. diva-portal. org/ smash / record. jsf?pid-diva 2:9578

Chauhan, B. C.; McCormick, T. A.; Nicolela, M. T.; LeBlanc, R. P. (2001). Comparison of scanning laser tomography with conventional perimetry and optic disc photography, *Arch. Ophthalmol.*, Vol. 119, pp.1492–1499

Ding, Z. H.; Ren, H. W.; Zhao, Y. H.; Nelson, J. S.; Chen, Z. P. (2002). High-resolution optical coherence tomography over a large depth range with an axicon lens, *Opt. Letters*, Vol. 24, No. 4, pp.243–245

Dresel, T.; Schwider, J.; Wehrhahn, A.; Babin, S. (1995). Grazing-incidence interferometry applied to the measurement of cylindrical surfaces, *Opt. Eng.*, Vol. 34, pp.3531–3535

Fadeyeva, T. A. & Volyar, A. V. (2010). Nondiffracting vortex-beams in a birefringent chiral crystal, *J. Opt. Soc. Am. A*, Vol. 27, Issue 1, pp. 13–20

Fercher, A. F.; Drexler, W; Hitzenberger, C. K.; Lasser, T. (2003). Optical coherence tomography-principles and applications, *Rep. Prog. Phys.*, Vol. 66, pp. 230–303

Garces-Chavez, V.; McGloin, D.; Melville, H.; Sibbett W.; Dholakia, K. (2002). Simultaneous micromanipulation in multiple planes using a self self-reconstructing light beam, *Nature*, Vol. 419, pp.145–147.

Goncharenko, A. M.; Khilo, N. A.; Petrova, E. S. (2001). Evanescent Bessel light beams, *Proceeding of SPIE 2001 SPIE International Conference Lightmetry: Metrology, Spectroscopy, and Testing Techniques Using Light,* Vol. 4517, pp. 95 - 99, Pultysk, Poland, June 5–8, 2001

Grosjean, T.; Courjon, D; Labeke, D. Van. (2003). Bessel beam as virtual tips for near-field optics, *J. Microscopy*, Vol. 210, pp. 319–323

Jaroszewicz, Z. & Morales, J. (1998). Lens axicon: system composed of a diverging aberrated lens ad a perfect converging lens, *J. Opt. Soc. Am. A.*, Vol. 15, No. 9, pp.2383–2390

Kazak, N.; Khilo, N.; Ryzhevich, A. (1999). Generation of Bessel beam under the conditions of internal conical refraction, *Quantum Electronics*, Vol. 29, pp. 1020–1024

Khilo, N. A.; Kramoreva, L. I.; Petrova, E. S. (2005). Reflection and absorption of conical and Bessel light beams by cylindrical objects, *Journal of Applied Spectroscopy*, Vol. 72, No. 5, pp. 663–669

Kramoreva, L. I. & Rozhko, Yu. I. (2010). Optical Coherence Tomography (Review), *Journal of Applied Spectroscopy*, Vol.77, No. 4, pp. 485–506

Kramoreva, L. I. & Rozhko Yu. I. (2010). Visualization of eye structure under the condition of tissue scattering in optical coherence tomography, *Contributed papers 2010 of International Conference Optical Techniques and Nano–Tools for Material and Life Science*, Vol. 2, pp.204–209, ISBN 978–985–6950–31–5, Minsk, Belarus, June 15–19, 2010

Kurilkina, S. N.; Belyi, V. N.; Kazak, N. S.; Al–Saud, Turki S. M.; Al–Khowaiter, Soliman H.; Al–Muhanna, Muhanna. (2010). Application of Evanescent Bessel beams superposition for testing quality of surfaces and thin dielectric layers, *Contributed papers 2010 of International Conference Optical Techniques and Nano–Tools for Material and Life Science*, Vol. 1, pp.38–48, ISBN 978–985–6950–31–5, Minsk, Belarus, June 15–19, 2010

Lee, Kye–Sung & Rolland, J. P. (2008). Bessel beam spectral–domain high–resolution optical coherence tomography with micro–optic axicon providing extended focusing range, *Opt. Letters*, Vol. 33, No. 15, pp.1696–1698

Leitgeh, R. A.; Villiger, M.; Bachmann, A. H.; Steinmann, L.; Lasser, T. (2006) Extended focus depth for Fourier domain optical coherence microscopy, *Opt. Letters*, Vol.31, No. 16, pp.2450–2452

McGloin, D. & Dholakia, K. (2005). Bessel beams: diffraction in a new light, *Contemp. Phys.*, Vol. 46, pp.15-28

Petrova, E. S. (2001). Bessel light beams in gyrotropic medium, *Proceeding of SPIE 2001 International Conference Optics of Crystals,* Vol.4358, pp. 265–271, Mozyr, Belarus, Sept. 26–30, 2006

Petrova E. S. & Kramoreva, L. I. (2010). Features of tissue probing by conic light beams, *Contributed papers 2010 of International Conference Optical Techniques and Nano–Tools for Material and Life Science*, Vol. 2, pp.160–165, ISBN 978–985–6950–31–5, Minsk, Belarus, June 15–19, 2010

Rushin, S. & Leiser, A. (1999). Evanescent Bessel Beam, *J. Opt. Soc. Am. A.*, Vol.15, pp. 1139–1143

Schmitt, J. M. & Knuttel, A. (1993). Measurement of optical-properties of biological tissues by low-coherence reflectometry, *Appl. Opt.*, Vol.32, pp.6032–6042

Turchin, I. V.; Sergeeva, E. A.; Dolin, L. S.; Kamensky, V. A. (2003). Estimation of biotissue scattering properties from OCT images using a small-angle approximation of transport theory, *Laser Phys.*, Vol.13, pp.1524–1529

Zamboni-Rached, M. (2006). Diffraction-Attenuation resistant beams in absorbing media, *Opt. Express*, Vol.14, pp.1804–1809

Zamboni-Rached, M.; Ambrosio, L. A.; Hernandez-Figueroa, H.E. (7Jul 2010). Diffraction-Attenuation Resistant Beams: their Higher Order Versions and Finite-Aperture Generations, In: Arxiv. org., 07.04.2011, Available from http: // arxiv.org/abs/1007.1046v1 [physics.optics]

Zhan, Q. (2006). Evanescent Bessel beam generation via surface plasmon resonance excitation by a radially polarized beam, *Opt. Letters*, Vol.31, pp.1725-1728

Part 2

OCT Applications

6

Neoatherosclerosis Within the Implanted Stent

Hironori Kitabata and Takashi Akasaka
Wakayama Medical University
Japan

1. Introduction

Although it is generally recognized that the long-term clinical outcome of bare-metal stents (BMS) is favorable, a late luminal narrowing with restenosis of BMS can occur during the extended follow-up (beyond 5 years), resulting in clinical events such as stent thrombosis and myocardial infarction. Regarding the mechanisms of progressive late luminal renarrowing, a persistent and remarkable foreign body inflammatory reaction to the metal may promote new atherosclerotic changes and consequent plaque vulnerability of the neointimal tissue around the stent struts. However, neointimal atherosclerotic change (neoatherosclerosis) after BMS implantation is rarely reported. Although drug-eluting stents (DES) have dramatically reduced restenosis and target lesion revascularization compared with BMS, long-term safety remains a clinical major concern due to persistent increase in the incidence of very late stent thrombosis (VLST). While stent thrombosis is a multifactorial process, it has shown that tissue coverage over stent struts is an important determinant of late stent thrombosis. Furthermore, the development of neoatherosclerosis inside the DES may be another rare mechanism of late thrombotic events. Neoatherosclerosis in DES (two years after implantation) can occur earlier than in BMS. Because of high resolution up to 10 μm, it has been described that optical coherence tomography (OCT) has the potential to identify the features of unstable plaques such as thin fibrous cap, large lipid core, thrombus, macrophage infiltration, and neovascularization. Furthermore, even in the evaluation of stent, OCT has been reported to be able to demonstrate the stented lesion morphology in detail including tissue protrusion, thrombus formation, incomplete apposition, late acquired malaposition, edge dissection, tissue coverage over struts, and so on. This chapter describes about the assessment of neoatherosclerosis within BMS and DES by OCT.

2. Late vascular healing response to bare-metal stent

Coronary stenting is an effective strategy to prevent restenosis in atherosclerotic lesions as compared to balloon angioplasty. Bare-metal stent (BMS) is widely used in the interventional cardiology. It has been reported that in-stent restenosis (ISR) after BMS implantation, especially late ISR, is not always benign and late ISR is closely associated with mortality. Furthermore, progressive increases in the incidence of late target lesion revascularization (TLR) is observed beyond 4 years and up to 15 to 20 years after BMS implantation. A serial angiographic follow-up study of BMS has demonstrated several phases, with early restenosis phase until the first 6 months, stabilization and regression phase from 6 months to 3 years, and late luminal renarrowing phase beyond 4 years. With regard to the mechanisms of progressive late luminal renarrowing, Inoue et al. reported the pathological findings within the BMS. Three years after BMS implantation, apparent chronic inflammatory cell infiltration (mainly T lymphocytes) and neovascularization are recognizable around the stent struts, and beyond 4 years, heavy infiltration of foamy cells (lipid-laden macrophages) is observed. The authors concluded that stainless steel stents evoke a remarkable foreign body inflammatory reaction to the metal and persistent peri-strut chronic inflammatory cells may accelerate new atherosclerotic changes and consequent plaque vulnerability of the neointimal tissue around the stent struts. Although the precise incidence of new atherosclerosis during an extended follow-up after BMS implantation is unknown, several papers report the features in neointima (Table 1).

Yokoyama et al serially evaluated the detailed changes inside the BMS by using angioscopy. Between the first follow-up (6 to 12 months) and the second follow up (≥ 4 years), the frequencies of lipid-laden yellow plaque and thrombus increased from 12% (3 of 26 patients) to 58% (15 of 26 patients) and from 4% to 31%, respectively. BMS segments with yellow plaque were significantly associated with late luminal narrowing.

OCT (LightLab Imaging, Westford, MA, USA) is an intracoronary imaging modality with a high-resolution of 10 to 20 μm, providing detailed information about microstructures such as thin fibrous cap as well as the histology. Furthermore, OCT has the greatest advantage in its accuracy of tissue characterization compared with other coronary imaging modalities. Recently, using OCT, Takano et al observed the differences in neointima between early phase (< 6 months) and late phase (≥ 5 years). When compared with normal neointima (Fig. 1) proliferated homogeneously in the early phase, neointima within the BMS ≥ 5 years after implantation was characterized by marked signal attenuation and a diffuse border, suggesting lipid-laden intima (Fig. 2). Its frequency was 67% and lipid-laden intima was not observed in the early phase. Thin-cap fibroatheroma (TCFA)-like intima (Fig. 3) was observed in 29% of the patients in the late phase. Intimal disruption (Fig. 4) and thrombus (Fig. 5) were found frequently in the late phase as compared with the early phase (38% vs. 0% and 52% vs. 5%, respectively; $p < 0.05$). However, there was no significant difference in terms of calcification (Fig. 6) between the 2 phases (10% vs. 0%). Although there was no significant difference with respect to the incidence of peristent neovascularization (Fig. 7A) between the 2 phases (81% vs. 60%, $p = 0.14$), intraintima neovascularization (Fig. 7B) was observed more frequently in the late phase than in the early phase (62% vs. 0%, $p < 0.01$) and in segments with lipid-laden intima than those in without lipid-laden intima (79% vs. 29%, $p = 0.026$). Furthermore, lipid-laden intima was more frequent in "symptomatic" patients than in asymptomatic patients. The frequencies of late ISR (62% vs. 0%, $p < 0.001$) and late TLR (62% vs. 0%, $p < 0.001$) were higher in patients with lipid-laden intima as compared with those without lipid-laden intima. Four patients with acute coronary syndrome in the late phase had both intimal disruption and thrombus. The authors speculated that neovascularization expanding from the peristent area into the intima with time might play a key role in atherosclerosis progression and the instability of neointimal tissue, as well as plaque neovascularization of nonstent segments in native coronary arteries. Hou et al also performed angiographic and OCT examinations in 39 patients with recurrent ischemia among 1636 patients who underwent BMS implantation. The average time interval between initial BMS implantation and OCT imaging was 6.5±1.3 years. Of 60 stents in 39 patients, 20 stents (33.3%) in 16 patients had OCT-derived lipid-rich plaques inside the stents. In 13 of these 20 stents, angiographic ISR was observed, and 7 restenotic lesions with lipid-rich

Studies	Stent	Imaging device	Implant duration (month)	Lipidic tissue	TCFA	Intimal disruption	Neovascularization		Thrombus
							peri-stent	intra-intima	
Yokoyama et al. (2009)	BMS (26 lesions)	Angioscopy	94.7±34.2	58%	N.A.	*31%	N.A.	N.A.	31%
Takano et al. (2010)	BMS (21 lesions)	OCT	91.5±25.9	67%	29%	38%	81%	62%	52%
Hou et al. (2010)	BMS (60 stents)	OCT	78±15.6	33.3%	N.A.	30%	N.A.	N.A.	5%
Nakazawa et al. (2011)	BMS (197 lesions) DES (209 lesions)	Pathology	BMS 72 (60 to 96) DES 14 (12 to 22.8)	†BMS 16% DES 31%	BMS 4% DES 1% (TCFA/plaque rupture)	-	N.A.	N.A.	N.A.
Kang et al. (2011)	DES (50 ISR lesions)	OCT	32.2 (9.2 to 52.2)	90%	52%	58%	60% (peristent and intraintima)	-	58%
Habara et al. (2011)	BMS (43 ISR lesions)	OCT	113.8±29.6	**90.7% (heterogeneous intima)	N.A.	**13.9%	**25.6%	**16.3%	**16.2%

Table 1. Neoatherosclerosis inside the implanted stent. BMS, bare-metal stent; DES, drug-eluting stent; ISR, in-stent restenosis; N.A., not applicable; OCT, optical coherence tomography; TCFA, thin-cap fibroatheroma; * Surface irregularity; ** Minimum lumen area site; †Any neoatherosclerosis.

plaque manifested clinical presentations of unstable angina. Six lipid-rich plaques had evidence of intimal disruption. However, thrombus was found in only one stent (5%). Notably, 7 (35%) of 20 lipid-rich plaques had features consistent with macrophage infiltration (Fig. 8). More recently, Habara et al evaluated the difference of tissue characteristics between early (within the first year) and very late (> 5 years, without restenosis within the first years) restenostic lesions after BMS implantation by OCT. The mean follow-up period of early and very late ISR was 8.7±4.1 months and 113.8±29.6 months, respectively. The morphological characteristics of restenostic tissue (characterized by heterogeneous intima) in very late ISR

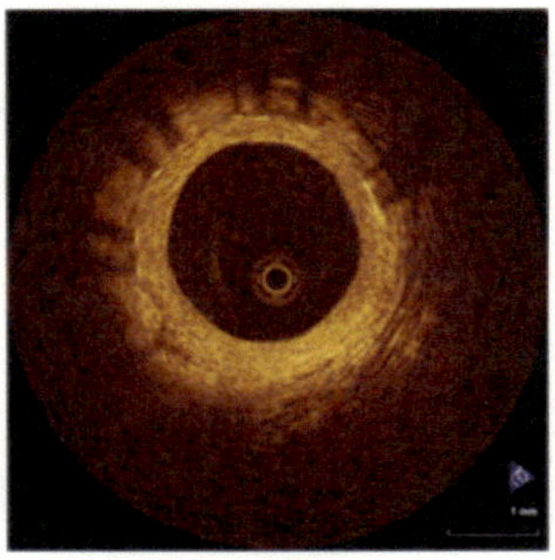

Fig. 1. Normal neointima inside the stent. OCT image of normal neointima showing a homogenous signal-rich band without signal attenuation.

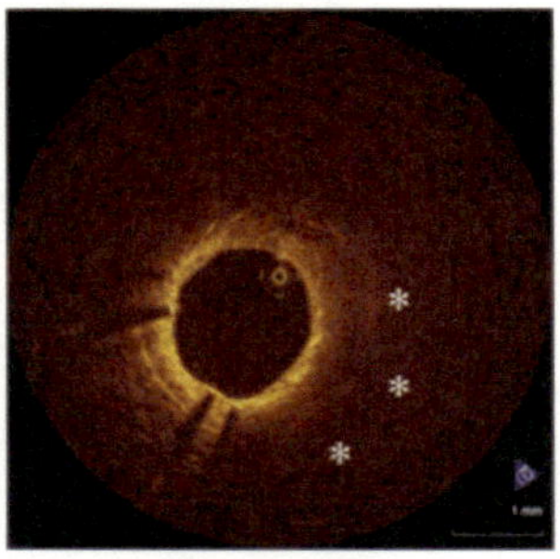

Fig. 2. Lipid-laden neointima inside the stent. OCT image of a neointima with lipid component showing a signal-poor region with poorly delineated border (*). In this area, the stent struts are invisible.

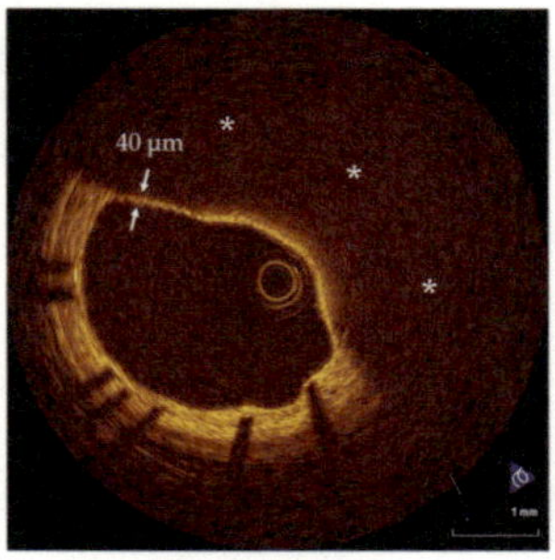

Fig. 3. Thin-cap fibroatheroma-like neointima inside the stent. Thin-cap fibroatheroma-like intima is defined as a lipidic tissue (*) with a thin fibrous cap measuring < 65 μm.

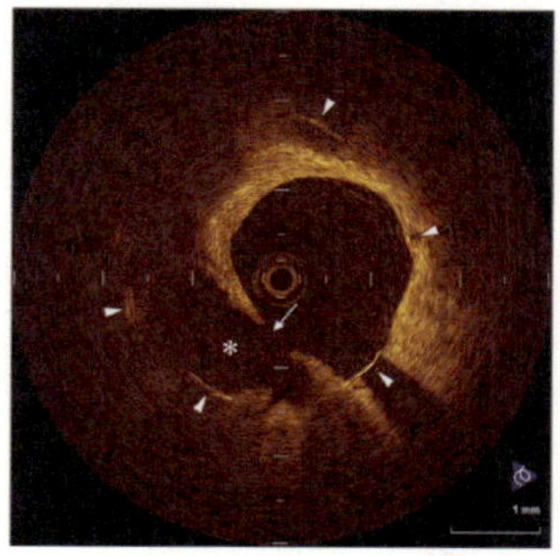

Fig. 4. Neointimal rupture inside the stent. OCT image of a neointimal rupture showing the disruption of fibrous cap (arrow) and cavity formation (*) within well expanded struts (arrowheads).

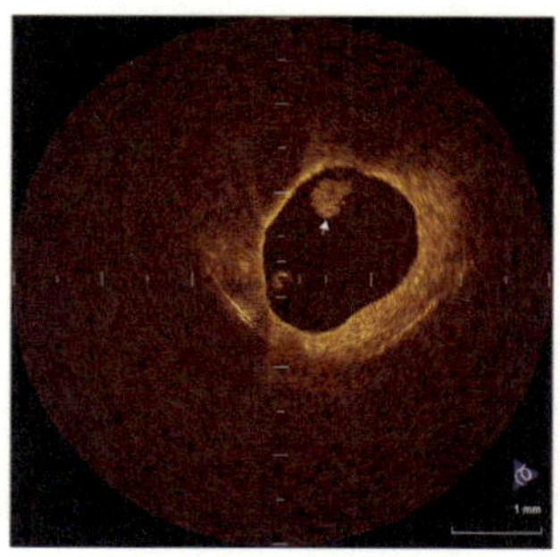

Fig. 5. Intracoronary thrombus inside the stent. OCT image of an intracoronary thrombus (arrow) showing a mass protruding into the vessel lumen.

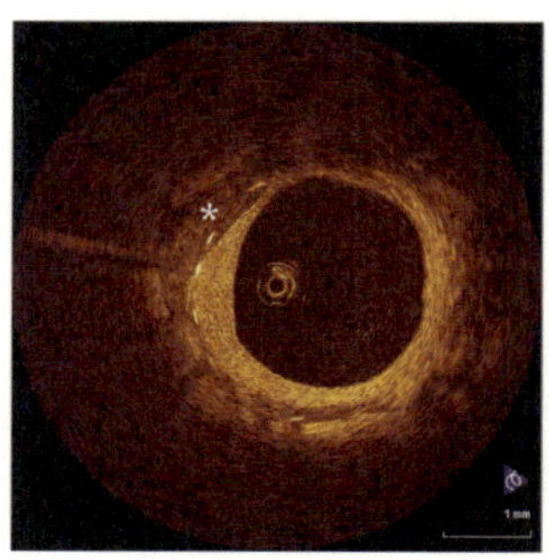

Fig. 6. Calcification inside the stent. OCT image of a calcification (*) showing a signal-poor region with sharply delineated border.

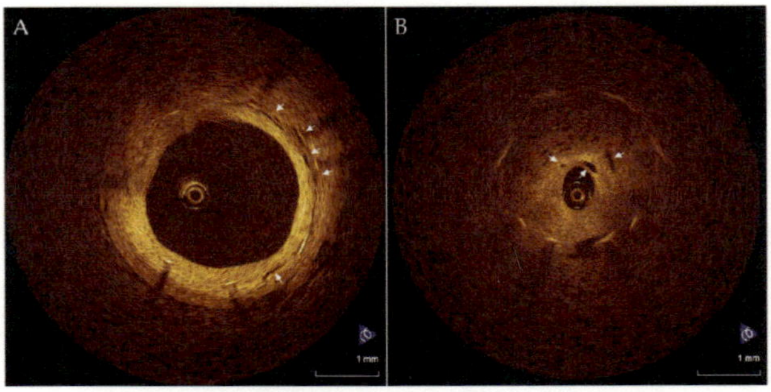

Fig. 7. Neovascularization inside the stent. (A) OCT image of peristent micro-vessels (arrows) showing a cluster of no-signal small vesicular and tubular structures locating around the struts. (B) OCT image of intraintima micro-vessels (arrows) showing small black holes locating near the vessel lumen within the neotintimal tissue.

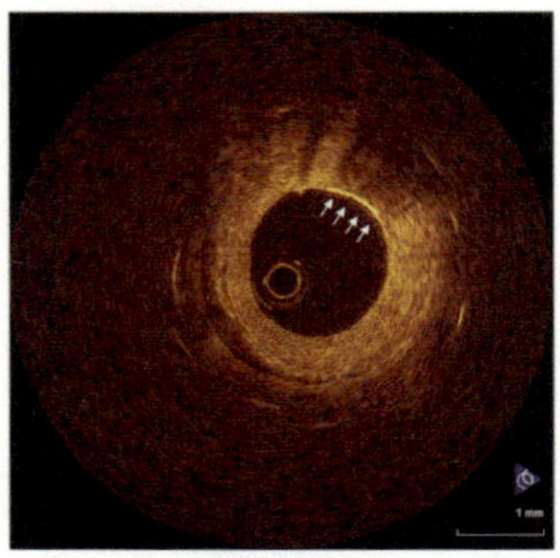

Fig. 8. Macrophage infiltration in neointima inside the stent. OCT image of macrophage infiltration showing a linear high-brightness region with shadowing behind (arrows).

were different from those (characterized by homogeneous intima) in early ISR and consistent with atherosclerotic plaque. In the very late ISR group, 31 (72.1%) of 43 patients underwent TLR. Notably, 17 patients (39.5%) had been asymptomatic until the follow-up angiography. These previous studies suggest that new atherosclerotic plaque formation in neointima may occur during an extended follow-up period after BMS implantation and contribute to clinical coronary events such as very late stent thrombosis. Even when the patients remain clinically stable and asymptomatic until their late follow-up presentations, unstable features such as TCFA and rupture may develop within the implanted BMS (Fig. 9). Therefore, a long-term optimal medical therapy including statins and a good control of coronary risk factors for secondary prevention will be needed to prevent such complications in patients who have previously undergone BMS implantation.

3. Vascular healing response to drug-eluting stent

Although drug-eluting stents (DES) have dramatically reduced restenosis and target lesion revascularization compared with BMS, long-term safety remains a clinical major concern because of persistent increase in the incidence of very late stent thrombosis (VLST). VLST in DES, after the first year, was reported at rates of 0.2-0.6% per year up to 3 years and the recommendations for dual antiplatelet therapy consisting of aspirin and thienopyridines

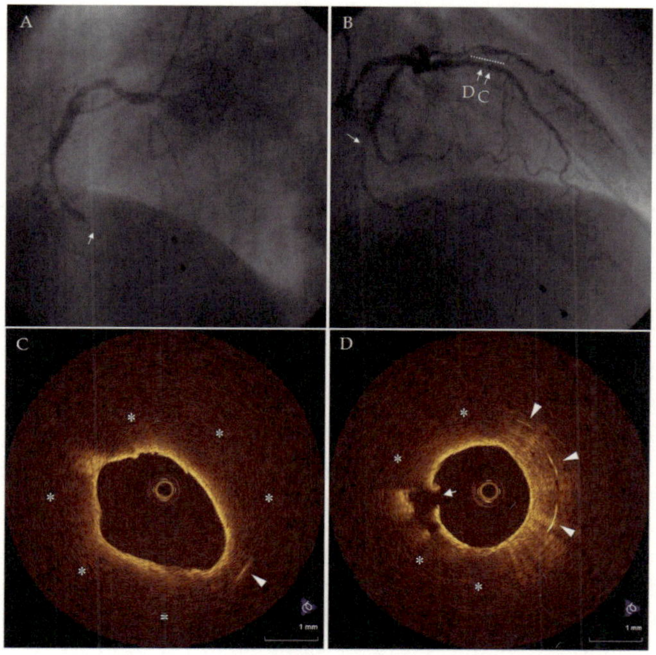

Fig. 9. A case with thin-cap fibroatheroma-like intima and neointimal rupture inside the bare-metal stent. A 57-year-old man was given a diagnosis of anterior ST-segment elevation myocardial infarction and treated with a 4.0X18 mm bare-metal stent (BMS) implanted to the proximal-portion of the left anterior descending artery (LAD) 6 years ago. A scheduled follow-up coronary angiography at 6 months after the index procedure demonstrated no restenosis. Six years after stent implantation, he suddenly presented with chest pain at rest and was admitted to the hospital. An emergent coronary angiography showed total occlusion of the right coronary artery (A, arrow), severe stenosis in the mid-portion of the left circumflex artery (B, arrow), and no in-stent restenosis of the previously implanted BMS of the LAD (B, dotted line). After successful reperfusion therapy of the RCA, optical coherence tomography (OCT) was performed in the LAD. OCT revealed thin-cap fibroatheroma-like intima (C) and neointimal rupture (D) inside the previous BMS. Many stent struts are invisible due to marked signal attenuation, representing lipid component (*). In this patient, medical control for secondary prevention was insufficient (low-density lipoprotein cholesterol level was 174mg/dL and hemoglobin A1c was 11.8%). Arrowheads indicate stent struts.

were extended to ≥ 12 months after DES implantation without a clear evidence wether this extension would reduce the rates of VLST. Although stent thrombosis is a multifactorial, Finn et al has reported that inadequate stent coverage (the ratio of uncovered struts to total struts) is a powerful histological predictor of late stent thrombosis. OCT can reliably distinguish thin neointimal hyperplasia (< 100 μm) on stent struts and uncovered struts, which is undetectable by intravascular ultrasound (IVUS). It has also been reported that OCT imaging can accurately assess the extent and thickness of neointimal coverage on stent struts after stent implantation with good histological correlation. Xie et al. performed OCT imaging at 3 months after sirolimus-eluting stent (SES) implantation. In this study, the frequencies of uncovered struts and struts with neointimal coverage < 100 μm were 15 % and 94 %, respectively. Matsumoto et al. also investigated 34 patients with SES who underwent OCT examination at 6 months after implantation. Eleven % of struts still remained uncovered. Only 9 SESs (16%) demonstrated full coverage by neointima, whereas the remaining stents had partially uncovered struts. Yao et al, by using OCT, evaluated the time course of neointimal coverage in SES after implantation. Between 6 months and 12 months, the frequency of uncovered struts decreased from 9.2% to 6.6%. Katoh et al also reported a comparison of OCT findings in identical SES at 6 months and 12 months. As a result, the frequency of struts without neointimal coverage (10.4% to 5.7%) was similar to the results of Yao's study. Furthermore, Takano et al. serially performed OCT imaging at 2 and 4 years after implantation in 17 patients treated with 21 SESs. The frequency of patients with uncovered struts significantly decreased from 88% to 29% ($p = 0.002$). The presence of mural thrombus might be one of risk factors for stent thrombosis. Otake et al reported that mural thrombus was detected in 14 (26%) of 53 lesions by OCT at 6 months after SES implantation. Subclinical thrombus was associated with larger number of uncovered struts, uneven neointimal thickness, greater asymmetric stent expansion, and longer SES. However, in this small study, the presence of mural thrombus did not lead to clinical stent thrombosis during follow-up period (median 485 days). Kim et al also reported a large-scale OCT registry data of 226 patients with various DESs. The frequencies of intracoronary thrombus were 28% in SES, 11% in paclitaxel-eluting stent (PES), and 1% in zotarolimus-eluting stent (ZES), respectively. Although the presence of intracoronary thrombus was associated with longer stent length (≥ 28mm), smaller stent diameter (< 3.0 mm), and more uncovered struts (≥ 8 uncovered struts in each stent), major adverse cardiac events including stent thrombosis were not found in patients with intracornary thrombus during follow-up period (mean 8 months). These studies demonstrate that there is a relationship between uncovered stent struts and thrombus formation. However, to obtain clear conclusion about clinical implications of subclinical thrombus detected by OCT, further studies with long-term clinical follow-up and larger population are warranted.

Late-acquired incomplete stent apposition (ISA) may also be one of main mechanisms of VLST of DES. One IVUS observational study demonstrated its possible association with VLST after DES implantation. The mechanism of late-acquired ISA is widely accepted to typically be the result of either positive arterial remodeling and/or thrombus dissolution behind the stent struts (especially in myocardial infarction). Although the clinical association of late-acquired ISA and stent thrombosis remains controversial and is under intense investigation, Ozaki *et al.* assessed the fate of ISA post-SES implantation by using OCT. The frequency of incompletely apposed struts post-intervention was 7.2% (309 struts). Of 309 struts, 202 (65%) struts remained persistent ISA without neointimal coverage even at 10-month follow-up. Mural thrombus was observed more frequently in struts with ISA (20.6%) compared with struts with a good apposition (only 2.0%). Thus, it has been suggested that the underlying mechanism of VLST may be different between BMS and DES. However, chronic inflammatory can occur in DES as well as BMS and may be more pronounced with DES due to the presence of the polymer carrying therapeutic drug. This high degree of inflammation can develop neoatherosclerosis with shorter implant duration in DES than in BMS. More recently, it has been reported that the development of neoatherosclerosis may be an additional contributing factor to very late thrombotic events in DES. Kang et al demonstrated the results of OCT analysis of in-stent neoatherosclerosis in 50 patients with ISR after DES implantation. The median follow-up period was 32.2 months (9.2 to 52.2). Twenty (40%) of 50 patients presented with unstable angina and the remaining 30 (60%) patients with stable angina. Despite clinical presentations of unstable or stable angina, 90% of the lesions had lipid-laden neointima. Fifty-two % of the lesions had at least 1 TCFA-like neointima and 58% had at least 1 neointimal rupture. Compared with DES < 20 months after implantation, DES ≥ 20 months after implantation had a greater incidence of TCFA-like neointima (69% vs. 33%, $p = 0.012$) and red thrombi (27% vs. 0%, $P = 0.007$). Notably, there was a negative correlation between the thickness of the fibrous cap and follow-up period ($r = -0.318$, $p = 0.024$). Furthermore, unstable patients showed a thinner fibrous cap (55 μm vs. 100 μm, $p = 0.006$) and higher incidence of TCFA-like intima (75% vs. 37%, $p = 0.008$), intimal disruption (75% vs. 47%, $p = 0.044$), and thrombi (80% vs. 43%, $p = 0.01$) than stable patients. The authors concluded that in-stent neoatherosclerosis may be an important mechanism of DES failure, especially late after implantation. However, the majority (70%) of DES evaluated in this study were first-generation DES (SES and PES). Nakazawa et al reported on pathological change in a registry series of 299 autopsies with 406 coronary stented lesions, including 197 BMS and 209 DES. Neoatherosclerosis was defined as clusters of peristrut lipid-laden foamy macrophages within the neointima with or without necrotic core formation. The overall incidence of neoatherosclerosis was significantly higher in DES (31%) than in BMS (16%) lesions ($p < 0.001$). Neoatherosclerosis was found to be more frequent in DES than in BMS and to occur earlier in DES than in BMS. In addition, multiple logistic regression analysis revealed younger age, longer implant durations, DES usage, and underlying unstable plaques as independent predictors of neoatherosclerosis. However, all DES included in this pathological study were also SES (49%) and PES (51%). Because the vascular healing response after implantation may be influenced by the types of DES (different stent material, strut thickness, design, and polymer), long-term follow-up OCT studies with a large number of second-generation DES (ZES and everolimus-eluting stent) are needed to understand the differences in neointimal atherosclerotic change between the DES types.

4. Limitation

OCT abnormal findings inside the BMS and DES observed in these studies above may be similar to the features of vulnerable plaque in a native coronary artery. However, a direct comparison of OCT findings with histology is not done. In fact, there is a discrepancy in the frequency of neoatherosclerosis between OCT findings and pathological findings (Table 1). Therefore, histological data that properly validate OCT findings within the stents are required in the near future.

5. Conclusion

Neointima within the stent in both BMS and DES can transform into atherosclerotic tissue with time although it occurs earlier in DES than BMS. Neoathrosclerosis progression inside the implanted stents may be associated with very late coronary events such as VLST after BMS and DES implantation.

6. Acknowledgment

The authors thank Kenichi Komukai, MD; Takashi Kubo, MD; Yasushi Ino, MD; Takashi Tanimoto, MD; Kohei Ishibashi, MD; Kunihiro Shimamura, MD; Makoto Orii, MD; Yasutsugu Shiono, MD for assitance with OCT imgae acquisition and analysis.

7. References

Chen, MS.; John, JM. & Chew DP. (2006). Bare metal stent restenosis is not a benign clinical entity. *Am Heart J*, Vol. 151, No. 6, (June), pp. 1260-1264.

Cook, S.; Wenaweser, P. & Togni, M. (2007). Incomplete stent apposition and very late stent thrombosis after drug-eluting stent implantation. *Circulation*, Vol. 115, No. 18, (May), pp. 2426–2434.

Doyle, B.; Rihal, CS. & O'Sullivan, CJ. (2007). Outcomes of stent thrombosis and restenosis during extended follow-up of patients treated with bare metal coronary stents. *Circulation* Vol. 116, No. 21, (November), pp. 2391-2398.

Doyle, B. & Caplice, N. (2007). Plaque neovascularization and antiangiogenic therapy for atherosclerosis. *J Am Coll Cardiol,* Vol. 49, No. 21, (May), pp. 2073-2080.

Finn, AV.; Joner, M. & Nakazawa, G. (2007). Pathological correlates of late drug-eluting stent thrombosis: strut coverage as a marker of endothelialization. *Circulation,* Vol. 115, No. 18, (May), pp. 2435-2441.

Habara, M.; Terashima, M. & Nasu, K. (2011). Difference of tissue characteristics between early and very late restenosis lesions after bare-metal stent implantation: an optical coherence tomography study. *Circ Cardiovasc Interv,* (Jun), Vol. 4, No. 3, pp. 232-238.

Hasegawa, K.; Tamai, H. & Kyo, E. (2006). Histopathological findings of new instent lesions developed beyond five years. *Catheter Cardiovasc Interv,* Vol. 68, No. 4, (October), pp. 554-558.

Hou, J.; Qi, H. & Zhang, M. (2010). Development of lipid-rich plaque inside bare metal stent: possible mechanism of late stent thrombosis? An optical coherence tomography study. *Heart,* (August), Vol. 96, No. 15, pp. 1187-1190.

Inoue, K.; Abe, K. & Ando K. (2004). Pathological analyses of long-term intracoronary Palmaz-Schatz stenting; Is its efficacy permanent? *Cardiovasc Pathol,* Vol. 13, No. 2, (March-April), pp. 109-115.

Jang, IK.; Tearney, GJ. & MacNeill, B. (2005). In vivo characterization of coronary atherosclerotic plaque by use of optical coherence tomography. *Circulation,* Vol. 111, No. 12, (March), pp. 1551-1555.

Kang, SJ.; Mintz, GS. & Akasaka, T. (2011). Optical coherence tomographic analysis of in-stent neoatherosclerosis after drug-eluting stent implantation. *Circulation,* Vol. 123, No. 25, (Jun), pp. 2954-2963.

Kashiwagi, M.; Kitabata, H. & Tanaka, A. (2010). Very late cardiac event after BMS implantation: In vivo optical coherence tomography examination. *J Am Coll Cardiol Img,* Vol. 3, No. 5, (May) pp. 525-527.

Katoh, H.; Shite, J. & Shinke, T. (2009). Delayed neointimalization on sirolimus-eluting stents: 6-months. and 12-month follow up by optical coherence tomography. *Circ J,* Vol. 73, No. 6, (Jun), pp. 1033-1037.

Kimura, T.; Abe, K. & Shizuta, S. (2002). Long-term clinical and angiographic follow-up after coronary stent placement in native coronary arteries. *Circulation*, Vol. 105, No. 25, (Jun), pp. 2986 -2991.

Kitabata, H.; Tanaka, A. & Kubo, T. (2010). Relation of microchannel structure identified by optical coherence tomography to plaque vulnerability in patients with coronary artery disease. *Am J Cardiol*, Vol. 105, No. 12, (Jun), pp. 1673-1678.

Kubo, T.; Imanishi, T. & Takarada, S. (2007). Assessment of culprit lesion morphology in acute myocardial infarction: ability of optical coherence tomography compared with intravascular ultrasound and coronary angioscopy. J Am Coll Cardiol Vol. 50, No. 10, (September), pp. 933-939.

Kume, T.; Akasaka, T. & Kawamoto, T. (2006). Assessment of coronary arterial plaque by optical coherence tomography. *Am J Cardiol*, Vol. 97, No. 8, (April), pp. 1172-1175.

Kume, T.; Akasaka, T. & Kawamoto, T. (2006). Assessment of coronary arterial thrombus by optical coherence tomography. *Am J Cardiol*, Vol. 97, No. 12, (Jun), pp. 1713-1717.

Kume, T.; Akasaka, T. & Kawamoto, T. Measurement of the thickness of the fibrous cap by optical coherence tomography. *Am Heart J*, Vol. 152, No. 4, (October), pp. 755e1-4.

Lemesle, G.; Pinto Slottow, TL. & Wakasman, R. (2009). Very late stent thrombosis after bare-metal stent implantation: case reports and review of the literature. J Invasive Cardiol, Vol. 21, No. 2, (February), pp. e27-32.

Lee, CW.; Kang, SJ. & Park, DW. (2010). Intravascular ultrasound findings in patients with very late stent thrombosis after either drug-eluting or bare-metal stent implantation. *J Am Coll Cardiol*, Vol. 55, No. 18, (May), pp. 1936-1942.

Nakazawa, G.; Otuska, F. & Nakano, M. (2011). The pathology of neoatheroscrelosis in human coronary implants: bare-metal and drug-eluting stents. *J Am Coll Cardiol*, Vol. 57, No. 11, (March), pp. 1314-1322.

Ozaki, Y.; Okumura, M. & Ismail, TF. (2010). The fate of incomplete stent apposition with drug-eluting stents: an optical coherence tomography-based natural history study. *Eur Heart J*, Vol. 3, No. 12, (Jun), pp. 1470-1476.

Takano, M.; Yamamoto, M. & Inami, S. (2008). Long-term follow-up evaluation after sirolimuseluting stent implantation by optical coherence tomography: do uncovered struts persist? *J Am Coll Cardiol*, Vol. 51, No. 9, (March), pp. 968-969.

Takano, M.; Yamamoto, M. & Inami, S. (2010). Appearance of lipid-laden intima and neovascularization after implantation of bare-metal stents. *J Am Coll Cardiol*, Vol. 55, No. 1, (January), pp. 26-32.

Waksman, R. (2007). Late stent thrombosis--the "vulnerable" stent. *Catheter Cardiovasc Interv*, (July), Vol. 70, No. 1, pp. 54-56.

Xie, Y.; Takano, M. & Murakami, D. (2008). Comparison of neointimal coverage by optical coherence tomography of a sirolimus-eluting stent versus a bare-metal stent three months after implantation. *Am J Cardiol*, Vol. 102, No. 1, (July), pp. 27-31.

Yokoyama, S.; Takano, M. & Yamamoto, M. (2009). Extended follow-up by serial angioscopic observation for bare-metal stents in native coronary arteries: from healing response to atherosclerotic transformation of neointmal. *Circ Cardiovasc Intervent*, Vol. 2, No. 3, (Jun), pp. 205-212.

Yamaji, K.; Kimura, T. & Morimoto, T. (2010). Very long-term (15 to 20 years) clinical and angiographic outcome after coronary bare metal stent implantation. *Circ Cardiovasc Interv*, Vol. 3, No. 5, (October), pp. 468-475.

Yabushita, H.; Bouma, BE. & Houser, SL. (2002). Characterization of human atherosclerosis by optical coherence tomography. *Circulation*, Vol. 106, No. 13, (September), pp. 1640 -1645.

Yao, ZH.; Matsubara, T. & Inada, T. (2008). Neointimal coverage of sirolimus-eluting stents 6 months and 12 months after implantation: evaluation by optical coherence tomography. *Chin Med* J, Vol. 121, No. 6, (March), pp. 503-507.

7

Cellular Level Imaging of the Retina Using Optical Coherence Tomography

Cherry Greiner and Stacey S. Choi
New England College of Optometry
USA

1. Introduction

Low-coherence interferometry was first demonstrated, in the early 1990s, in imaging the eye due its tissue transparency and minimal attenuation of the input light. For this reason, ophthalmic imaging is the most successful application of optical coherence tomography (OCT). Since its first demonstration, advancements in technology and OCT designs have resulted in higher resolution images of the retinal layers including retinal photoreceptors, retinal pigment epithelium (RPE), and retinal nerve fiber layer (RNFL) thus improving the potential for early diagnosis, the understanding of disease pathology, as well as the assessment of therapeutic response. This chapter will mainly discuss improvements in OCT systems over time, particularly developments towards cellular level imaging and their clinical applications in ophthalmology in the present and in the future.

The success of OCT is in part due to its ability to obtain high structural information at reasonable depths, bridging the capabilities of confocal and ultrasound imaging. OCT is analogous to ultrasound pulse echo imaging, using light instead of acoustic waves. Since the signal from OCT is traveling considerably fast, i.e. at the speed of light, OCT detects optical echoes from tissue surfaces using low coherence interferometry technique. As a result, higher resolution cross-sectional images of tissue structures are possible compared to ultrasound imaging (Fercher et al., 1988; Fujimoto et al., 1986). Early OCT images were based on time domain approaches with axial and lateral resolutions of less than 20 μm (Huang et al., 1991; Swanson et al., 1993). Interests in OCT increased resulting in the use preliminary in clinical studies and eventually to the development of commercial OCT system for ophthalmic imaging in the mid-1990s. The development of high speed scanners increased imaging speed capabilities of time domain OCT (TD-OCT). Nonetheless, dramatic improvements in scan speed was not attained until the development of Fourier domain detection, i.e. spectral domain (SD-OCT) or swept source OCT. By removing the need to mechanically scan the reference mirror increased scan speeds by an order of magnitude from a few thousand to ten to hundred thousand axial scans per second while also improving sensitivity (de Boer et al., 2003; Lietgeb et al., 2003, Potsaid et al., 2008). In addition to speed and sensitivity, other important parameters that should be considered for cellular level imaging are high axial and lateral resolutions.

Developments of wider band light sources ≥ 80 nm, which we referred to as "ultrawideband" in this chapter, have dramatically improved the axial resolution to ≤ 5 μm at 800 nm. In addition, ultrawideband light source at other wavelengths, such as those over 1000 nm, provide structural imaging beyond the retinal layers (Povazay et al., 2003; Puvanathasan et al., 2008). The lower scattering at longer wavelengths is an important design consideration since it can extend the applicability of OCT technique to certain patient populations with pre-existing afflictions (Povazay et al., 2003). In parallel to light source developments to improve axial resolutions, researchers continue to improve lateral resolutions in OCT ophthalmic imaging. A vital technological advancement in improving lateral resolution in OCT is the use of adaptive optics (AO) to correct for ocular aberrations. Multiple variations of AO-OCT currently exist; as AO-OCT systems continue to develop, they offer great clinical potential for improved clinical assessment of retinal pathologies great clinical potential for improved clinical assessment of retinal pathologies.

OCT systems have proven its effectiveness in detecting small retinal changes in patients with various retinal diseases from age-related macular degeneration (AMD) to retinal detachment. Hence it has become an integral part of diagnostic paradigm in clinical practice in ophthalmology. By incorporating ultrawideband source and AO in OCT systems, it is now possible to resolve individual photoreceptors as well as nerve fiber bundle. The power of cellular level in-vivo imaging is that it allows clinicians to follow retinal and optic nerve changes over time in patients, which ultimately results in earlier detection and intervention. Current applications of both OCT and AO-OCT will be reviewed and future direction will be discussed.

2. Ultrahigh resolution OCT designs

2.1 Ultrawideband light sources

For ophthalmic imaging, high axial resolution in OCT images is particularly important due to the stratified organization of the retina. In OCT, the interference signal detected is the field autocorrelation of the light source. Since the envelope of the autocorrelation is the Fourier transform of the source power spectrum, the axial resolution is determined by coherence length, l_c, of the light source:

$$\Delta z = l_c = \frac{2\ln 2\,\lambda_c^2}{\pi\Delta\lambda} \tag{1}$$

where λ_c is the center wavelength and $\Delta\lambda$ is the spectral bandwidth. Axial resolutions can therefore be improved by using lower wavelengths and/or increasing the spectral bandwidth. In selecting the choice of wavelength, it is also important to consider tissue absorption and scattering that influence OCT imaging contrast and penetration depth. Hemoglobin and melanin are main tissue absorbers that limit penetration depth of wavelengths in the visible to near infra-red regime. At longer wavelengths but less than 1800 nm, tissue scattering dominates, which decreases with increasing wavelength. At wavelength greater than 1800 nm and around 1400 nm, imaging is limited by the absorption of water. For these reasons and available laser at certain wavelengths, OCT typically uses 800 and 1300 nm center wavelengths. Ultrawideband sources such as superluminscent diodes (SLD), femtosecond Titanium:Sapphire (Ti:Sapph) lasers and photonic crystal fiber (PCF) based sources, are typically designed in either wavelength regime. Another important consideration is the attainable resolution for a given spectral bandwidth at a given center wavelength. Fig. 1 shows the required optical bandwidths to achieve axial resolutions at 800 and 1300 nm. Assuming similar spectral shape, the axial resolution is better with 800 nm light source for the same spectral bandwidth. In addition, the shallower slope for 1300 nm compared to 800 nm, indicates that the use of longer wavelength will require a larger increase in bandwidth in order to reach the same axial resolution as with shorter wavelengths.

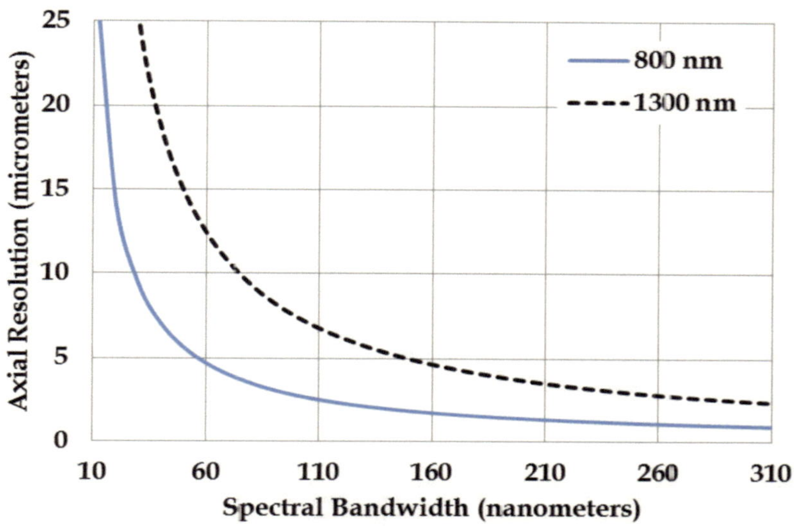

Fig. 1. Comparison of optical bandwidths and axial resolutions at two center wavelengths, 800 and 1300 nm.

2.1.1 SLD sources

Light source for conventional OCT imaging is typically SLDs with spectral bandwidths of 20-30 nm resulting in OCT axial resolutions of 10-15 μm. Though this resolution is sufficient to image retinal layers, identification of individual cells or sub-cellular structures is not possible. Pushing towards cellular imaging, advanced SLDs have been developed with wide spectral bandwidths ≥ 80 nm by multiplexing 2 or more SLDs, providing OCT axial resolutions of < 10 μm (Adler et al., 2004; Cense et al., 2009a; Hong et al., 2007; Ko et al., 2004; Potsaid et al., 2008; Zawadzki et al., 2005). A prototype of this ultrawideband SLD for OCT imaging was first demonstrated by Ko et al. in 2004. Two independent SLD sources at center wavelengths 840 and 920 nm were combined with a custom designed fiber coupler based on fiber GRIN microlenses and miniature dielectric coated mirrors (Adler et al., 2004; Ko et al., 2004). OCT imaging in the retina with this SLD, which had a 155 nm bandwidth, resulted in axial resolutions of ~ 3.2 μm. Fig. 2 shows a comparison between images obtained with an ultrawideband SLD OCT system and a conventional commercial system from the same subject. As shown, multiple retinal layers were better defined with the ultrawideband SLD. Moreover, retinal features such as photoreceptor segments, external limiting membrane and ganglion cell layers were better visualized (Ko et al., 2004). With a 170 nm SLD source, more choroidal vessels were visualized, allowing one to find connecting vessels between adjacent imaging areas (Hong et al., 2007).

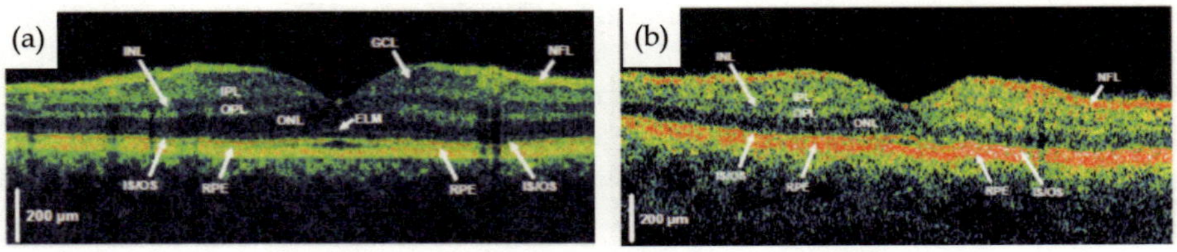

Fig. 2. Comparison of in-vivo images acquired with (a) an OCT sytem with an ultrawideband SLD source with an axial resolution of 3.2 µm and(b) a standard resolution OCT with an axial resolution of 10 µm. Images from Ko et al., 2004.

One of the drawbacks of SLD is that its spectral shape can be less Gaussian-like and more spectrally modulated. As a result, the axial point spread function (PSF) has sidelobes that can result in image artifacts. Despite this limitation, spectral shaping may be applied digitally to approximate a Gaussian envelope and reduce the sidelobes (Potsaid et al., 2008; Tripathi et al., 2002). SLDs, however, offer advantages over other sources, which can be key in transitioning high resolution OCT systems from the laboratory and into the clinic. In particular, they are highly efficient, reliable and portable. Moreover, SLDs are lower in cost, as much as an order of magnitude in comparison to femtosecond lasers.

In assessing the imaging quality between SLDs and femtosecond sources, a comparative study has recently been performed by Cense et al. (2009). They used a Femtolasers Integral Ti:Sapph laser with a spectral bandwidth, center wavelength and power of 135 nm, 800 nm, and 60 mW, respectively (Cense et al., 2009a). In comparison, the BroadLighter, a multiplexed SLD, has 110 nm spectral bandwidth, 840 nm center wavelength and 12 mW of input power (Cense et al., 2009a). The output spectrums from each source are shown in Fig. 3a. Both sources were used on the same OCT system and imaged the same patient on different days. In-vivo measurements showed similar axial resolutions in tissue specifically, 3.2 µm with the Ti:Sapph laser and 3.3 µm with the SLD (Fig. 3b) (Cense et al., 2009). Despite more pronounced sidelobes in the axial PSF with the SLD compared to that with the Ti:Sapph laser (Fig. 3b), the difference in the dynamic range was ≤ 5 dB, which the group expected to be within the range of variability between individual measurement sessions (Cense et al., 2009). Finally, a comparison of acquired volumetric images showed that the wideband SLD can image individual cone photoreceptors, retinal capillaries and nerve fiber bundles as well as the Ti:Sapph laser source (Fig. 3c-d) (Cense et al., 2009).

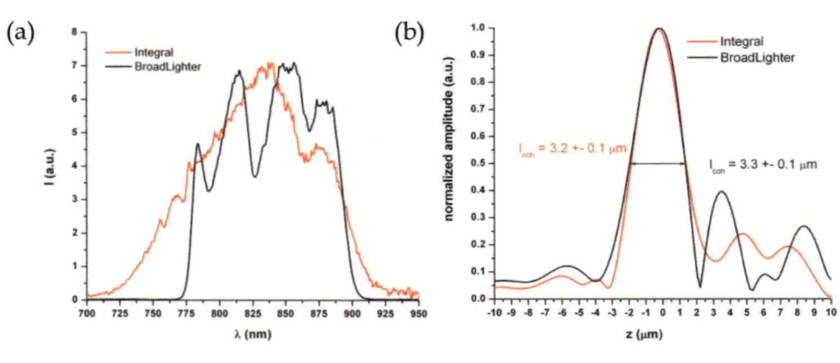

(c) (d)

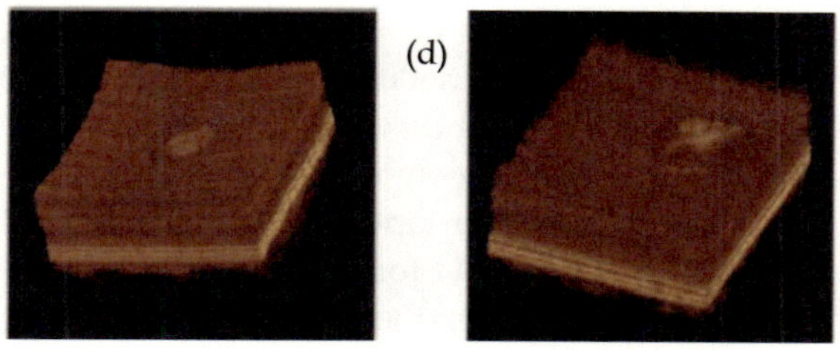

Fig. 3. (a) Comparison of spectra from ultrawideband Ti:Sapph (Integral) and multiplexed SLD (BroadLighter). (b) Normalized coherence function from both sources. (c,d) Comparison of high resolution imaging with the ultrawideband SLD (c) and Ti:Sapph (d) light sources. Images from Cense, et al., 2009.

2.1.2 Titanium:Sapphire laser sources

Since OCT was developed in research laboratories, it is not surprising that the first sub-10 µm axial resolution OCT imaging was demonstrated using a laboratory source, femtosecond Ti:Sapph laser, as opposed to a commercial SLD source (Clivaz et al., 1992). Femtosecond mode-locked lasers can generate not only wide spectral bandwidth, but also provide sufficient power for high speed imaging. A novel design is a high power Kerr-lens mode-locked Ti:Sapph laser with a spectral bandwidth of up to 350 nm at 800 nm center wavelength developed by Drexler et al. (1999). High performance was obtained with custom designed chirped mirrors with high reflective bandwidth and intracavity dispersion compensating prims (Drexler et al., 1999). In-vivo ophthalmic imaging of a normal subject showed axial resolutions of ~ 2-3 µm (Drexler et al., 2001; Wojtkowski et al., 2004). Later, improvements resulted in less complex, more compact and lower cost Ti:Sapph laser with 135-176 nm spectral bandwidth (Unterhuber et al., 2003). Spectral broadening was accomplished by specially designed low dispersive mirrors and the footprint was reduced by asymmetric folding of the resonator and some double pass configurations (Unterhuber et al., 2003). In-vivo imaging of patients with macular pathologies showed images with ~ 3 µm axial resolutions (Unterhuber et al., 2003).

2.1.3 PCF based sources

Another class of wideband light sources for high resolution OCT imaging is based on nonlinear propagation of pulsed laser into PCF. PCFs are optical fibers made with pure silica core surrounded by air holes throughout the length of the fiber. The large difference in refractive index between the air and the silica leads to nonlinear effects resulting in supercontinuum generation, i.e. extreme broadening of narrow band incident pulse into a spectrally broadband continuous output. Just a few pulses with nJ of energy are sufficient to generate supercontinuum (Humbert et al., 2006). Moreover, fiber dispersion can be engineered to control temporal broadening. Hartl et al. (2001) reported the first supercontinuum based OCT system. A femtosecond Ti:Sapph laser was launched into a PCF resulting in a spectral bandwidth of 450 nm in the 1300 nm wavelength region resulting in an axial resolution of 2 µm in tissue (Hartl et al., 2001). Even higher resolutions have been demonstrated. Modifications including fiber lengths, core sizes and polarization states can be used to optimize the performance of PCF based sources (Apolonski et al., 2002). With some optimization, a PCF based source was developed with a spectral bandwidth ~ 400 nm centered at 750 nm resulting in an axial resolutions of ~ 0.5 μm (Povazay et al., 2002). OCT cross-sectional imaging was demonstrated using monolayers of human colorectal adenocarcinomas on coverslips with OCT images showing subcellular structures, such as the nucleoli (Povazay et al., 2002). Humbert et al. (2006) later demonstrated that supercontinuum can also be generated by launching Ti:Sapph laser into tapered PCF. Controlled tapering involved the heating and stretching of a section of the fiber forming a narrow waist (Birks et al., 2000). The decrease in the fiber pitch or distance between the air holes from the tapering process increases the non-linear process (Humbert et al., 2006). Using tapered PCF, a maximum spectral bandwidth of 194 nm centered at 809 nm was developed, resulting in OCT images with an axial resolution of 1.5 μm in air (Humbert et al., 2006).

OCT imaging with PCF based light source centered at 1100 nm has also been demonstrated. This wavelength regime is of interest since the absorption of melanin in RPE decreases with wavelength, therefore imaging with wavelengths greater than 800 nm should allow for better imaging of the choroid below the RPE layer. In a study by Povazay et al., (2003) a Ti:Sapph laser was launched into a PCF generating a supercontinuum source from 400 to 1200 nm which was then passed through long pass filter, resulting in a spectrum with a 165 nm bandwidth centered around 1050 nm (Povazay et al., 2003). OCT images of ex-vivo pig retina were acquired and also compared with OCT images using a 165 nm bandwidth Ti:Sapph laser at 800 nm (Povazay et al., 2003). As expected, better visualization of intraretinal layer was noted with the lower center wavelength source, i.e. Ti:Sapph laser (Fig. 4a) (Povazay et al., 2003). However, the PCF based light source showed improved penetration in the choroid, as evident by more visible choroidal blood vessels as shown in Fig. 4b (Povazay et al., 2003).

(a) (b)

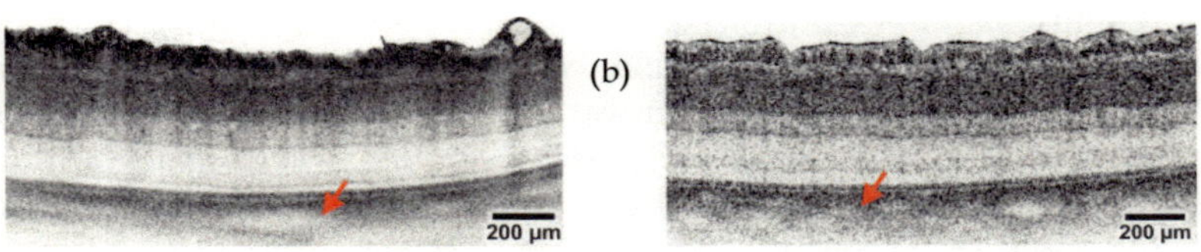

Fig. 4. (a,b) Comparison of OCT images acquired with (a) a Ti:Sapph laser and (b) a PCF fiber source. Red arrows indicates blood vessels in the choroid. Images from Povazay, et al., 2003.

More recently, 1064 nm was pumped into PCF generating both 800 and 1300 nm wavelengths simultaneously. Near complete depletion of the pump wavelength created a double peak spectrum with bandwidth and average power of 116 nm and ~ 30 mW, respectively at 800 nm center wavelength and 156 nm and ~ 48 mW at 1300 nm center wavelength (Aguirre et al., 2006). However, coupling loss reduced the power by nearly 50% (Aguirre et al., 2006). Additionally, power stability was found to be sensitive to environmental condition (Aguirre et al., 2006). Fiber end facet protection was recommended to improve long term power stability (Aguirre et al., 2006). The supercontinuum source was integrated into a TD-OCT system with different couplers, sample arm optics and photodiode detector for each center wavelength but with a common galvometric scanner and scanning stage (Aguirre et al., 2006). OCT imaging in hamster cheek pouch showed axial resolutions of 2.2 μm at 800 nm and 4.7 μm at 1300 nm. Some blurring of the image was observed at both wavelengths due to side lobe coherence artifacts on the PSF as a result of spectral modulation at 800 and 1300 nm (Aguirre et al., 2006). To address this issue, further work will investigate spectral smoothing (Aguirre et al., 2006).

Another dual band OCT imaging was demonstrated with 840 and 1230 nm center wavelength with 1060 nm pump wavelength (Spoler et al., 2007). The spectral shape of the supercontinuum source was tailored with a double pass prism, razor blades and an end mirror (Spoler et al., 2007). Resulting bandwidths were > 200 nm after spectral filtering with > 100 mW average power for each wavelength (Spoler et al., 2007). The source was incorporated in a free space OCT system to launch both wavelengths simultaneously (Spoler et al., 2007). Dichroic filters separated the two wavelength channels prior to detection (Spoler et al., 2007). In-vitro OCT imaging of a rabbit eye was performed and showed axial resolutions <2 and < 4 um at 840 and 1230 nm in tissue, respectively (Spoler et al., 2007). As expected, 840 nm imaging yielded higher resolution while higher penetration was achieved with the longer 1230 nm wavelength (Fig. 5a & 5b) (Spoler et al., 2007). Simultaneous measurements allowed the feasibility to extract spectroscopic information, since differences in image contrast are influenced by wavelength dependent scattering and absorption of different types of tissue (Spoler et al., 2007). Differences in intensities are used to construct spectroscopy images (Fig. 5c) that provided tissue differentiation, such as the conjunctiva and sclera (Spoler et al., 2007).

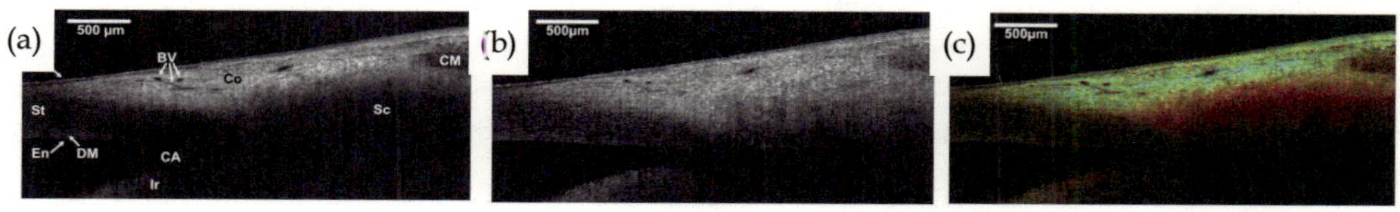

Fig. 5.(a-c) OCT imaging at (a) 840 nm and (b)1230 nm (c) Differential color image based on scattering intensity from each wavelength range. Higher scattering in 840 nm is shown in shades of blue while those 1230 nm is in shades of red. Ep: Epithelium; BV: Blood vessel; CM: Ciliary muscle; St: Stroma; Sc: Sclera; En: Endothelium; DM: Descement's membrane; CA: Chamber angle; Co: Conjunctiva. Images from Spoler et al., 2007.

2.2 Adaptive Optics (AO)

In OCT, axial and lateral resolutions are decoupled. The lateral resolution in OCT is similar to that in standard microcopy:

$$\Delta x = \frac{4\lambda f}{\pi D} \tag{2}$$

where f is the focal length of the focusing lens and the D is the beam diameter on the lens. Therefore, lateral resolution can be improved by increasing the numerical aperture of the beam delivery optics by decreasing the focal length and/or increasing the beam diameter. In ophthalmic imaging, the focusing optics is limited by the eye itself. A 3mm pupil diameter will yield a lateral resolution of 10–15 µm diffraction limited spot at 800 nm center wavelength (Drexler, 2004). Increasing the pupil diameter by 1 mm will reduce the focused beam spot diameter to 4.3 µm, in theory. However with larger pupil size, the ocular aberrations will limit the achievable size of the focus beam. Additionally, the use of broadband light sources to improve axial resolution will further contribute to chromatic aberrations.

Adaptive optics (AO) in OCT has been shown to be a successful approach in correcting ocular and system's aberrations to improve lateral resolutions. The two essential components of an AO system for retinal imaging are a wavefront sensor and a corrector placed conjugate to the pupil plane of the eye as shown in Fig. 6a. To measure ocular aberrations, a Shack- Hartmann wavefront sensor containing a 2D array of lenslets, each of which with the same diameter and focal length is used. Light reflected from the retina are distorted by aberrations of the eye particularly from corneal surfaces and crystalline lens (Yoon et al., 2006). This reflected light is spatially sampled by the 2D lenslet array on the wavefront sensor, forming multiple beams focused at the focal plane of the lenses and imaged onto a camera. Light reflected from a perfect eye, i.e., free of aberrations, emerges as a collimated beam. Therefore, Shack-Hartmann spots will be imaged at the focal point of each lenslet, forming a regularly spaced grid (Fig. 6b, left). In comparison, wavefront error from a real eye, i.e., with aberrations such as defocus and astigmatism, will displace the Shack-Hartmann spots from the optical axis of each lenslet, resulting in an image of an irregular grid (Fig. 6b, right). Since the displacement is proportional to the wavefront slope sampled by the lenslet at a particular location, the aberrations from the eye can be determined. The aberration information is then used to alter the phase profile of the incident wavefront by changing the physical length that the light propagates to correct the wavefront error. Different types of wavefront correctors or deformable mirrors (DMs) have been used including those based on bimorph, piezoelectric and micro-electro-mechanical systems (MEMS) technologies (Doble & Miller, 2006). An example of a MEMs based mirror with piston/tip/tilt capability per mirror segment is shown in Fig. 6c.

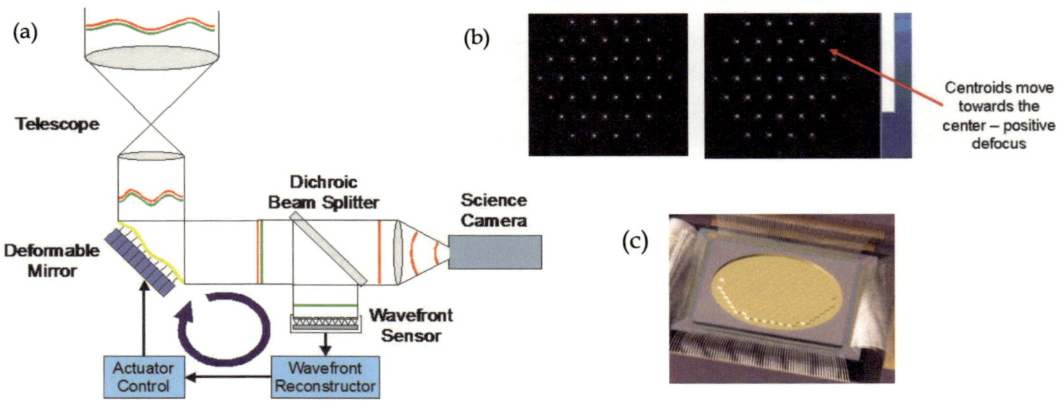

Fig. 6.(a)A schematic of an AO system for retinal imaging. (b) Example of a Shack-Hartmann wavefront sensor images from a perfect eye (left) and from a real eye (right). (c) Scanning electron microscope of a 163 segment MEMs based mirror. Images courtesy of Iris AO, Inc.

The first attempt to improve retinal images from scanning laser ophthalmoscope with AO was shown by Dreher et al. (1989). Using a DM, the group corrected the astigmatism in one eye based on the patient's spectacle prescription (Dreher et al., 1989). Several years later, the Hartmann-Shack wavefront sensor was implemented to measure the wavefront error of the eye (Liang et al., 1997). With the DM, aberrations from the system and the eye were also corrected (Liang, 1997). Initially, wavefront compensation was achieved with a closed loop feedback system. At each loop, images were acquired and the aberrations of the system and eye were calculated. The DM partially, ~10%, corrected the wavefront error and loop iterations were performed until a minimum wavefront error was reached. Later, closed loop AO systems were developed with faster and automated wavefront sensing and dynamic correction of ocular aberrations (Hofer, 2001; Fernandez 2001). To date, AO has been successfully combined with ophthalmic imaging systems such as flood illuminated fundus camera, scanning laser ophthalmoscope (SLO) and OCT systems for improved lateral resolution and image contrast (Choi et al., 2005; Choi et al., 2006; Jonnal et al., 2007; Roorda et al., 2002a; Roorda et al., 2002b; Thorn et al., 2003; Wolfing et al.,2006; Xue et al.,2007).

2.2.1 AO with ultrawideband source OCT

Cellular level OCT imaging can be realized by combining AO with ultrawideband sources to achieve high lateral and axial resolutions. Hermann et al. (2004) first applied AO with a 130 nm bandwidth Ti:Sapph laser in a TD-OCT system. With AO, the Strehl ratio was improved by at least a factor of 10 (Hermann et al., 2004). The axial resolution with this system was 3μm while the lateral resolution was ~ 5-10 μm, 2-3 times better than similar systems without AO (Hermann et al., 2004). In later developments, AO was combined with SD-OCT systems, taking advantage of the higher sensitivity, enabling faster data acquisition. Fig. 7 shows an example design of a SD-OCT system with an AO sub-system.

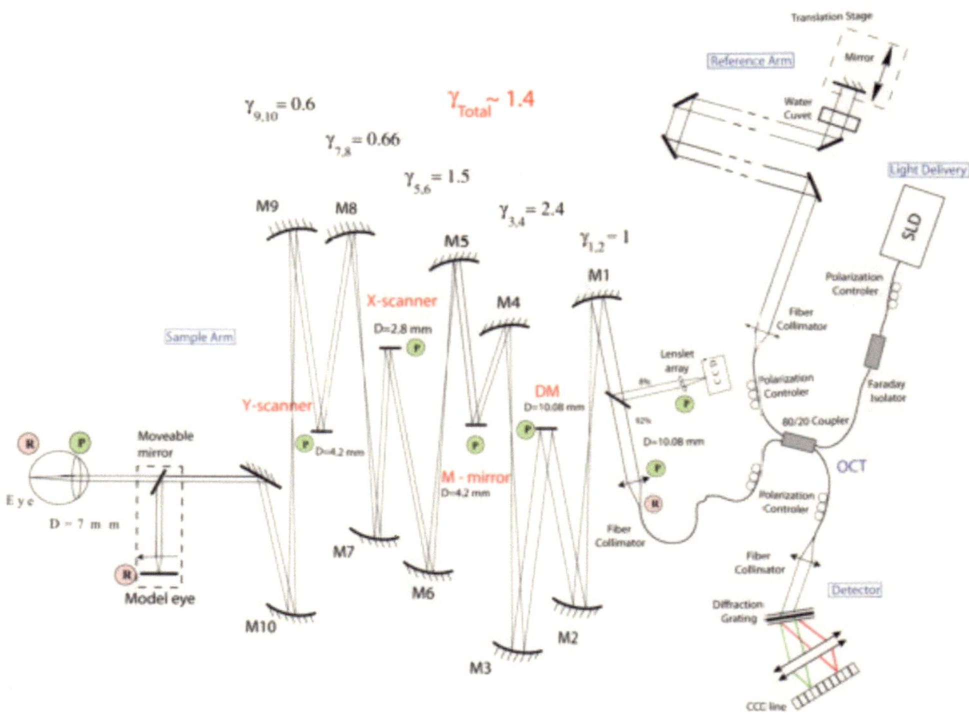

Fig. 7. A schematic of an AO-OCT system. P: Pupil plane; R: Retinal plane; M: Spherical mirror; γ: Telescope magnification. Image from Zawadzki et al., 2005.

The system was designed with a series of telescopes that relayed the pupil conjugate plane to the Shack Hartmann, bimorph DM and two scanning mirrors, while the retinal conjugate plane is relayed to the OCT detector. The SLD source used had a spectral bandwidth of 140 nm centered at 890 nm. Axial and lateral resolutions were 6 μm and 4 μm, respectively. With AO, it was found that image brightness was improved which the group attributed to be due to astigmatism and defocus correction. Overall improvements allowed for better visualization of retinal structures and cone photoreceptors (Zawadzki et al., 2005).

Although AO-OCT systems are mostly used to image the photoreceptor layer, it can also be used to image the RNFL, which is important in the clinical management of glaucoma. With an AO-OCT system, Kocaoglu et al. (2011) were able to easily visualize individual axonal bundles in both enface and cross-sectional views due to improved image contrast, as a result of wavefront error correction. For the first time, the researchers were able to quantify individual nerve fiber bundles, i.e. width and thickness, from acquired OCT images (Kocaoglu et al., 2011).

2.2.2 Dual-DM AO-OCT systems

Since wavefront correctors have a limited dynamic range, the use of trial lenses may be necessary particularly in correcting subjects with large refractive errors. Others, however, have developed alternative designs to increase the range of wavefront correction of AO-OCT systems. One example is the addition of a Badal to coarsely correct for large defocus (Chen et al., 2008). Another design alternative is to incorporate two wavefront correctors with the first DM (DM1) mainly used to correct for large stroke, low order aberrations while the second DM (DM2) used to correct for low stroke, high order aberrations (Cense et al., 2009; Mujat et al., 2010; Zawadzki et al., 2007,2008). DM1 is first used to correct for aberrations, as calculated by the wavefront sensor, then held static after reaching minimum wavefront error. The remaining aberrations are again determined by the wavefront sensor, and then corrected by DM2. Fig. 8 shows the time course of the dual DM AO implementation. Though DM1 corrected most of the aberrations, these were further reduced after both DMs were implemented (Zawadzki et al., 2007).

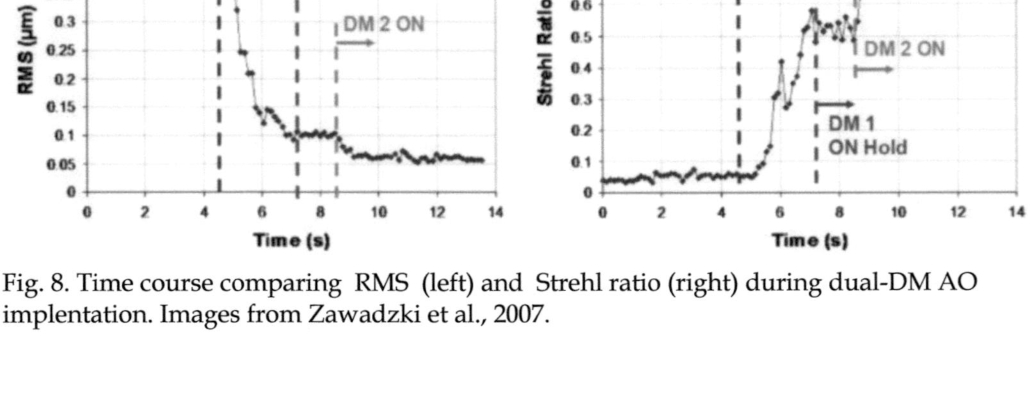

Fig. 8. Time course comparing RMS (left) and Strehl ratio (right) during dual-DM AO implentation. Images from Zawadzki et al., 2007.

2.2.3 Correcting motion artefacts in AO-OCT

Despite faster image acquisition, involuntary head and eye movements still occur, despite the use of bite bars and head restraints, resulting in motion artefacts that distort volumetric OCT images. Though motion artefacts can be corrected via post-processing software, hardware based implementations have also been demonstrated. For example, Fergueson et al. were able to track and correct for retinal motion during or after data acquisition using a low power tracking beam projected onto a retinal feature, such as a blood vessel junction (Ferguson et al., 2004). Real time signal processing is used to determine the position and orientation of the targeted retinal feature to correctly steer the tracking beam (Ferguson et al., 2004). Since the OCT imaging and the tracking beam share the same pair of scanners, the OCT beam similarly follows the retina (Ferguson et al., 2004).

More recently, an alternative system design to correct for motion artifact was demonstrated by Zawadzki et al. by integrating SLO with an AO-OCT. In this combined system, SLO and OCT retinal images were acquired simultaneously, since both modalities share the same AO sub-system and vertical scanner, as shown in the optical schematic diagram, Fig. 9a (Zawadzki et al., 2009). In this system, separate light sources are used for the OCT and SLO optical paths. The SLO imaging beam is combined into and filtered out of the OCT imaging path using dichroic filters. Similarly, a dichroic filter is used to separate SLO and OCT signal in the detection path. To determine motion, the scanning frequencies are such that an SLO frame is acquired for every OCT B-scan, therefore the researchers were able to correlate features in the SLO images with disruption of layers from the B-scan images due to lateral and transverse eye motion (Zawadzki et al., 2009). Fig. 9 b-d show an example of a co-registered AO-OCT B-scan and AO-SLO frame (Zawadzki et al., 2009).

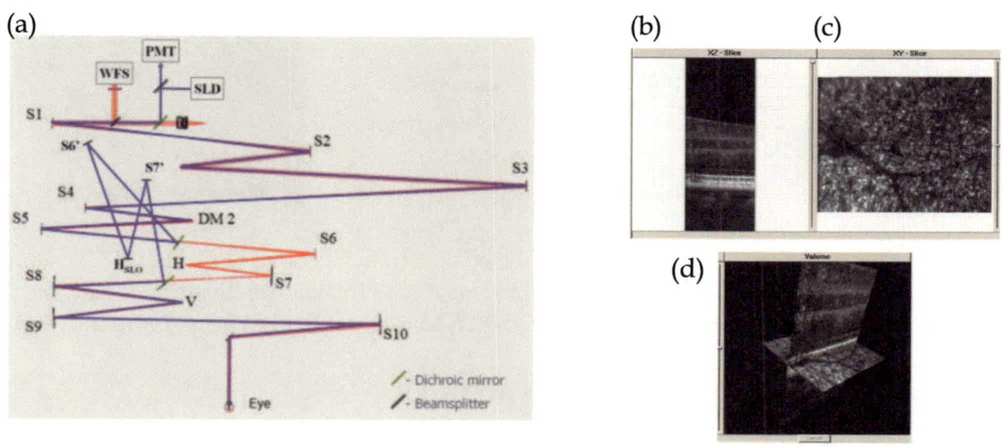

Fig. 9. (a) Optical schematic diagram of combined AO-SLO-OCT system. (b-d) Example of a B-scan (b)acquired at the same time as a SLO frame (c) and resulting co-registered image from both modalities (d). Images from Zawadzki et al., 2011.

Another variation of the combined SLO-OCT system, but without AO, is based on interlacing spectrally encoded SLO frame with OCT B-scans. In spectrally encoded SLO, the illumination beam is dispersed by a diffractive element that spectrally encodes each spatial position (Tao, 2010). The back scattered light is then recombined and directed into a fiber, which acts as a confocal detection pinhole (Tao et al., 2010). Spatial information is then decoded by a spectrometer, the same detector used for OCT imaging (Tao et al., 2010). A schematic diagram of the system is shown in Fig. 10. The slow galvanometer of the OCT scan (Gy,S) acts as a switch between the spectrally encoded SLO (red) and the OCT path (blue), directing the beam towards the combined path (green) (Tao et al., 2010). As shown, the same light source and detector are used by both imaging modalities. During SLO imaging, the galvanometer switch is flipped to its maximum angle, through the grating then along the OCT optical path (Tao et al., 2010). The driving signals for the scanning mirrors are such that a SLO frame is interlaced with an OCT B-scan (Fig. 10 b-c) (Tao et al., 2010). De-interlacing of SLO and OCT frames were performed prior to image registration (Tao et al., 2010). Although this imaging technique has yet to be demonstrated with AO sub-system or the use of ultrawideband light sources, this design has the advantages of potentially allowing for motion tracking while minimizing cost and footprint.

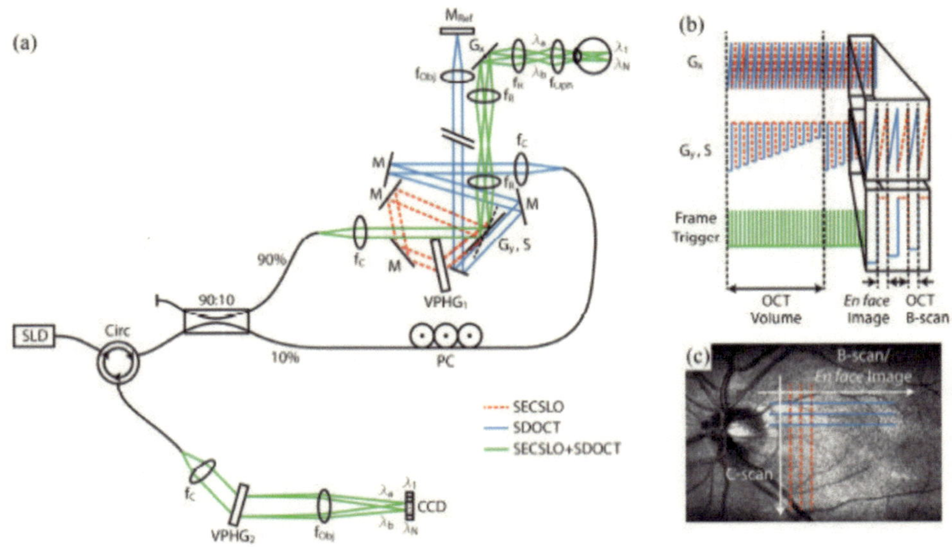

Fig. 10. (a) Optical schematic diagram of combined spectrally encoded SLO and OCT system. (b) Timing diagram showing interlacing of SLO and B-scan images. (c) Illustrated scanning geometry. f: lens, VPHG: Grating, G: Galvanometer, M: Mirror. Images from Tao et al., 2010.

2.2.4 Correcting chromatic aberrations in AO-OCT

In spite of the efforts for increasing transverse resolution, AO-OCT systems are still limited in correcting for axial (or longitudinal) and lateral (or transverse) chromatic aberration of the eye, particularly in dilated pupils in combination with the use of broader spectral bandwidth sources. Axial chromatic aberration is manifested as a change in the focus plane with wavelength, while lateral chromatic aberration appears from off-axis illumination laterally shifting the focus with wavelength. The use of an achromatizing lens to correct for axial chromatic aberration was first proposed by Fernandez et al. (2006). This concept was later demonstrated in AO-OCT systems with wide spectral bandwidth sources (Fernandez et al., 2008, Zawadzki et al., 2008). Custom design achromatizing lens was integrated by

Fernandez et al. in a conjugate pupil plane between the scanning mirrors and the DM, while Zawadzki et al. placed the achromatizing lens immediately after collimating the input laser. Both designs showed improved imaging of the individual photoreceptors with the addition of the achromatizing lens. Fernandez et al. showed that with chromatic aberration correction, photoreceptor structures between the inner and outer segment junctions appear elongated, as opposed to rounded as in standard AO, resembling axial morphology of cones in histology.

Although, an achromatizing lens can correct for axial chromatic aberrations, it does not correct for lateral chromatic aberrations. Zawadzki et al. (2008) theoretically investigated the extent of lateral chromatic aberration and its impact on retinal imaging. The group found that the main contributors to this type of aberration are errors in the lateral positioning of the eye and off-axis imaging (Zawadzki et al., 2008). Proper alignment of the eye relative to the OCT camera optical axis should result in lateral chromatic aberration free imaging (Zawadzki et al., 2008). Based on their system design, the group expects that lateral chromatic aberration is smaller than the lateral resolution that can be achieved by the AO in their system and therefore have little impact on image quality (Zawadzki et al., 2008).

2.2.5 AO in functional-based OCT systems

Adaptive optics has also transitioned into functional extensions of OCT, specifically polarization sensitive OCT (PS-OCT). PS-OCT measures the intensity and polarization state in tissue, thus allowing depth resolve imaging of birefringent retinal structures such as the RNFL. The PS-OCT system designed by Cense et al. (2009b) utilized a dual DM AO-subsystem. The group deduced the improvement in signal contrast and resolution with AO allowed for a more sensitive measurement of change in phase retardation and hence birefringence (Cense et al., 2009b). With this system, the group was able to quantify birefringence of thin retinal nerve fiber bundles in the macula lutea, not measurable with standard PS-OCT (Cense et al., 2009b). As AO becomes widely implemented, it is expected that more AO will be integrated in other forms of OCT.

3. Clinical applications

OCT has become an integral part of routine diagnostic paradigm in ophthalmology. Due to its non-invasive nature and the ability to extract quantitative morphological information, it has been extensively used in the diagnosis of retinal and optic nerve diseases as well as in the monitoring of their progression with treatments over time. Here, only some of the selected representative papers on limited topics are briefly reviewed due to space limitation.

3.1 Ultrahigh resolution OCT

OCT has been able to reveal various microscopic changes ranging from macular edema to disruptions in photoreceptor layer in patients with various retinal diseases and reduction of RNFL in patients with glaucoma and other types of optic neuropathy.

3.1.1 Macular edema

OCT imaging is readily used to diagnose and follow macular edema. It occurs in many disorders including diabetic retinopathy, age-related macular degeneration, retinal vein occlusion, uveitis and macular hole. Macular edema is the result of an accumulation of fluid in the retinal layers around the fovea with an increase in retinal thickness, which contributes to vision loss. Fluorescein angiography (FA) has been and still is the critical diagnostic tool for macular edema by identifying the characteristic stellar pattern of cystoid macular edema (CME). Fig. 11 illustrates the appearance of CME through different diagnostic modalities, namely, conventional fundus photography, FA and OCT.

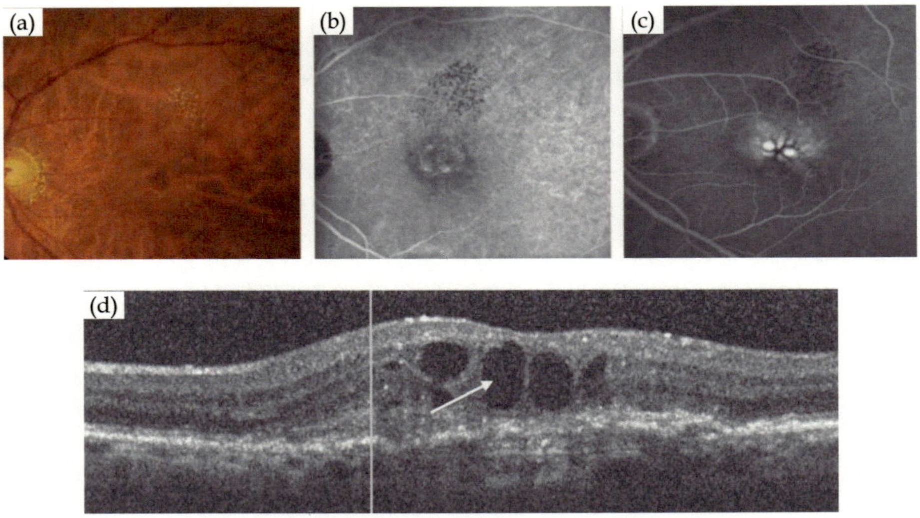

Fig. 11. Cystoid Macular Edema (CME) imaged by 3 different diagnostic modalities. (a) Conventional fundus picture (b, c) Fluorescein angiography (early and late stages respectively) - dilation and leakage of capillary are revealed. Fluorescein dye pools in cystoid spaces and arranged radially from the fovea. (d) OCT image - cystoid spaces are shown. The central macula is indicated with an arrow. Images from Cunha-Vaz, et al., 2010.

In the early stage of macular edema, a diffuse swelling of the outer retinal layer is observed, and then leads to the development of cystoid spaces. In the later stage, the large cystoid spaces can extend from the RPE to the internal limiting membrane, which then eventually rupture causing macular holes. In diabetic patients, macular edema involves three structural changes - most commonly, sponge-like retinal swelling (88%), then CME (47%) and then serous retinal detachment (15%) (Ontani et al., 1999). Fig. 12 shows the fundus pictures and corresponding OCT images of retinal swelling and serous retinal detachment seen in diabetic macular edema.

In sponge-like retinal swelling, the OCT image showed low reflective areas in the outer retinal layers with relatively preserved inner retinal layer with interspersed low reflective areas. The inner retinal layers were displaced anteriorly by the swollen outer retinal layers. In serous retinal detachment, the OCT image clearly showed detached retina as a highly reflective line with the formation of sub-retinal space underneath.

A good correlation has been found between OCT images and visual acuity and FA findings (Hee et al., 1998; Jaffe & Caprioli, 2004; Ontani et al., 1999). Larger area of increased retinal thickness and the involvement of the macular area correlated with greater loss of vision. Fig. 13 shows the correlation curve between visual acuity (VA) and retinal thickness

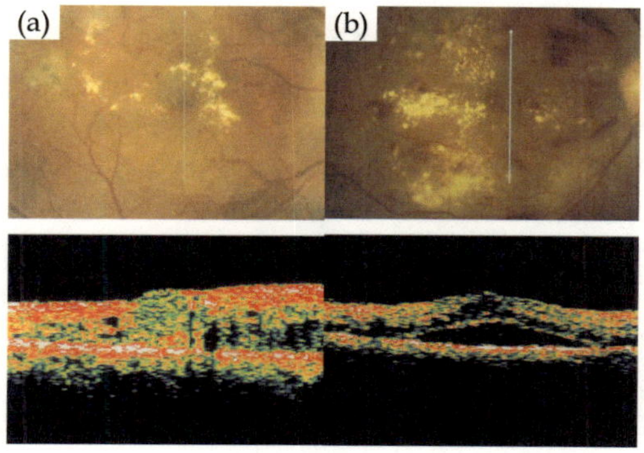

Fig. 12. (a) Retinal swelling. The retinal thickness at the fovea is 560 μm. (b) Serous retinal detachment with retinal swelling. The thickness of the sub-retinal space is 420 μm. The vertical arrow on the fundus picture indicates the line and direction of scanning. Scan length = 5 mm. Images from Otani, et al., 1999.

at the fovea in the eyes with CME (Ontani et al., 1999). Twenty eight of 59 eyes (47%) developed CME, and the foveal retinal thickness and the VA were found to be negatively correlated with the correlation coefficient of -0.64, P < 0.01.

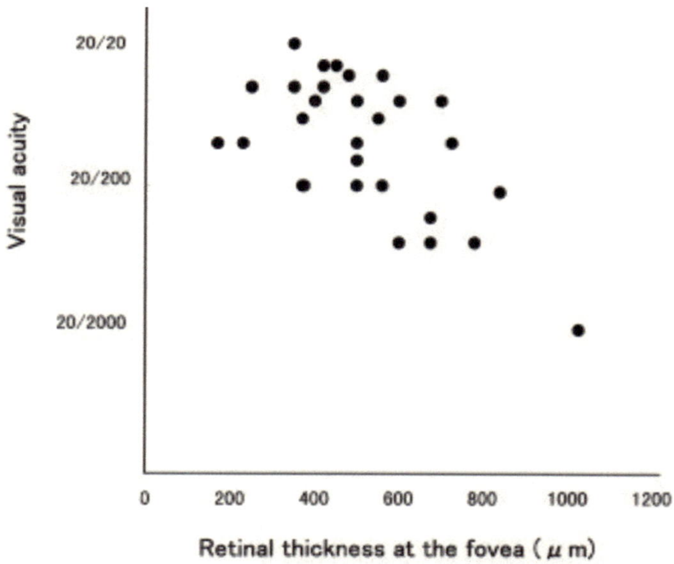

Fig. 13. Correlation between VA and retinal thickness at the fovea in patients with CME. Correlation coefficient = -0.64, P < 0.01. Figure from Otani, et al., 1999.

When compared with FA, OCT findings also correlated well with the pattern of edema noticed in FA. Diffuse leakage is associated with nonspecific retinal swelling in the OCT image, whereas petaloid-pattern hyper fluorescence is associated with large cystic spaces in outer plexiform layer (OPL) and outer nuclear layer (ONL) and honeycomb hyper fluorescence is associated with cystic changes in the OPL, ONL, inner nuclear layer (INL) and inner plexiform layer (IPL) (Al-latayfeh et al., 2010).

3.1.2 Age related Macular Degeneration (AMD)

OCT has proven extremely useful in both the diagnosis and treatment of AMD. It is even more so in the initial diagnosis of AMD lesion, as it is less hindered by blood or lipid as it is in FA (Singh & Kaiser, 2007). A study compared the diagnostic accuracy of OCT with that of FA in predicting the angiographic pattern of choroidal neovascularization, and found the sensitivity and specificity to be 94% and 89% respectively when stereo fundus images were added (Sandhu & Talks, 2005).

OCT has been used to update the drusen classification system; one group identified 3 drusen patterns whereas another group identified 17 different patterns (Khanifar et al., 2008; Pieroni et al., 2006). Drusen were classified based on shape (concave, convex saw-toothed), reflectivity (low to high), homogeneity (present or absent, with or without core), and foci of hyper-reflectivity (present or absent). Soft indistinct drusen were mostly found to be convex and homogenous with medium internal reflectivity and without overlying hyper-reflective foci (Khanifar et al., 2008). Another study showed that basal laminar drusen exhibited a moderately hyper-reflective and saw-toothed pattern on OCT images, and there was an associated sub-retinal fluid in the macula which could be monitored by using automated segmentation software in OCT (Leng et al., 2009). Fig. 14 shows FA, infrared and OCT images of both eyes of a patient with familial drusen. The OCT images show a saw-tooth appearance of the RPE-Bruch's membrane complex consistent with the presence of basal laminar drusen seen on the corresponding FA and infrared images.

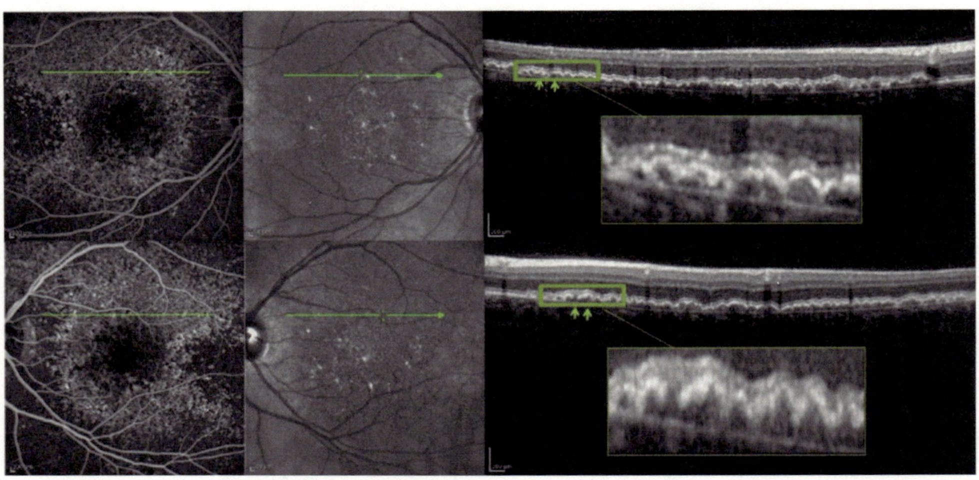

Fig. 14. Early-frame FA (left), infrared (center) and OCT (right) images of both eyes of a patient with familial drusen. Top row = right eye, bottom row = left eye. FA images show early hyperfluorescence characteristic of basal laminar drusen. Green line on FA and infrared images marks the area of OCT scans. In OCT images, the green arrows indicate a saw-tooth appearance of basal laminar drusen. Images from Sohrab, et al., 2011.

The effect of drusen on the overlying retina was investigated using OCT and it was found that the photoreceptor layer was thinned over 97% of drusen while inner retinal thickness was unaffected and over at least one druse in 47% of eyes, photoreceptor outer segments were absent. Furthermore, two types of hyper-reflective abnormalities were observed in the neurosensory retina over drusen: (1) distinct hyper-reflective speckled pattern over drusen (41% of AMD eyes) and (2) prominent hyper-reflective haze in the photoreceptor nuclear layer over drusen (67% of AMD eyes) (Schuman et al., 2009). Fig. 15 shows the two types of hyper-reflective abnormalities.

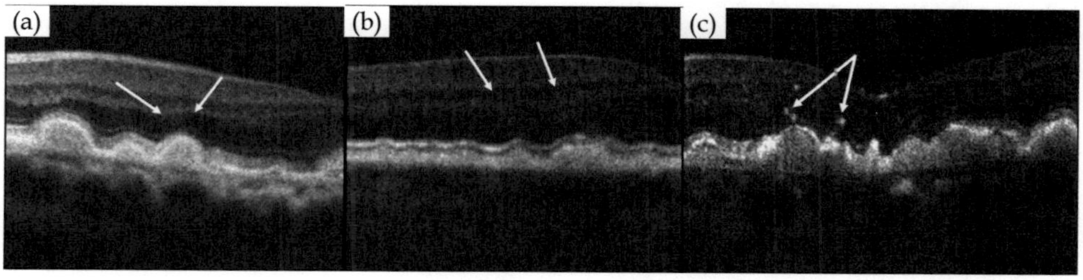

Fig. 15. (a,b) The sites of prominent diffuse hyper-reflective haze were observed over drusen in 2 different eyes (shown with arrows). (c) Focal hyper-reflective speckling (arrows) was visible over drusen. Images from Schuman, et al., 2009.

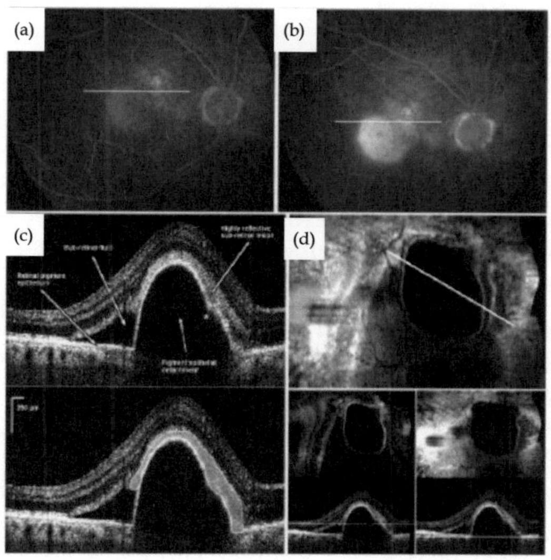

Fig. 16. FA and OCT images of the right eye in case 17. (a) Early-phase of FA. (b) Late-phase of FA. (c) OCT image (top) and the extent of the hyper-reflective lesion is outlined (bottom). (d) OCT C-scan was used to measure the greatest linear diameter (GLD) of the CNVM (top). OCT B-scans with white lines represent the cut depicted by the C-scan shown above (bottom). Images from Park, et al., 2010. Copyright [2010] ARVO.

The hyper-reflective foci overlying drusen are thought to represent progression of disease with RPE cell migration into the retina and possible photoreceptor degeneration or glial scar formation. The reduction in photoreceptor layer thickness suggests degeneration of photoreceptors which eventually leads to vision loss.

The choroidal neovascular membranes (CNVMs) have also been detected in all 21 eyes with exudative AMD by OCT and the anatomic growth pattern of the CNVM was determined based on the OCT images (Park et al., 2010). A highly reflective sub-retinal and/or sub-RPE lesion was visualized in the macula. Of twenty eyes, 7 eyes (33%) had > 90% sub-RPE growth pattern (type 1), 10 eyes (48%) had > 90% sub-retinal growth pattern (type 2) and 3 eyes (14%) had a combined growth pattern. When the size of the CNVM was compared between FA and OCT images, a good correlation was found between these modalities (i.e., for classic CNVM, $r = 0.99$, $P < 0.0001$ and for non-classic CNVM, $r = 0.78$, $P < 0.001$). Fig. 16 shows FA and OCT images from the right eye of a patient (case 17) with an occult CNVM associate with exudative AMD. The FA images showed hyper-fluorescence centered over the macula in the early-phase followed by an intense pooling of the dye into the pigment epithelial detachment (PED) with ill-defined leakage at the superonasal edge in the late-phase. The OCT image showed a large PED with an adjacent area of sub-retinal fluid. A highly reflective sub-retinal lesion above the PED (consistent with type 2 CNVM) and a focal spot of discontinuity in the RPE (indicated with *) with a possible small extension of the hyper-reflectivity into the sub-RPE space were observed.

3.1.3 Glaucoma

OCT has shown the greatest potential for imaging glaucomatous structural changes such as the RNFL. A cross-sectional observational study involving 160 control subjects and 134 patients with primary open-angle glaucoma (POAG) was conducted to evaluate the accuracy of OCT in detecting differences in peripapillary RNFL thickness between normal and glaucomatous eyes as well as between different severity groups (Sihota et al., 2006). The POAG patients were divided into early (n=61), moderate (n=31), severe (n=25) and blind (n=17) groups. The OCT was reliable in detecting changes in the RNFL thickness between normal and all glaucoma subgroups. The RNFL thickness was significantly thinner in the POAG patients compared to the control subjects and also the RNFL thickness continued to reduce with an increase in the severity of POAG with $P < 0.001$.

The reproducibility of the RNFL thickness measurements was tested on 51 stable glaucoma patients using Stratus OCT (Budens et al., 2008). For the mean RNFL thickness, the intra-session and inter-session intraclass correlation coefficient (ICC) for the standard and fast scans were 0.98 and 0.96 respectively. The coefficient of variation (COV) ranged from 3.8 to 5.2% (Carpineto et al., 2003). Other study has reported lower ICC of 0.5 and higher COV of 10%. However, the reproducibility is still sufficient to be useful clinically as a measure of glaucoma progression. Fig. 17 shows a picture of glaucomatous optic nerve head (ONH) with a dense superior visual field defect. A circle concentric OCT scan around the ONH shows thinning of the RNFL in the inferiortemporal quadrant, which corresponds to both the visual field defect and loss of the neural rim of the ONH.

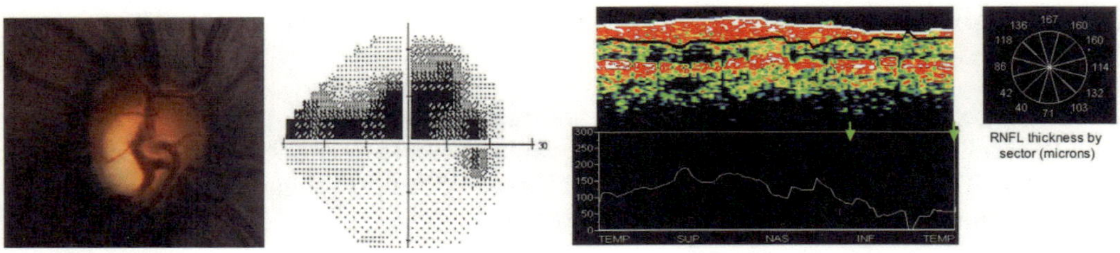

Fig. 17. An ONH picture, a visual field plot and a circle concentric OCT scan around the ONH from a glaucomatous eye. Green arrows indicate the area of thinning of the RNFL. Images from Jaffe, et al., 2004.

3.2 Adaptive optics - OCT

With further improvement in lateral resolution of the system, it is possible to resolve even smaller details in the retina.

As previously mentioned, Kocaoglu et al. (2011) have shown the first measurements of RNFL axonal bundles (RNFB) in the living human eyes using their AO-OCT system. Four normal subjects and one subject with an arcuate RNFL defect were imaged and they were able to visualize individual RNFB in all subjects. Fig. 18 shows the individual RNFB in one of the normal subjects (S4). As the RNFB approach fovea, they become thinner and separate.

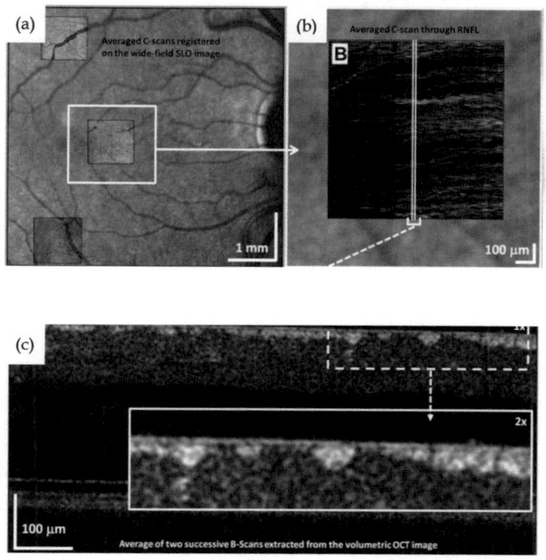

Fig. 18. (a) A wide field SLO, (b) An averaged C-scan and (c) An averaged B-scan images acquired from subject, S4, at 3° nasal retina (indicated with a white square). The white lines in (b) denote the area where the B-scans in (c) were obtained. The white solid rectangle in (c) represents 2x magnification of the area outlined with white dotted rectangle. Images from Kocaoglu, et al., 2011.

In conjunction with the expected inner retinal changes such as, thinning of the RNFL in glaucoma and optic neuropathy, AO-OCT imaging has revealed outer retinal changes as well at the retinal locations with reduced visual function, specifically shortening of cone outer segments and blurring of the junction between the tip of the cone outer segments and RPE. These outer retinal changes only occurred when there was a permanent visual field loss. The same findings were observed in all types of optic neuropathy patients including glaucoma (Choi et al., 2008; Choi et al., 2011).

Fig. 19 shows AO-OCT images obtained from a nonarteritic anterior ischemic optic neuropathy (NAION) patient. The AO-OCT images were taken at 2 retinal locations, 2° temporal 2° superior retina and 4° nasal 4° superior retina. The 4° nasal 4° superior retina had better visual function than 2° temporal 2° superior retina, hence, the layer labeled 3 (the junction between the cone outer segment tip and RPE) was better defined and distinct at that location, and it was not visible at 2° temporal 2° superior retina.

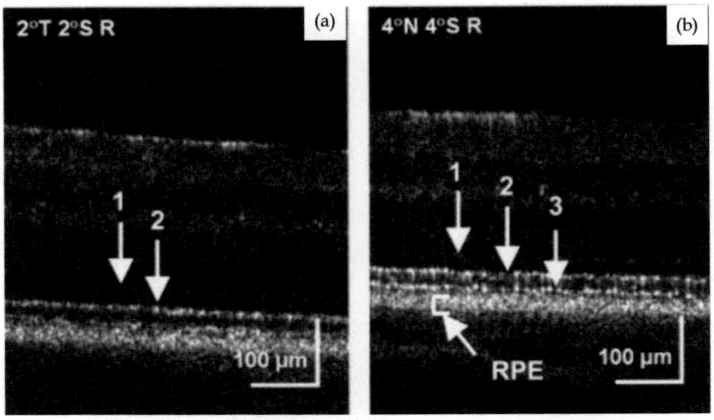

Fig. 19. AO-OCT images at two retinal locations in the right eye of the patient with NAION. (a) 2° temporal 2° superior retina and (b) 4° nasal 4° superior retina. 1: ELM, 2: IS/OS, 3: OS/RPE. Images from Choi, et al., 2008. Copyright [2008] ARVO.

4. Summary and future directions

With technological advancements, OCT has undergone substantial changes towards high resolution cellular level OCT imaging. Light sources with ≥ 80 nm spectral bandwidth paved the way for sub-10 µm axial imaging. At the same time, the adoption of AO in OCT system's addressed ocular and systems aberrations, improving lateral resolutions. Various research groups have shown the potential of high resolution imaging with ultrawideband sources with AO in OCT systems. However for these systems to be widely implemented into the clinic, additional improvements are needed. Ultrawideband sources must provide sufficient power and stability, and are compact and inexpensive. Similarly, AO-OCT systems will also need to consider cost and size in addition to patient comfort and ease of use. Finally, by understanding and addressing the limitations of AO-OCT systems, can researchers and clinicians fully exploit the capabilities of AO to better image patients with various forms of retinal diseases.

The advent of OCT technology has allowed extensive amounts of new anatomic, physiologic, and pathologic data for the practice of ophthalmology. The ability to image retinal and ONH structures in detail in-vivo makes OCT an ideal modality for detection of early disease in screening and prevention for differential diagnosis of various diseases as well as for quantifying therapeutic effects and identifying recurrence during follow-up. The practicality of OCT in terms of obtaining motion artifact free images and presentation of quantified data in a user friendly way requires further improvement. Also, with an increase in the number of OCT users and commercial systems, there is a need to establish adequate normative data and common clinical standards to allow for consistency across devices and comparison between patients and diseases.

5. Acknowledgment

Financial support is acknowledged to the Department of Defense (DOD) Telemedicine and Advanced Technology Research Center (TATRC), W81XWH-10-1-0738.

6. References

Adler, D.; Ko, T.; Konorev, A. et al. (2004). Broadband Light Source Based on Quantum-well Superluminescent Diodes for High-resolution Optical Coherence Tomography. *Quantum Electronics*, Vol. 34, No. 10, pp. 915-918, ISSN 1063-7818

Aguirre, A.; Nishizawa, N. & Fujimoto, J. (2006) Continuum Generation in a Novel Photonic Crystal Fiber for Ultrahigh Resolution Optical Coherence Tomography at 800 nm and 1300 nm. *Opt Express*, Vol. 14, No. 3, (Feb 2006), pp. 1145-1160, ISSN 1094-4087

Al-latayfeh, M.; Sun, J. & Aiello, L. P. (2010). Ocular coherence tomography and diabetic eye disease. *Semin Ophthal*, Vol. 25, No. 5-6, (Sept – Nov, 12010), pp. 192-197, ISSN 1744-5205

Apolonski, A.; Povazay, B.; Unterhuber, A. et al. (2002) Spectral shaping of supercontinuum in a cobweb photonic-Crytal Fiber with Sub-20-fs-pulses. *J Opt Soc Am A*, B Vol. 19, No.9, (Sept 2002), pp.2165-2170, ISSN 1084-7529

Birks, T.; Wadsworth, J. & Russel, P. (2000). Supercontinuum Generation in Tapered Fibers. *Opt Letters*, Vol. 25, No. 19, (Oct, 2000), pp. 1415-1417, ISSN 0146-9592

Budenz, D., Fredette, M., Feuer, W. et al. (2008). Reproducibility of peripapillary retinal nerve fiber thickness measurements with Stratus OCT in glaucomatous eyes. *Ophthalmology*, Vol. 115, No. 4, (Apr 2008), pp 661-666, ISSN 1549-4713

Carpineto, P.; Ciancaglini, M.; Zuppardi, E. et al. (2003). Reliability of nerve fiber layer thickness measurements using optic coherence tomography in normal and glaucomatous eyes. *Ophthalmol*, Vol. 110,No 1, (Jan 2003) pp 190-195, ISSN 1549-4713

Cense, B.; Koperda, E.; Brown, J. et al. (2009a). Volumetric Retinal Imaging with Ultra-high Resolution Spectral-Domain Optical Coherence Tomography and Adaptive Optics Using Two Broadband Light Sources. *Opt Express*, Vol. 17, No. 5, (Mar 2009), pp. 4095-4111, ISSN 1094-4087

Cense, B.; Gao, W.; Brown, J. et al., D.(2009b). Retinal Imaging with Polarization-Sensitive Optical Coherence Tomography and Adaptive Optics, *Opt Express*, Vol. 17. No. 24, (Nov 2009), pp. 21634-21651, ISSN 1094-4087

Choi, S.; Doble, N.; Lin, J. et al. (2005). Effect of Wavelength on in Vivo Images of the Human Cone Mosaic. *J Opt Soc Am A*, Vol. 22, No. 12, (Dec, 2005), pp. 2598–2605, ISSN 1084-7529

Choi, S.; Doble, N.; Hardy, J. et al. (2006) In vivo imaging of the photoreceptor mosaic in retinal dystrophies and correlations with visual function. *Invest Ophthalmol Vis Sci*, Vol. 47, No. 5, (May 2006), pp. 2080-2092, ISSN 1552-5783

Choi, S.; Zawadzki, R.; Keltner, J. et al. (2008). Changes in cellular structures revealed by ultra-high resolution retinal imaging in optic neuropathies. *Invest Ophthalmol Vis Sci*, Vol. 49, No. 5, (May 2008), pp. 2103-2119, ISSN 1552-5783

Choi, S.; Zawadzki, R.; Lim, M. et al. (2011). Evidence of outer retinal changes in glaucoma patients as revealed by ultrahigh-resolution in vivo retinal imaging. *Br J Ophthalmol*, Vol. 95, No. , (Jan 2011), pp. 131-141, ISSN 0007-1161

Clivaz, X.; Marquis-Weible, F. & Salathe, R. (1992). Optical Low Coherence Reflectometry with 1.9 μm Spatial Resolution. *Elect Letters*, Vol. 28, No. 16, (Jul 1992), pp.1553-1555, ISSN 0013-5194

Coen, S. & Haelterman, M. (2001). Continuous-wave Ultrahigh-repetition-rate Pulse-train Generation Through Modulational Instability in a Passive Fiber Cavity. *Opt Letters*, Vol. 26, No. 1, (Jan 2001), pp. 39-41 , ISSN 0146-9592

de Boer, J.; Cense, B.; Park, B. et al. (2003). Improved Signal-to-Noise Ratio in Spectral Domain Compared with Time-Domain Optical Coherence Tomography. *Opt Letters*, Vol. 28, No. 21 , (Nov 2003), pp. 2067-2069, ISSN 0146-9592

Dreher, A.; Billie, J. & Weinreb, R. (1989). Active Optical Depth Resolution Improvement of the Laser Tomographic Scanner. *Appl Opt*, Vol. 28, No. 4, (Apr 1989), pp. 804–808, ISSN 0003-6935

Drexler, W.; Mogner, U.; Kartner, F et al. (1999). In vivo Ultrahigh-resolution Optical Coherence Tomography. *Opt Letters*, Vol. 24, No. 17, (Sept 1999), pp. 1221-1223, ISSN 0146-9592

Drexler, W.; Morgner, U.; Ghanta, R. et al. (2001). Ultrahigh-resolution Ophthalmic Optical Coherence Tomography. *Nat Med*, Vol. 7, No. 4, (Apr 2001), pp. 502-507, ISSN 1078-8956

Drexler, W.; Sattman, H.; Hermann B. et al. (2003). Enhanced Visualization of Macular Pathology With the Use of Ultrahigh-Resolution Optical Coherence Tomography. *Arch of Ophthalmol*, Vol. 121, No. 5, (May 2003), pp. 695-706, ISSN 0003-9950

Drexler, W. (2004). Ultrahigh-resolution Optical Coherence Tomography. *J Biomed Opt*, Vol .9, No. 1, (Jan/Feb 2004), pp. 47-74, ISSN 1083-3668

Doble, N. & Miller, D. (2006). Wavefront Correctors for Vision Science, In: *Adaptive Optics for Vision Science*, J. Porter, H. Queener, J. Lin, K. Thorn, A. Awwal (Ed) , pp. 82-117, ISBN 978-0-471-67941-7, Hoboken, NJ, USA.

Fercher, A.; Mengedoht, K. & Werner, W. (1988) Eye-length Measurement by Interferometry with Partially Coherent Light. *Opt Letters*, Vol. 13, No. 3, (Mar 1988), pp. 186-188, ISSN 0146-9592

Fernandez, E.; Iglesias, I. & Artal, P. 2001. Closed-loop Adaptive Optics in the Human Eye. (2001). *Opt Express*, Vol. 26, No. 10, (May, 2001), pp. 746-748, ISSN 0146-9592

Ferguson, R.; Hammer, D.; Paunescu, L. et al. Tracking Optical Coherence Tomography. *Opt Letters*, Vol. 29, No. 18, (Sept 2004), pp. 2139-2141, ISSN 0146-9592

Fujimoto, J; De Silvestri, S.; Ippen, E. et al. (1986). Femtosecond Optical Ranging in Biological Systems. *Opt Letters*, Vol. 11, No. 3, (Mar 1986), pp. 150-152, ISSN 0146-9592

Hartl, I.; Li, X.; Chudoba, C. et al. (2001). Ultrahigh-resolution Optical Coherence Tomography Using Continuum Generation in a Air-Silica Microstructure Optical Fiber. *Opt Letters*, Vol. 26, No. 9, (May 2001), pp. 608-610, ISSN 0146-9592

Hee, M.; Puliafifito C.; Duker, J. et al. (1998). Topography of diabetic macualr edema with optical coherence tomography. *Ophthalmology*, Vol. 105, No. 2, (Feb 1998), pp. 360-370, ISSN 1549-4713

Hofer, H.; Chen, L.; Yoon, G. et al. (2001). Improvement in Retinal Image Quality with Dynamic Correction of the Eye's Aberrations. *Opt Express*, Vol. 8, No. 11, (May 2001), pp. 631–643, ISSN 0146-9592

Hong, Y.;Makita, S.; Yamanari, M. et al. (2007). Three-dimensional Visualization of Choroidal Vessels by Using SStandard and Ultra-high Resolution Optical Coherence Tomography. *Opt Express*, Vol. 15, No. 12, (Jun 2007), pp. 7538-7550, ISSN 0146-9592

Huang, D.; Swanson, E.; Lin, C. et al. (1991). Optical Coherence Tomography. *Science*, Vol. 254, No.5035 , (Nov 1991), pp.1178-1181, ISSN 0036-8075

Humbert, G.; Wadsworth, W.; Leon-Saval, G. et al. (2006). Supercontinuum Gneration System for Optical Coherence Tomography based on Tapered Photonic Crytal Fibre. *Opt Express*, Vol. 14, No. 4, (Feb 2006), pp. 1596-1603.

Jaffe, G. J. & Caprioli, J. (2004). Optical coherence tomography to detect and manage retinal disease and glaucoma. *Am J Ophthalmol*, Vol. 137, No. 1, (Jan 20044), pp. 156-169, ISSN 0002-9394

Jonall, R.; Rha, J.; Zhang, Y et al. (2007). In Vivo Functional Imaging of Human Cone Photoreceptors. *Opt Express*, Vol. 15, No. 24, (Nov 2007), pp 16141-16160, ISSN 0146-9592

Jungtae, R.; Jonnal, R.; Thorn, K., et al. (2006). Adaptive Optics Flood-Illumination Camera for High Speed Retinal Imaging. *Opt Express*, Vol. 14. No. 10, (May 2006), pp. 4552-4569, ISSN 0146-9592

Khanifar, A.; Koreishi, A.; Izatt, J. et al. (2008). Drusen ultrastructure imaging with spectral domain optical coherence tomography in age-related macular degeneration. *Ophthalmology*, Vol. 115, No. 11, (Nov 2008), pp.1883-1890, ISSN 1549-4713

Ko, T.; Adler, D.; Fujimoto, J. et al.. (2004). Ultrahigh Resolution Optical Coherence Tomography Imaging with a Broadband Superluminscent Diode Light Source. *Opt Express*, Vol 12, No. 10, (May 2004), pp. 2112-2119, ISSN 1094-4087

Kocaoglu, O.; Cense, B.; Jonnal, R. et al. (2011). Imaging Retinal Nerve Fiber Bundles Using Optical Coherence Tomography with Adaptive Optics. *Vision Res*, Vol. 51, No. 16, (Aug 2011), pp. 1835-1844, ISSN 42-6989

Leng, T.; Rosenfeld, P.; Puliafito, G. et al. (2009). Spectral domain optical coherence tomography characteriatics of cuticular drusen. *Retina*, Vol. 29, No. 7, (Jul-Aug 2009),pp. 988-993, ISSN 1539-2864

Liang, J.; Williams, D.; & Miller, D. (1997). Supernormal Vision and High-Resolution Retinal Imaging Through Adaptive Optics. *J Opt Soc Am A*, Vol. 14 No. 11, (May, 2007), pp. 2884–2892, ISSN 1084-7529

Lietgeb, R.; Hitzenberger, C. & Fercher, A. (2003). Performance of Fourier Domain vs. Time Domain Optical Coherence Tomography. *Opt Express*, Vol. 11, No. 8, (Apr 2003), pp.889-894, ISSN 0146-9592

Mujat, M.; Ferguson, D.; Patel, A. et al. (2010). High Resolution Multimodal Clinical Ophthalmic Imaging System. *Opt Express*, Vol. 18, No. 11, (May 2010), pp. 11607–11621, ISSN 0146-9592

Ontani, T.; Kishi, S. & Maruyama, Y. (1999) Patterns of diabetic macular edema with optical coherence tomography. *Am J Ophthalmol*, Vol. 127, No. 6,(Jun 1999) pp. 688-693, ISSN 0002-9394

Park, S.; Truong, S., Zawadzki, R. et al. (2010). High-resolution Fourier-domain Optical Coherence Tomography of Choroidal Neovascular Membranes Associated with Age-related Macular Degeneration. *Invest Ophthalmol Vis Sci.*, Vol. 51, No. 8, (Aug 2010), pp. 4200-4206, ISSN 1552-5783

Pieroni, C.; Witkin, A.; Ko, T et al. (2006). Ultrahigh resolution optical coherence tomographyin non-exudative age-related macular degeneration. *Br J Ophthalmol*, Vol. 90, No. 2, (Feb 2006), pp. 191-197, ISSN 0007-1161

Potsaid, B.; Gorczynska, I.; Srinivasan, V. et al. (2008). Ultrahigh Speed Spectra/Fourier Domain OCT Opthalmic Imaging at 70,000 to 312,500 Axial Scans per Second. *Ophthalmol Express*, Vol. 16, No. 19, (Sept 2008), pp. 15149–15169, ISSN 0146-9592

Povazay, B.; Bizheva, K.; Hermann, A. et al. (2003). Enhanced Visualization of Choroidal Vessels using Ultrahigh Resolution Ophthalmic OCT at 1050 nm. *Opt Express*, Vol. 11, No. 17, (Aug 2003), pp. 1980-1986, ISSN 0146-9592

Puvanathasan, P.; Forbes, P.; Ren, Z. et al. (2008). High-speed, high resolution Fourier-domain optical coherence tomography system for retinal imaging in the 1060 nm wavelength region. *Opt Letters*, Vol. 21, No. 21, (Nov 2008) pp. 2479-2481, ISSN 0146-9592

Roorda, A. & Williams D. (2002a). Optical Fiber Properties of Individual Human Cones. *J Vis*, Vol. 2, No. 5, (Apr, 2002), pp. 404–412, ISSN 1534-7362

Roorda, A.; Romero-Borja, F.; Donnely, W. et al. Adaptive Optics Laser Scanning Opthalmoscopy. (2002b). *Opt Express*, Vol. 10, No. (May 2002), pp. 405-412, ISSN 0146-9592

Sandhu, S. & Talks S. (2005). Correlation of optical coherence tomography, with or without additional colour fundus photography, with stereo fundus fluorescein angiography in diagnosing choroidal neovascular membranes. *Br J Ophthalmol*, Vol. 89, No. 8, (Aug 2005), pp. 967-970, ISSN 0007-1161

Schocket, L.; Wikins A.; Fujimoto, J. et al. (2006). Ultrahigh-Resolution Optical Coherence Tomography in Patients with Decreased Visual Acuity after Retinal Detachment Repair. *Ophthalmol*, Vol. 113, No. 4, (Apr 2006), pp. 666-692, ISSN 0161-6420

Schuman, S.; Koreishi, A.; Farsiu, S. et al. (2009). Photoreceptor layer thinning over drusen in eyes with age-related macular degeneration imaged in vivo with sepctral domain optical coherence tomography. *Ophthalmol*, Vol. 116, No. 3, (Mar 2009), pp. 488-496, ISSN 1549-4713

Sihota, R.; Sony, P.; Gupta, V. et al. (2006). Diagnostic Capability of Optical Coherence Tomography in Evaluating the Degree of Glaucomatous Retinal Nerve Fiber Damage. *Invest Ophthalmol Vis Sci*, Vol. 47, No. 5, (), pp 2006-2010, , ISSN 1552-5783

Singh, R. & Kaiser, P. K. (2007). Advances in AMD imaging. *Int Ophthalmol Clin*, Vol. 47, No. 1 (Winter 2007), pp. 65-74, ISSN 0020-8167

Spoler, F.; Kray, S.; Grychtol, P. et al. (2007). Simultaneous Dual-band Ultra-high Resolution Optical Coherence Tomography. *Opt Express*, Vol. 15, No. 17, (Aug 2007), pp. 10832-10841, ISSN 1094-4087

Srinivasan, V.; Monson, B.; Wojtkowski, M. et al. (2006). High-Definition and 3-dimensional Imaging of Macular Pathologies with High-speed Ultrahigh-Resolution Optical Coherence Tomography, *Ophthalmology*, Vol. 113, No. 11, (Nov 2006), pp. 2054-2065, ISSN 1549-4713

Srinivasan, V.; Monson, B.; Wojtkowski, M. et al. (2008). Characterization of Outer Retinal Morphology with High-Speed, Ultrahigh-Resolution Optical Coherence Tomography. *Invest Ophthalmol Vis Sci*, Vol. 49, No. 4, (Apr 2008), pp. 1571-1579, ISSN 0146-0404

Swanson, E.; Izatt, J.; Hee, M. et al. (1993). In Vivo Retinal Imaging by Optical Coherence Tomography. *Opt Letters*, Vol. 18, No. 21,(Nov 1993), pp. 1864-1866, ISSN 0146-9592

Tao, Y.; Farsiu, S. & Izatt, J. (2010). Interlaced Spectrally Encoded Confocal Scanning Laser Ophthalmoscopy and Spectral Domain Optical Coherence Tomography. *Biomed Opt Express*, Vol. 1, No. 2, (Sept 2010), pp. 431-440, ISSN 0146-9592

Unterhuber, A.; Povazay, B; Hermann, B. et al. (2003). Compact, Low-cost Ti:Al2O3 Laser for In Vivo Ultrahigh-resolution Optical Coherence Tomography. *Opt Letters*, Vol. 28, No. 11 (Jun 2003), pp. 905-907, ISSN 0146-9592

Witkin, A.; Ho, T.; Fujimoto, J, et al. (2006). Ultra-high Resolution Optical Coherence Tomography Assessment of Photoreceptros in Retinintis Pigmentosa and Related Diseases. *Am J Ophthalmol*, Vol. 142, No. 6, (Dec 2006), pp.945-952, ISSN 0002-9394

Wolfing, J.; Chung, M.; Carroll, J. et al. (2006). High Resolution Imaging of Cone-Rod Dystrophy with Adaptive Optics. *Ophthalmology*, Vol. 113, No. 6, (Jun 2006), pp. 1014-101, ISSN 1549-4713

Xue, B.; Choi, S.; Doble, N. et al. (2007). Photoreceptor counting and montaging of en-face retinal iamges from an adaptive optics fundus camera. *J Opt Soc Am A*, Vol. 24, Issue 5, (Apr 2007) , pp. 1364-1372, ISSN 1084-7529

Zawadazki, R.; Jones, S.; Olivier, S. et al. (2005). Adaptive-Optics Optical Coherence Tomography for High-Resolution and High-Speed 3D Retinal In Vivo Imaging. *Opt Express*, Vol. 13, No. 21, (Oct 2005), pp. 8532-8546, ISSN 0146-9592

Zawadzki, R.; Choi, S.; Olivier, S. et al. (2007). *J Opt Soc Am A*, Vol. 24, Issue 5, (May 2007) , pp. 1373-1383, ISSN 1084-7529

Zawadzki, R.; Cense, B.; Zhang, Y. et al. (2008). Ultrahigh-resolution Optical Coherence Tomography with Monochromatic and Chromatic Aberration Correction. *Opt Express*, Vol. 16, No. 11, (May 2008), pp. 8126-8143, ISSN 1094-4087

Zawadazki, R., Jones, S., Chen, D. et al. (2009). Combined Adaptive Optics - Optical Coherence Tomography and Adaptive Optics - Scanning Laser Ophthalmoscopy System for Retinal Imaging, *Proceed of SPIE*, ISBN 9780819474094, San Jose, CA, USA, Jan 24, 2009

Zawadzki, R.; Jone, S.; Pilli, S.; Balderas-Mata, S.; Kim, D.; Olivier, S. & Werner, J. (2011) Integrated Adaptive Optics Optical Coherence Tomography and Adaptive Optics Scanning Laser Ophthalmoscope System for Simultaneous Cellular Resolution In Vivo Retinal Imaging. *Biomed Opt Express*, Vol. 2, No. 6, (May 2011), pp. 1674-1686, ISSN 0146-9592

8

Spectral-Domain Optical Coherence Tomography in Hereditary Retinal Dystrophies

Isabelle Meunier et al.*
Centre national de Référence Maladies Sensorielles Génétiques, Hôpital Gui de Chauliac and INSERM U583, Institute for Neurosciences of Montpellier, France

1. Introduction

Inherited retinal diseases are rare disorders that affect 40 000 to 50 000 individuals in France. They represent 20% of cases of blindness in subjects younger than 20 years of age. There is great clinical and genetic diversity among these dystrophies: diversity at the clinical level ranging from mild maculopathies to Leber's congenital amaurosis; diversity among genes and modes of transmission (more than 150 known genes expressed in the retina). Non-syndromic retinitis pigmentosa is the most common among hereditary dystrophies (fig 1) (Berger et al, 2010).

Devices for time-domain optical coherence tomography and, more recently, spectral-domain optical coherence tomography (spectral OCT) with an improved depth resolution of 7µm (wavelength 840nm, scannong speed 27 000 to 40 000 scans per second) carry out a non-invasive and in vivo visualization of the retinal layers, particularly the outer nuclear layer (ONL), the photoreceptor inner segment/outer segment junction (IS/OS) and the retinal pigment epithelium (RPE) (fig 2). Hence, the integrity or abnormality of the retinal pigment epithelium, the inner/outer segment junction, and the external limiting membrane can be analyzed even during early stages of inherited retinal diseases, when the fundus appears normal on examination.

Several commercial spectral OCT are available for posterior segment imaging (Cirrus HD-OCT, Carl Zeiss Meditec, with a speed of 27 000 scans per second and a resolution of 5µ - Spectralis OCT, Heidelberg Engineering, with a speed of 40 000 scans per second and a resolution of 7µ - RTVue-100, Optovue, with a speed of 26 000 scans per second and a

---

* Carl Arndt[2], Xavier Zanlonghi[3], Sabine Defoort-Dhellemmes[4], Isabelle Drumare[4], Martine Mauget-Faysse[5], Benjamin Wolff[5], Aude Affortit[6], Christian Hamel[1] and Bernard Puech[4]

1 Centre national de Référence Maladies Sensorielles Génétiques, Hôpital Gui de Chauliac and INSERM U583, Institute for Neurosciences of Montpellier, France

2 Eye clinic, Hôpital Robert Debré, CHRU de Reims, France

3 Sourdille Clinic, Nantes, France

4 Service d'Exploration de la Vision et Neuro-ophtalmologie, Hôpital Robert Salengro, CHU de Lille, France

5 Centre d'Imagerie et de Laser Rabelais, Lyon, France

6 Rothschild Fondation, Pediatric Eye department, Paris, France resolution of 5μ - Copernicus HR, Optopol technologies, with a speed of 52 000 scans per second and a resolution of 3μ). OCT scans presented in this article were obtained with a Spectralis OCT, Heidelberg Engineering.

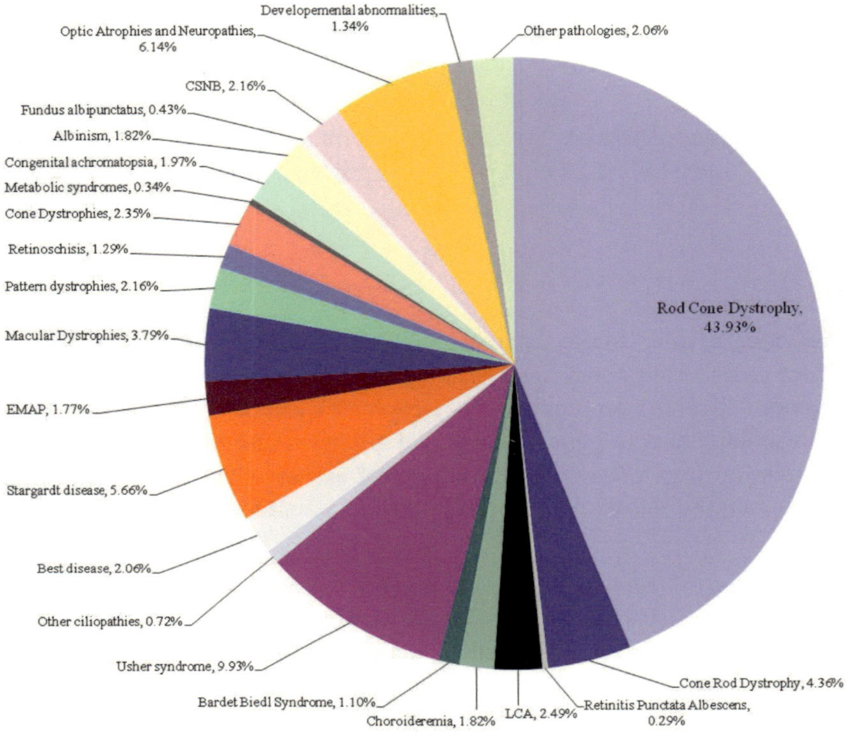

Fig. 1. Prevalence of retinal dystrophies by disease in terms of percentage of affected individuals, from the database of the National Center for Rare Sensory and Genetic Diseases, Montpellier, France. EMAP : Extensive macular atrophy with pseudo-drusen.

After this recapitulation of hereditary dystrophies and normal OCT scan, we will describe OCT anomalies in rod-cone (retinitis pigmentosa, RP), cone-rod (CRD) and progressive cone dystrophies (COD), followed by the principal hereditary maculopathies.

2. Definition and classifications of hereditary retinal dystrophies

A retinal dystrophy is to be considered when there is bilateral, symmetric (except in vitelliform dystrophies and pattern dystrophies) and evolutive visual damage in the absence of inflammatory, toxic or paraneoplastic causes. The evolutive character of the damage is an essential criterion related to the progressive degeneration of photoreceptors, which allows these disorders to be distinguished from other non-evolutive causes of loss of sight such as albinism, congenital essential night blindness and other congenital disorders (embryopathies). The notion of a familial disorder is an important argument, but its absence does not exclude a genetic cause (unique single cases of a recessive disorder).

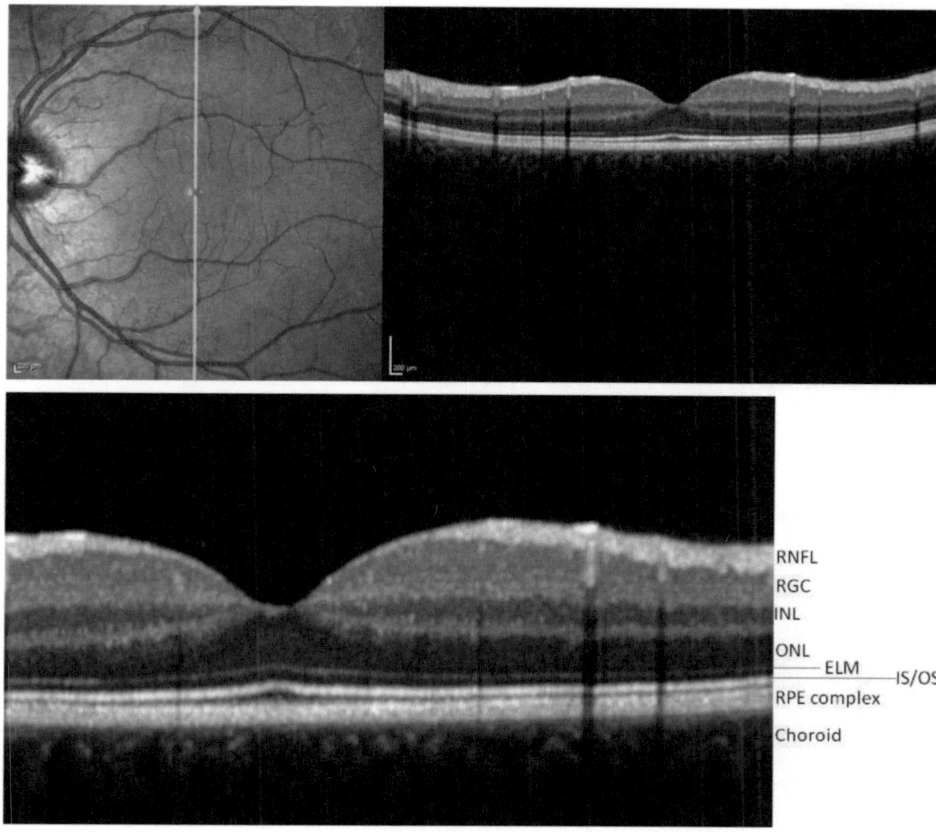

Fig. 2. Red free photography and corresponding OCT scan (top left and right) of a normal eye, in vivo visualization of the main retinal layers. Magnified OCT scan (bottom). RNFL: retinal nerve fiber layer. RGC: retinal ganglion cell layer, nuclei of the third set of neurons. INL: inner nuclear layer, nuclei of the second set of neurons. ONL: outer nuclear layer, nuclei of the first set of neurons, i.e. the photoreceptors. ELM: external limiting membrane. IS/OS: inner segment/outer segment. RPE: retinal pigment epithelium.

Macular diseases with or without autofluorescent deposits can be differentiated into progressive cone dystrophies, cone-rod dystrophies (cone-dominant diseases), retinitis pigmentosa (rod-dominant diseases), chorioretinal dystrophies and erosive vitroretinopathies. Macular diseases compromise central vision (loss of reading, writing and facial recognition functions), while mixed central and peripheral dystrophies can lead to a complete loss of vision.

From a genetic point of view, cones, rods or retinal pigment epithelial cells express the genetic dysfunction, but the damage may occur predominantly in the macular area due to differences in the level of metabolism or the deleterious accumulation of lipofuscin. In addition, a given gene could lead to different clinical profiles (macular damage, cone-rod dystrophy or rod-cone dystrophy) of varying severity, with inter- and intra-familial variations. For example, the genes involved in COD are also associated with CRD.

3. Spectral OCT in retinitis pigmentosa, cone-rod dystrophy and cone dystrophy

In these dystrophies related to photoreceptor and RPE apoptosis, OCT in combination with fundus autofluorescence imaging is of great use in the analysis of the pattern and extent of neurosensory retinal disorganization in the macular zone. These modifications are apparent right from the early stages of the disease, before any macular changes are visible on fundus examination.

3.1 Retinitis pigmentosa

Retinitis pigmentosa is characterized by night blindness, primary progressive visual field defects and, eventually, the loss of central vision and legal blindness.

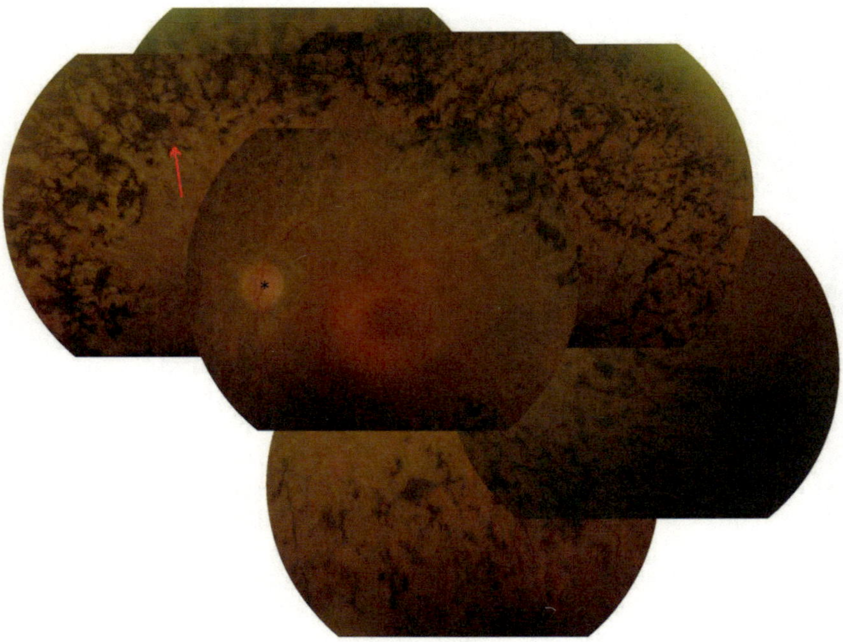

Fig. 3. A 32-year-old man with retinitis pigmentosa. Typical bony spicules of the peripheral retina (arrow), attenuation of retinal blood vessels. There is no pallor of the optic nerve head yet (*).

OCT reveals the disruption or disappearance of the inner segment/outer segment junction (IS/OS) at one or more extrafoveal locations from early stages, even though the macula is normal on fundus examination. Disorganization of the IS/OS junction is an early indication of dysfunction and loss of photoreceptors in retinitis pigmentosa. Progressive PR loss is subsequently reflected by a diminution of the thickness of the ONL (nuclei of photoreceptors) and RPE complex (fig 4-6).

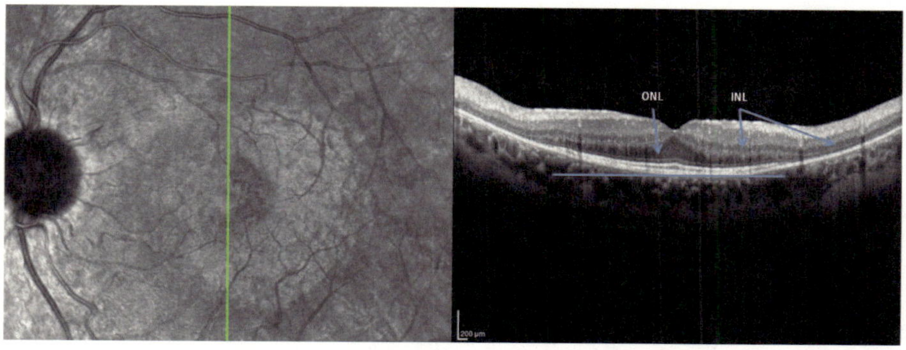

Fig. 4. Red free photography (left) and corresponding OCT scan of a 34-year-old man with retinitis pigmentosa. The IS/OS junction is only visible in the foveal zone, marked by a blue bar. Outside this zone, no IS/OS junction, ELM, or ONL is observed.

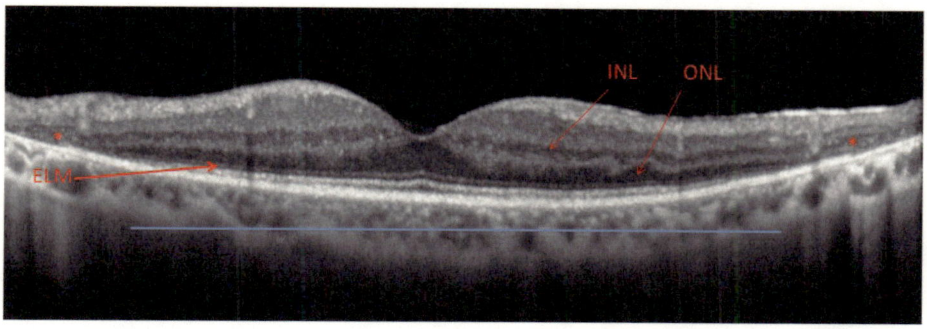

Fig. 5. OCT scan of a 20-year-old woman with retinitis pigmentosa. The IS/OS junction is visible in the entire foveal zone, marked by a blue bar. Outside the fovea, no IS/OS junction, ELM, or ONL is observed, and there is in addition a disorganization of the INL (*) with a marked reduction in total retinal thickness.

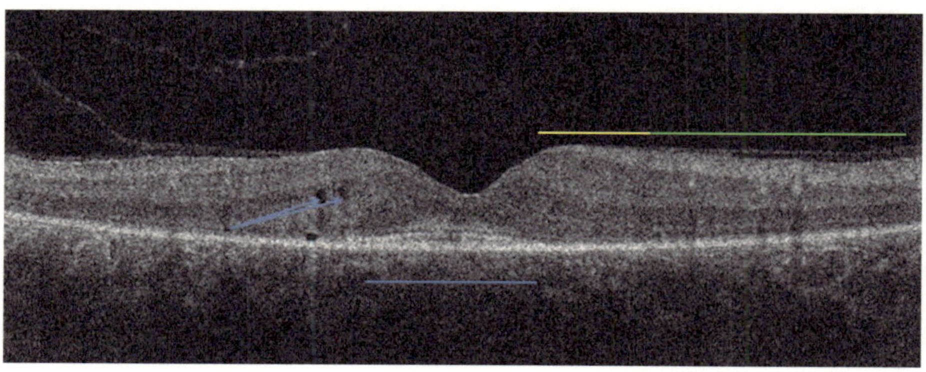

Fig. 6. OCT scan of a 32-year-old man with retinitis pigmentosa. Only the subfoveal part of the IS/OS junction is preserved (blue bar). Visual acuity is normal as long as the subfoveal IS/OS is present. Outside the macula, no IS/OS junction or ELM is observed (green bar). The ELM can still be noted in the perifoveal zone (yellow bar). Note several cystic spaces in the inner nuclear layer (blue arrows).

3.2 Progressive cone dystrophies

Affected individuals report decreased visual acuity. They mention progressive intense photophobia and variable degrees of color vision abnormalities. The degenerative process predominates in cones but not in rods, as in retinitis pigmentosa (fig 6).

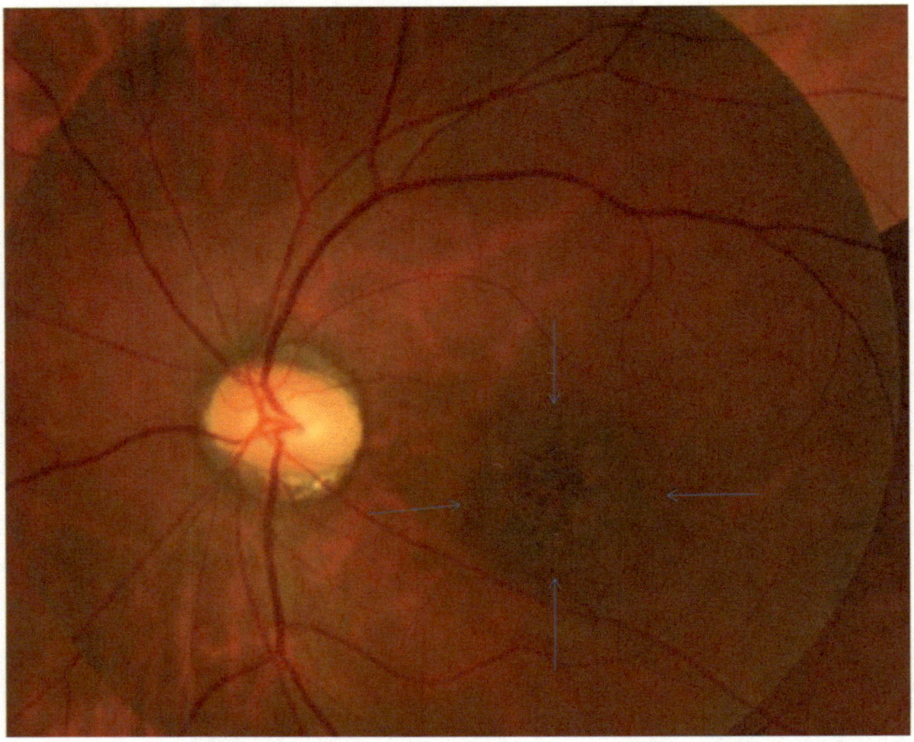

Fig. 7. Fundus photograph of a 17-year-old boy with progressive cone dystrophy. Visual acuity is 20/200. The patient is very photophobic. The macula is modified with a typical bull's eye pattern. The vessels are moderately attenuated. The peripheral retina is normal. An electroretinogram (ERG) is required to confirm that rod responses are within normal values.

The OCT pattern is reversed in cone dystrophies: the disorganization of the IS/OS junction is observed in and limited to the fovea and the perifoveal zone. The thinning of the ONL is progressive and easily recognized in the fovea where the INL and GCL are not present (fig 8, 9). OCT anomalies are again noted at early stages, and precede the reorganization of the macula on biomicroscopic examination (fig 8).

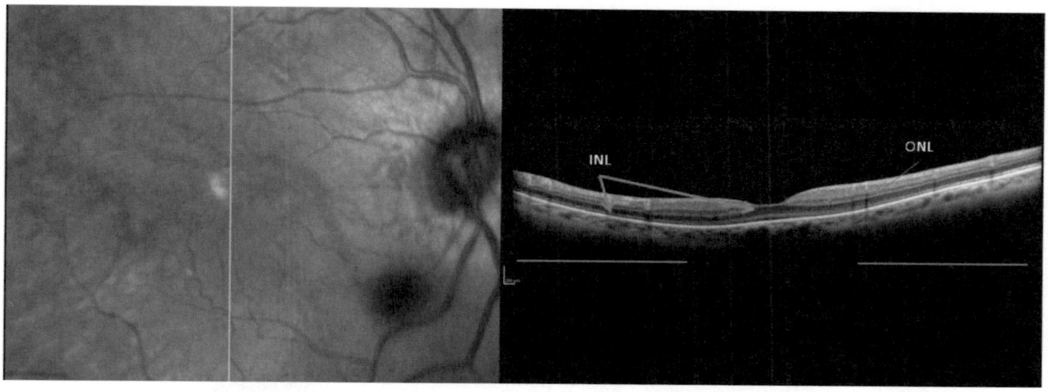

Fig. 8. Red free photography (left) and corresponding OCT scan of a young boy with a visual acuity of 20/200 in both eyes (right). The IS/OS junction is normal in the extrafoveal regions (blue bars). In the central zone, the IS/OS junction is disorganized, and the INL is not as developed as it should be in the foveola (compared with figure 2). The macula appears normal in the red free photograph (left).

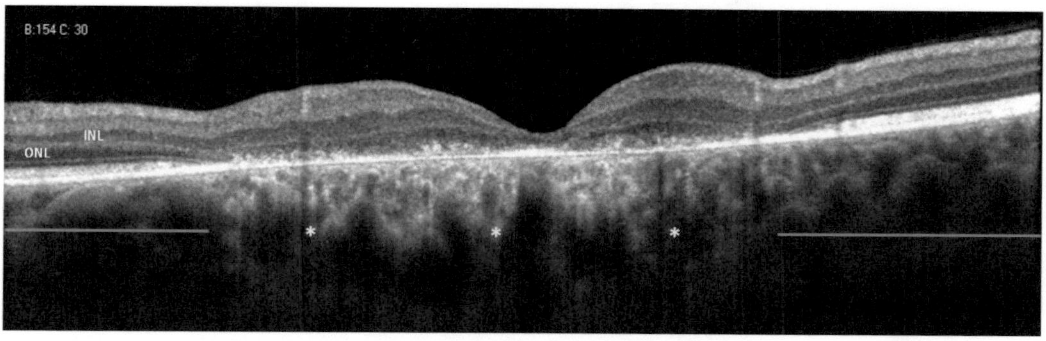

Fig. 9. OCT scan at a more advanced stage of cone dystrophy. Outside the fovea (blue bars), the ONL is very thin in comparison with the INL. In the fovea and perifoveal zone (between the blue bars), no IS/OS junction or ELM is observed. Note the hyperreflective signal of the choroid, related to RPE loss (*).

3.3 Cone-rod dystrophy

Cone-rod dystrophies (CRDs) belong to the group of pigmentary retinopathies (fig 10). They are characterized by the progressive damage of photoreceptors, predominantly cones. CRDs are remarkable for the precocity of the loss of visual acuity and the rapid evolution towards central and peripheral visual loss. The evolutive sequence here is the inverse of that in retinitis pigmentosa: night blindness and anomalies of the peripheral visual field appear after macular damage, and may remain of in the background. An ERG is unavoidable to distinguish the first stages of a CRD, in which the patient may not mention night blindness or problems with the peripheral visual field, from pure maculopathies (including cone dystrophies), which pose no threat to peripheral vision. The frequency of CRDs (1/40 000) is ten times less than that of retinitis pigmentosa (RCD).

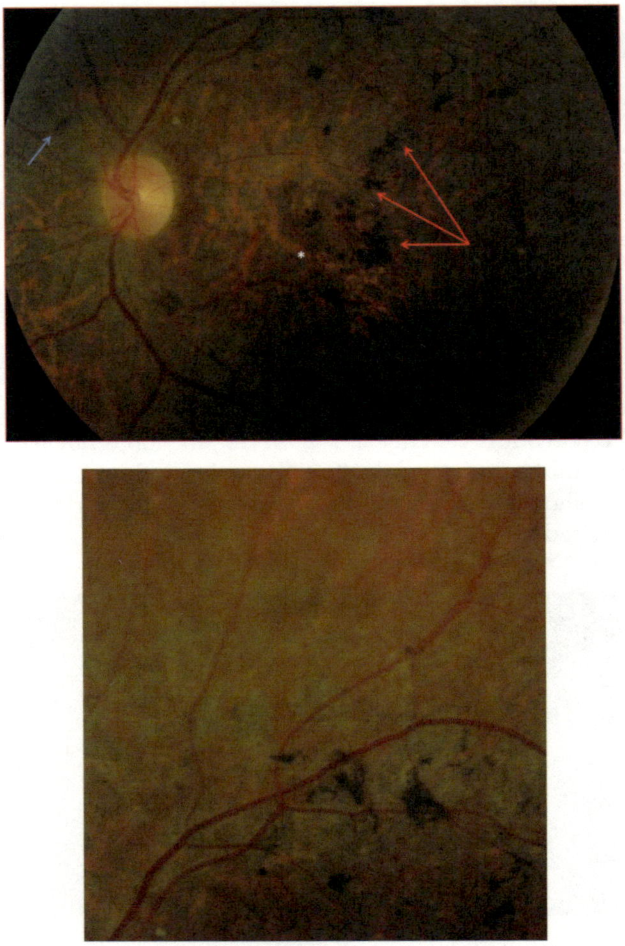

Fig. 10. Fundus of a 17-year-old girl with CRD linked to *ABCA4* (the Stargardt gene). Note the presence of pigment deposits of various shapes (red arrows) in the posterior pole with atrophy of the retina (left). The retina appears less damaged in the periphery (right).

The thinning of the neurosensory retina and the discontinuity or loss of the IS/OS junction are very early signs, occurring before any macular reorganization (fig 11). The loss of photoreceptors may predominate in the foveolar or perifoveolar zones (CRD related to *ABCA4*) or be diffuse as in retinitis pigmentosa. This is different from the case in pure cone dystrophies, in which the photoreceptor layer is still present and continues beyond the perifoveolar zone.

3.4 Final stages of RP, COD and CRD

The IS/OS junction and the EML are not observed and the ONL is extremely thin or even absent. Indeed, RP and CRD display the same pattern at this stage (fig 12). Cone dystrophies can be separated from CRD or RP, based on the fact that the IS/OS junction is still preserved outside the macula (fig 13).

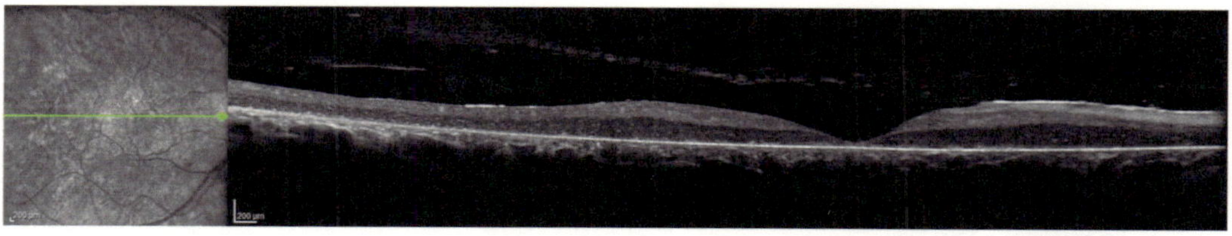

Fig. 12. Red free photography (left) and corresponding OCT, final stage of retinitis pigmentosa or cone-rod dystrophy. No IS/OS junction, EML or ONL can be observed at any point of the section.

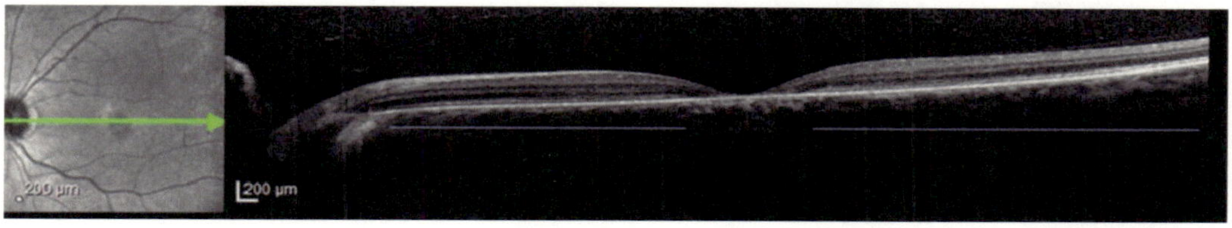

Fig. 13. Red free photography (left) and corresponding OCT, final stage of a cone dystrophy. Visual acuity is 20/100 in both eyes. The macula is atrophic. The defect is small, limited to the fovea (between blue bars). The retina is thin outside the fovea despite the presence of the IS/OS junction. Note that the INL and ONL are thin.

3.5 Macular edema in RP

The principal complication is the occurrence of macular edema, with an estimated frequency of 50% for autosomal dominant forms and 30% for recessive forms. Macular edema has been rarely observed in X-linked forms. OCT is relevant to the diagnosis of macular edema and for the evaluation of the therapeutic effectiveness of acetazolamide in patients with RP. The prognosis depends on the preservation of the IS/OS junction (fig 14-16) below the central cystic space corresponding to the foveola (Hyewon et al, 2006; Sandberg et al, 2008).

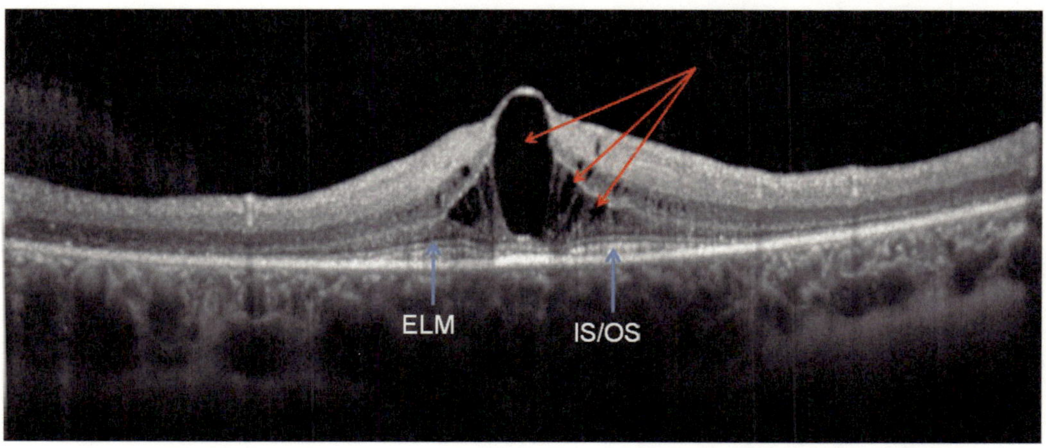

Fig. 14. Cystoid macular edema with large intraretinal cystic spaces. The IS/OS junction is present below the edema, with the exception of the central cyst.

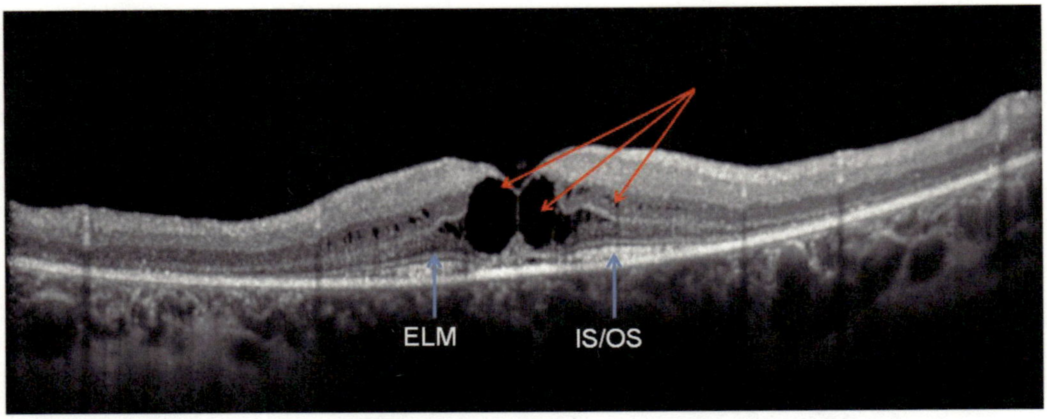

Fig. 15. Same patient as in figure 14, other eye. The thickening of the fovea is less pronounced than in the right eye. The IS/OS junction is present below the edema, with the exception of the two central cysts.

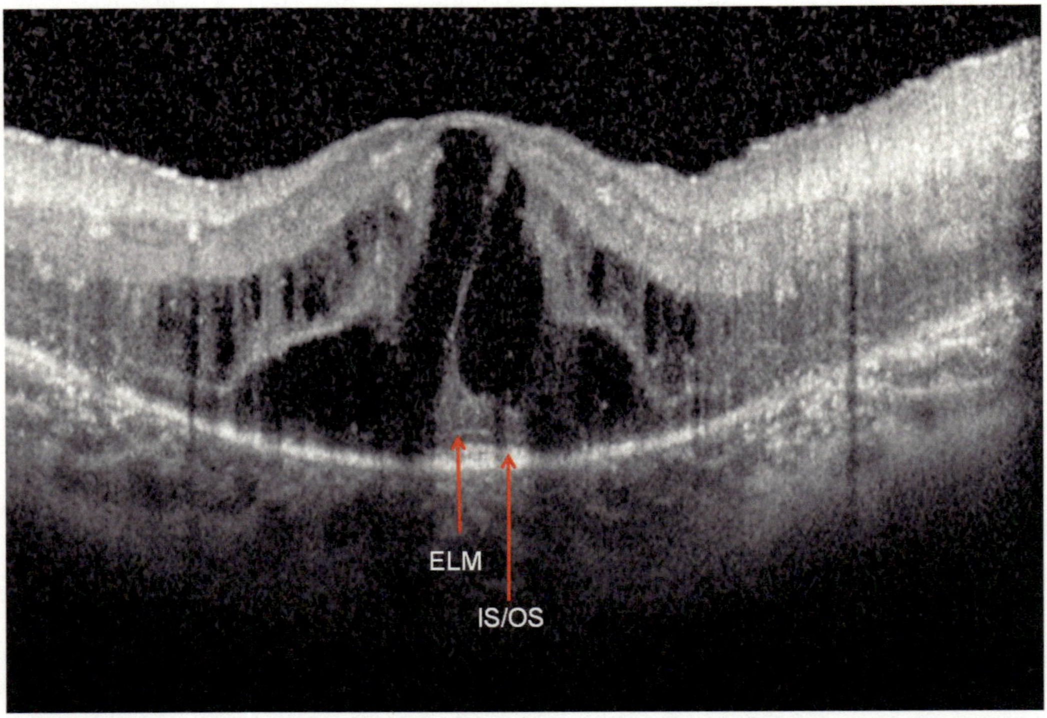

Fig. 16. Severe cystoid macular edema with preserved IS/OS junction below the central cystic space. Visual acuity could be improved by treatment with acetazolamide.

4. Inherited macular diseases

This term is used to indicate maculopathies with or without autofluorescent deposits and those with drusen (or drusen-like lesions). These maculopathies are for the most part non-syndromic. Photophobia, early anomalies of color vision and a decrease in central vision are the principal criteria characterizing these maculopathies. These signs are present to varying degrees: photophobia is a major sign in cone dystrophy, but less obvious in Best disease. Neither night blindness nor any substantial reduction in the peripheral visual field is seen. The loss of visual acuity may be asymmetric but the lesions are symmetric, except in vitelliform dystrophies and pattern dystrophies.

4.1 Stargardt disease

Described by Stargardt in 1909, Stargardt disease is a bilateral symmetric maculopathy, characterized by the presence of a variable number of fish-scale shaped, yellowish, autofluorescent deposits (fig 17,18). This maculopathy, which has an autosomal recessive transmission linked to the *ABCA4* gene, is the most frequent of juvenile maculopathies with a prevalence of 1 in 10 000, and represents 7% of hereditary diseases. In Stargardt disease, the degeneration of photoreceptors (PR) expressing a genetic abnormality is thus secondary to the loss of pigment epithelial cells. The preferential macular damage is explained by the high density of cones and rods in the perifoveolar and foveolar zones. There is an early and severe loss of visual acuity, even if the reorganization of the fundus appears to be slight. Visual acuity stabilizes at around 20/200 to 20/400.

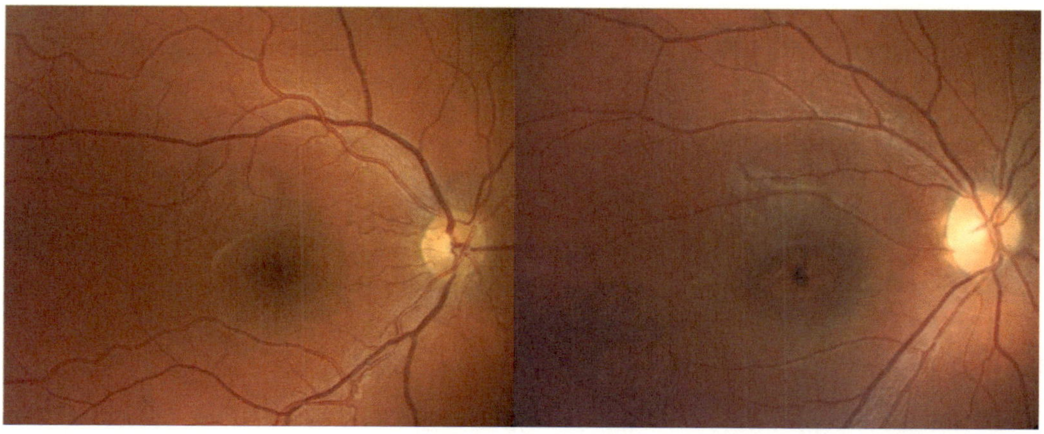

Fig. 17. Fundus photographs at different stages of Stargardt disease. Left: the macula appears normal in spite of a visual acuity of 20/100 in both eyes in a 12-year-old child. Note the absence of retinal flecks. Right: Oval reorganization of the macula (dark in appearance) along the major horizontal axis in a 9-year-old child with visual acuity limited to 20/200 in both eyes. Visual acuity was at 20/30 at the end of preschool. A few rounded yellowish deposits can be seen temporally.

OCT anomalies occur very early in Stargardt disease including loss of the foveal clivus, discontinuity or loss of the photoreceptor layer (Ergun et al, 2005; Querques et al, 2006). They precede the occurrence of fundus abnormalities. As the zone with the highest density of photoreceptors, the perifoveolar zone is preferentially affected. Thus, OCT reveals a premature loss of the clivus and the photoreceptor layer throughout the zone of macular reorganization defined by autofluorescence images, with a thinning of the retina (fig 19-22). This is very different from the aspect of cone dystrophies in OCT (initial and predominant

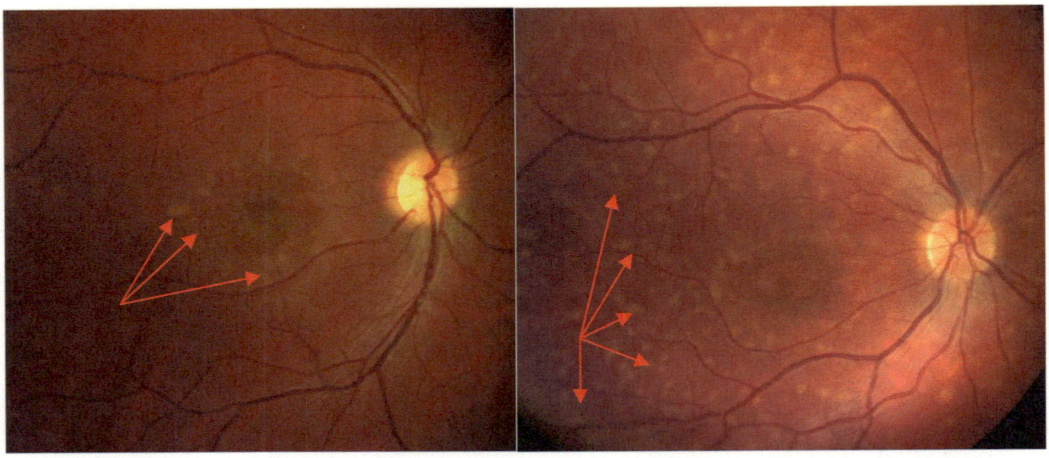

Fig. 18. Left: Macular reorganizations associated with yellowish perifoveolar retinal flecks immediately reminiscent of Stargardt disease in a 19-year-old subject with a visual acuity of 20/40 P2. Right: A 24-year-old subject with a visual acuity of 20/200 in both eyes. There are abundant yellow retinal specks spreading throughout the posterior pole. The macula is extremely disorganized with zones of perifoveolar atrophy.

damage of the retrofoveolar PR layer). Visual acuity is correlated more closely with PR loss than with retinal thinning as measured by OCT. Retinal flecks have the appearance of hyperreflective deposits apposed to the pigment epithelium, or more rarely, further away in the outer nuclear layer [5]. Type 1 flecks are dome-shaped deposits located within the retinal pigment epithelium and the outer segment of photoreceptors (fig 23). Type 2 flecks are deposits involving the outer nuclear layer as well. They are encountered in advanced or severe stages, with the loss of the photoreceptor layer within the central foveal zone.

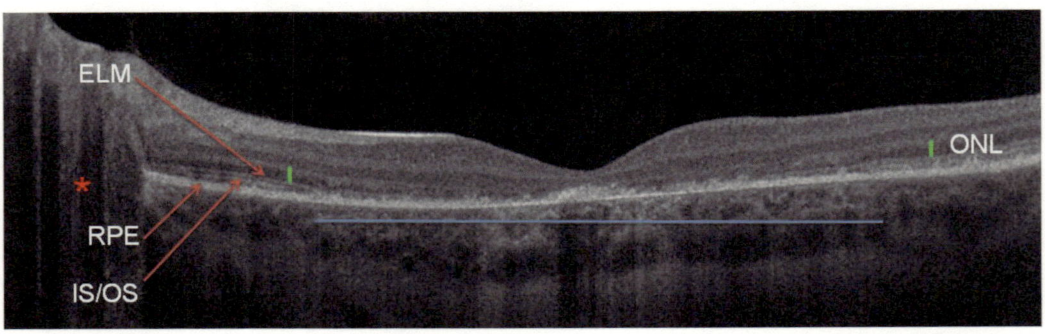

Fig. 19. Horizontal OCT section through the fovea and the optic nerve head. The following elements should be noted: alterations in the RPE and the OS/IS junction, loss of relief of the clivus, thinning of the retina. These alterations reflect the loss of pigment epithelial cells, followed by photoreceptors. In the macular zone (horizontal blue line) the loss of photoreceptors is severe and reflected by the disappearance of the IS/OS junction line, as well as the absence of the outer nuclear layer (ONL, i.e. the layer of photoreceptor nuclei). Retinal thickness is reduced in accordance with the disappearance of the outer layers of the retina. These anomalies are obvious and severe, although the fundus appears normal.

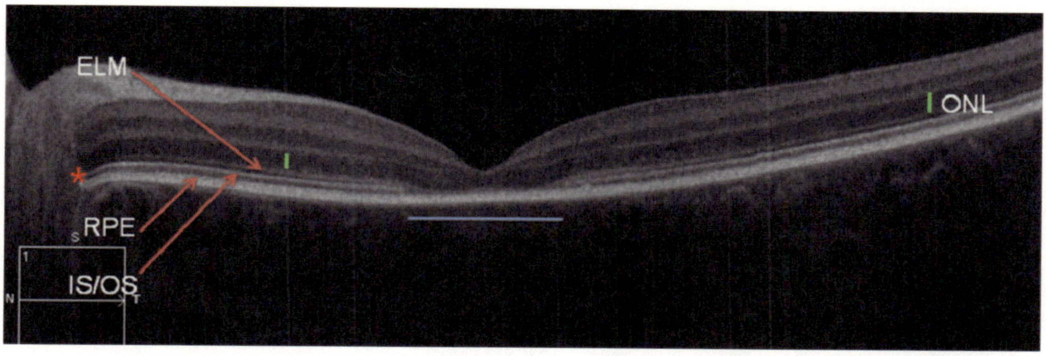

Fig. 20. Disappearance of the IS/OS junction line of photoreceptors, and the absence of the outer nuclear layer (ONL, i.e. the layer of photoreceptor nuclei) in the limited subfoveal zone.

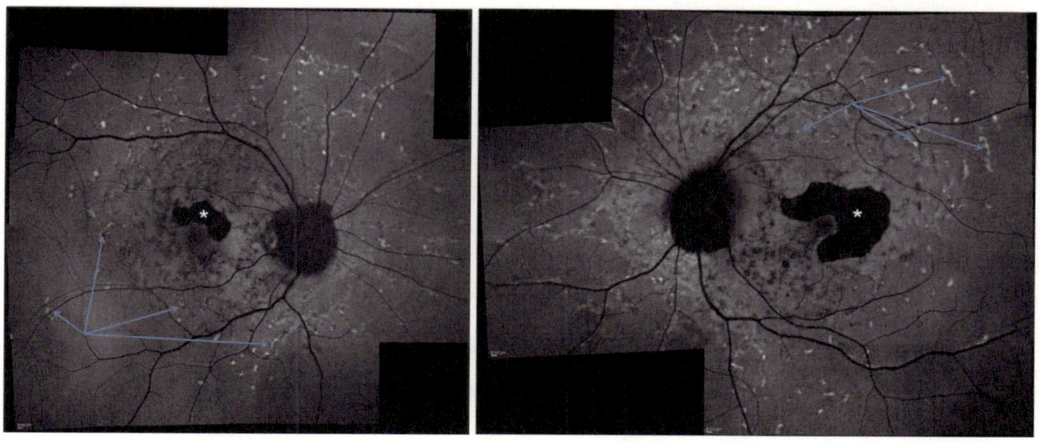

Fig. 21. Late-onset Stargardt disease with perifoveolar damage. Autofluorescence images: The bilateral and symmetric retinal flecks are autofluorescent (arrows). The perifoveolar atrophy appears dark black (*), and spares the fovea in both eyes.

4.2 Best disease

Initially described by Adams in 1883 and revisited by Best in 1905 from a genetic point of view (autosomal dominant transmission), Best disease is characterized by the present of autofluorescent vitelline deposits ("vitelliform deposits"). The sequence of evolution of the deposits is stereotypic (fig 24), from their appearance to the fragmentation of the material until its reabsorption. The deposits, single or multiple, macular or extramacular, can differ in their evolutive stage from one eye to the other, or even within the same eye. This asymmetry, both in the size of the lesions and in their stage, is particularly evocative of the vitelliform dystrophies, which are the only asymmetric unilateral or bilateral hereditary maculopathies. Best disease, the second most-widespread juvenile maculopathy, is linked to the *BEST1* gene. The visual prognosis for this dystrophy is relatively satisfactory, unlike that of other hereditary disorders: a majority of patients conserve visual acuity in one of the two eyes (71% of cases).

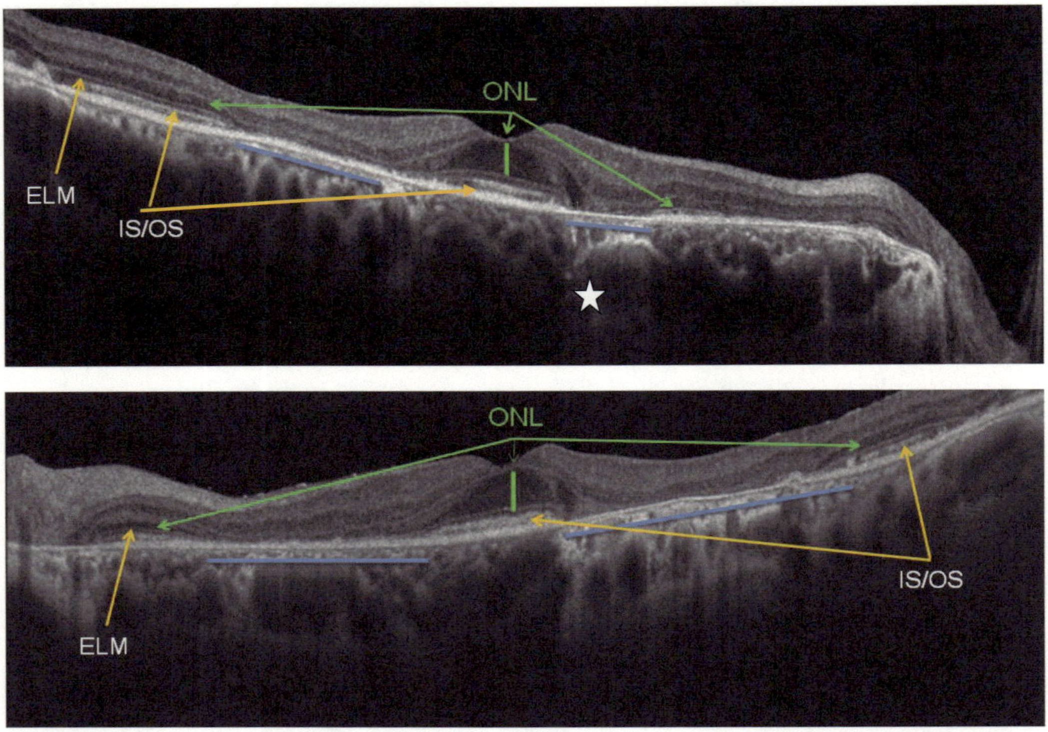

Fig. 22. Late-onset Stargardt disease with perifoveolar damage (same patient as figure 21). Top: right eye. Bottom: left eye. The IS/OS layer is totally absent in the perifoveolar zone only (blue line). The choroid displays a hyperreflective signal (star). The thickness of the fovea is normal, with a well-preserved photoreceptor layer, accounting for the conservation of visual acuity.

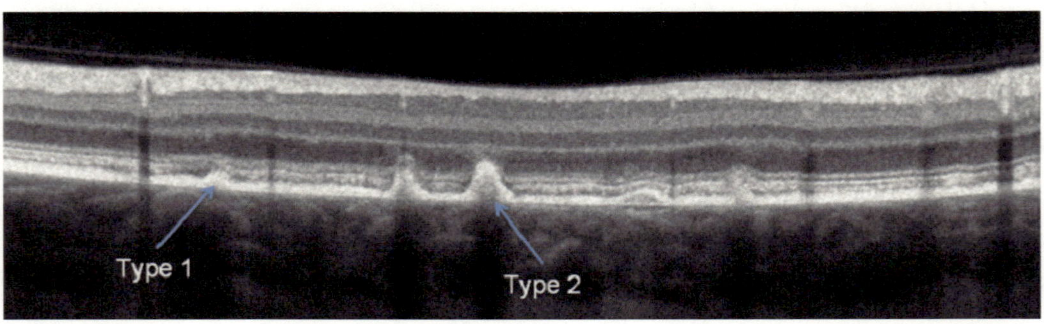

Fig. 23. Retinal flecks in Stargardt disease. Type 1 flecks are dome-shaped deposits located in the retinal pigment epithelial layer and the outer segment of the photoreceptors. Type 2 deposits also involve the outer nuclear layer.

In OCT, the vitelline material appears as a convex/dome-shaped, hyperreflective and homogenous lesion (Fig 25), located below the hyperreflective photoreceptor layer (Ferrara et al, 2010).

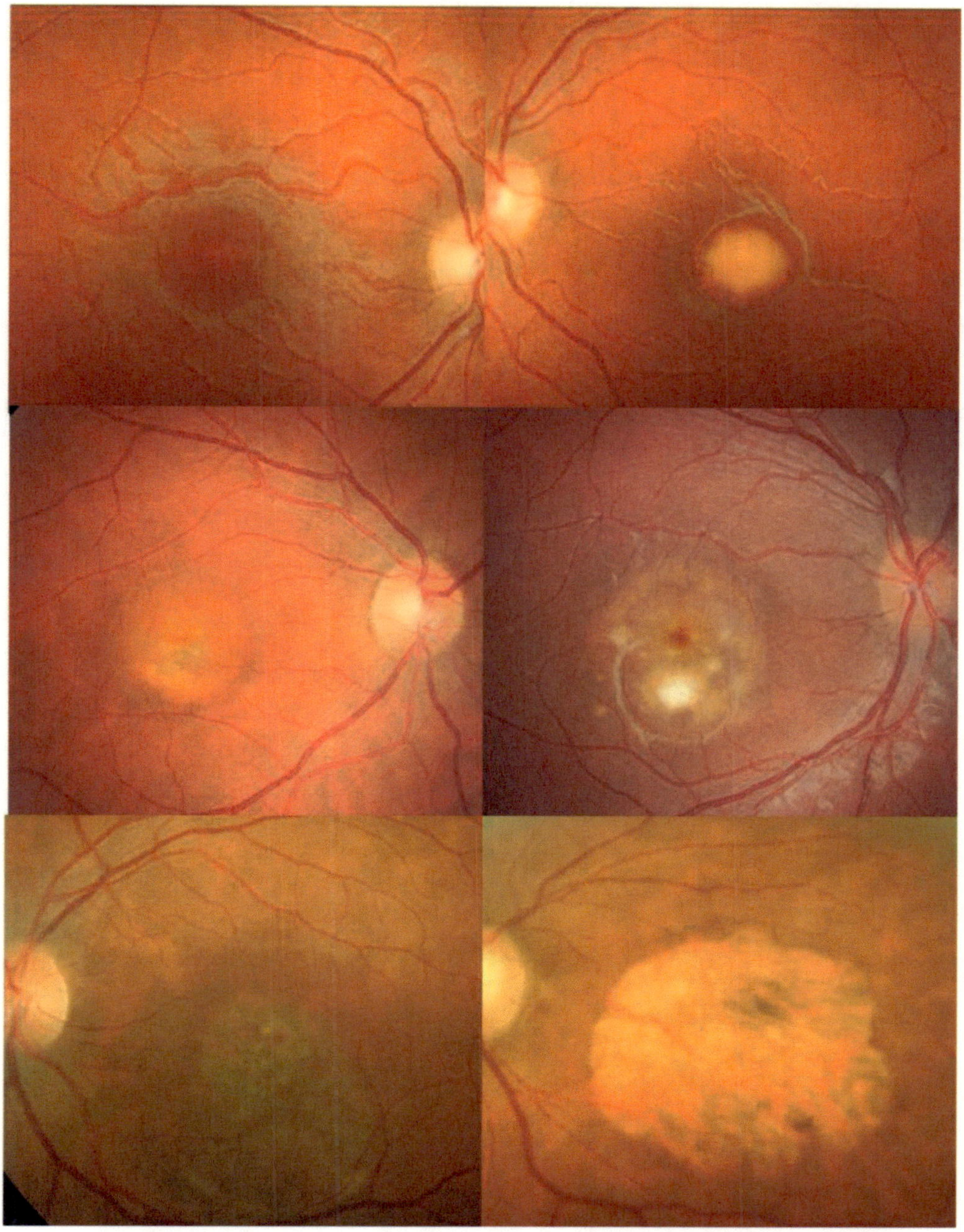

Fig. 24. Evolutive sequence of vitelliform lesions. A. Previtelliform stage. B. Vitelliform stage. C and D. Scrambled egg stage with (C) or without hypopyon (D). E. RPE alterations; the vitelline lesion has been resorbed. F. Atrophic stage.

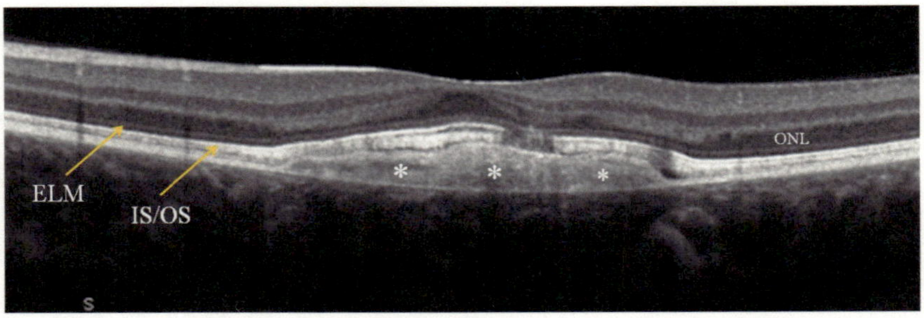

Fig. 25. Best disease, vitelliform stage. The subfoveal vitelliform deposit (*) is homogenous, situated at the level of the pigment epithelium and above it, touching the inner/outer segment (IS/OS) junction line and the external limiting membrane (ELM).

At the fragmentation stage, differences in the reflectivity of the material and the appearance of dark, optically empty zones resembling a false serous retinal detachment can be noted (fig 26-27). This last, pseudo-retinal detachment-like appearance associated with vitelline material should not be taken for a neovascular complication. Only exudative intraretinal modifications are a sign of neovascularization. The photoreceptor layer may be discontinuous with diminished visual acuity, or conserved with normal visual acuity.

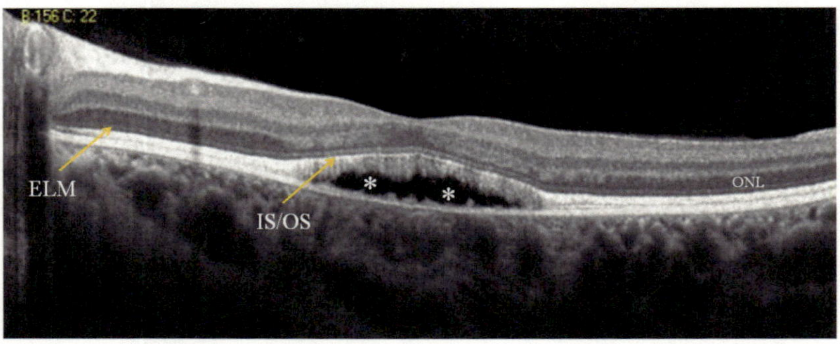

Fig. 26. Best disease, scrambled-egg stage. The deposit is optically empty and dark. Note the perfect conservation of the photoreceptor layer, including above the vitelline material. Visual acuity is 20/20.

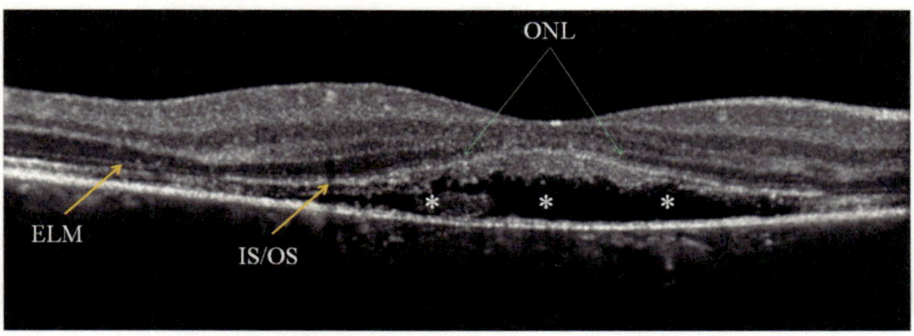

Fig. 27. Best disease, scrambled-egg stage. Visual acuity is 30/60. Extensive scrambling of the lesion except at the left extremity. The inner/outer segment (IS/OS) junction is altered and the outer nuclear layer has disappeared.

At later stages of atrophy and/or fibrosis, the lesion is hyperreflective, the overlying retina is disorganized and thin, and the photoreceptor layer may be completely absent (fig 28).

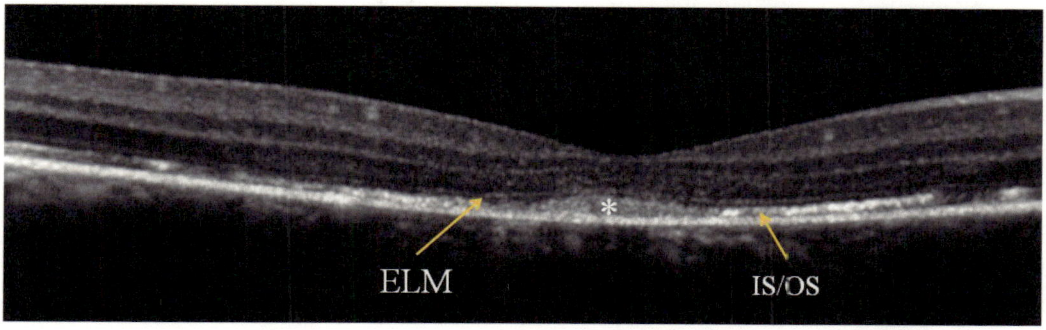

Fig. 28. Best disease, RPE alterations. Visual acuity is 20/30. The external limiting membrane is preserved (ELM). The subfoveal IS/OS line is ill-defined. The grey structure (*) corresponds to residual vitelline material.

4.3 Juvenile X-linked retinoschisis

X-linked juvenile retinoschisis is the most frequent form of macular retinoschisis (fig 29). The diagnostic signs are simple, with an appearance characteristic of macular schisis in OCT, confirmed by an electroretinogram (ERG). Prevalence is variable, with geographical differences ranging from 1/5000 in Finland to 1/25 000 elsewhere. X-linked juvenile retinoschisis is associated with mutations of the *RS1* gene (6 exons). This gene, expressed by photoreceptors and bipolar cells, codes for retinoschisin, a protein involved in adhesion and cohesion of the retina. This function depends on a conserved region of the protein, the discoidin domain, encoded by exons 4 to 6. Macular retinoschisis results in the progressive thinning of the retina with a slow and variable decrease in visual acuity after 50 years of age. Macular atrophy is the last stage.

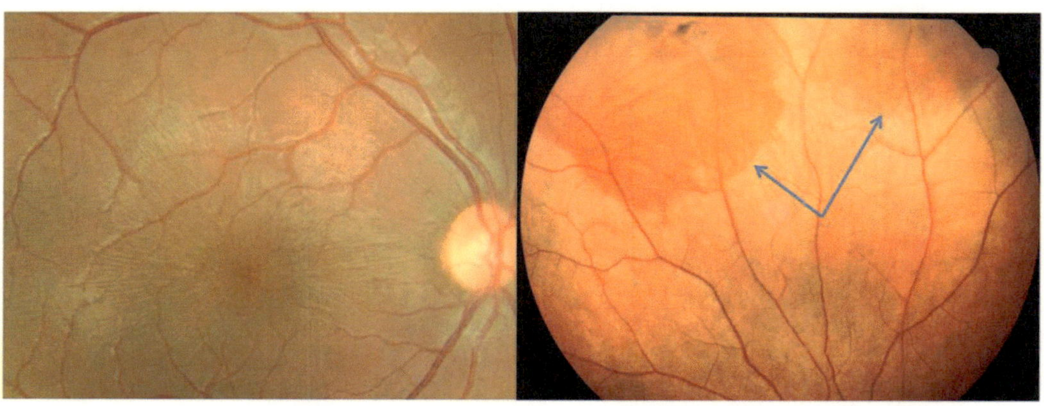

Fig. 29. X-linked juvenile retinoschisis. Left : Characteristic bilateral and symmetric wrinkling of the retina resembling the spokes of a wheel in a 7-year-old boy. Right: the two rounded darker-colored zones in the superior periphery are flat peripheral retinoschisis.

Spectral OCT is unavoidable for the visualization of a pathognomonic pattern of macular cysts that can extend up to the mid-periphery (Yu et al, 2010). Within the retina, the cysts can extend from the ganglion cell layer to the inner or outer nuclear layer (fig 30, 31). In the late stage of the disease, the zone corresponding to the schisis is thin or atrophic, and its appearance is aspecific.

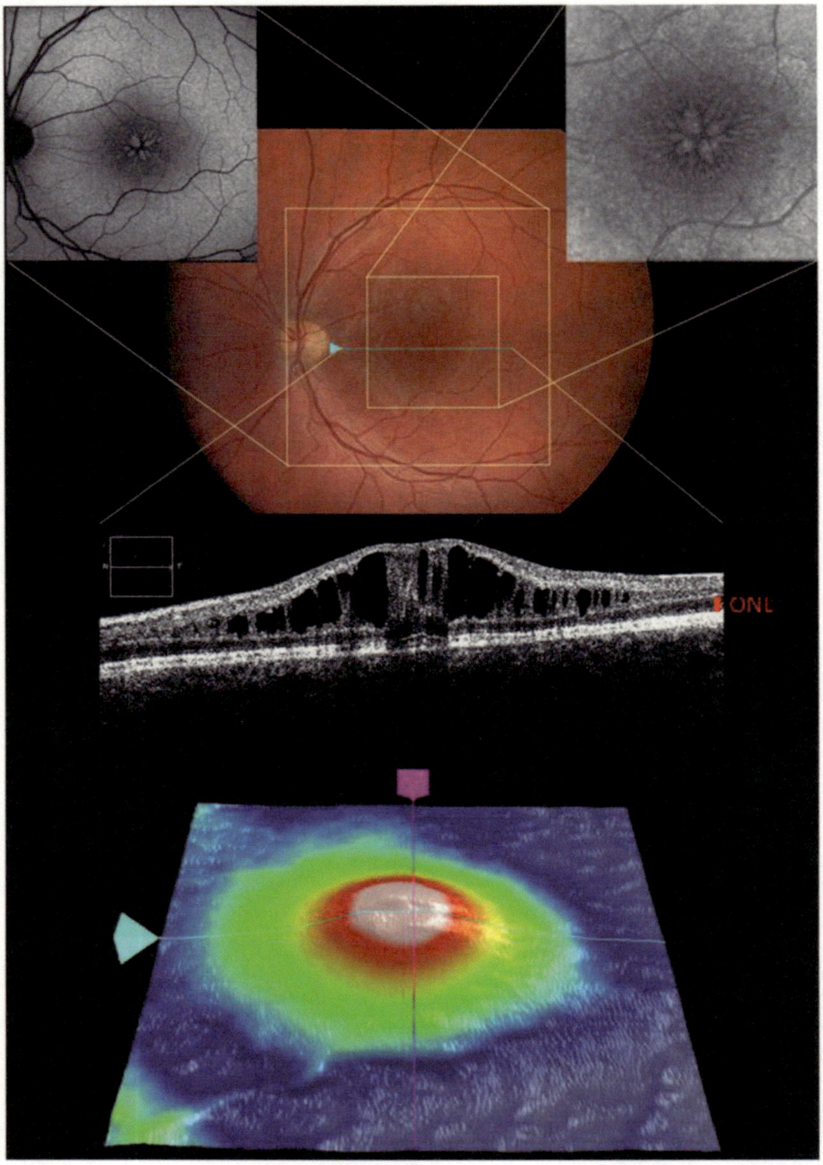

Fig. 30. Spectral-domain OCT of a macular retinoschisis in a young boy. The cysts extend throughout the perimacular retina and the ganglion cell layer up to the outer nuclear layer, which is not involved. Insets showing the typical autofluorescent pattern of retinoschisis (two top greyscale images; the one on the right is a magnification of the macular schisis).

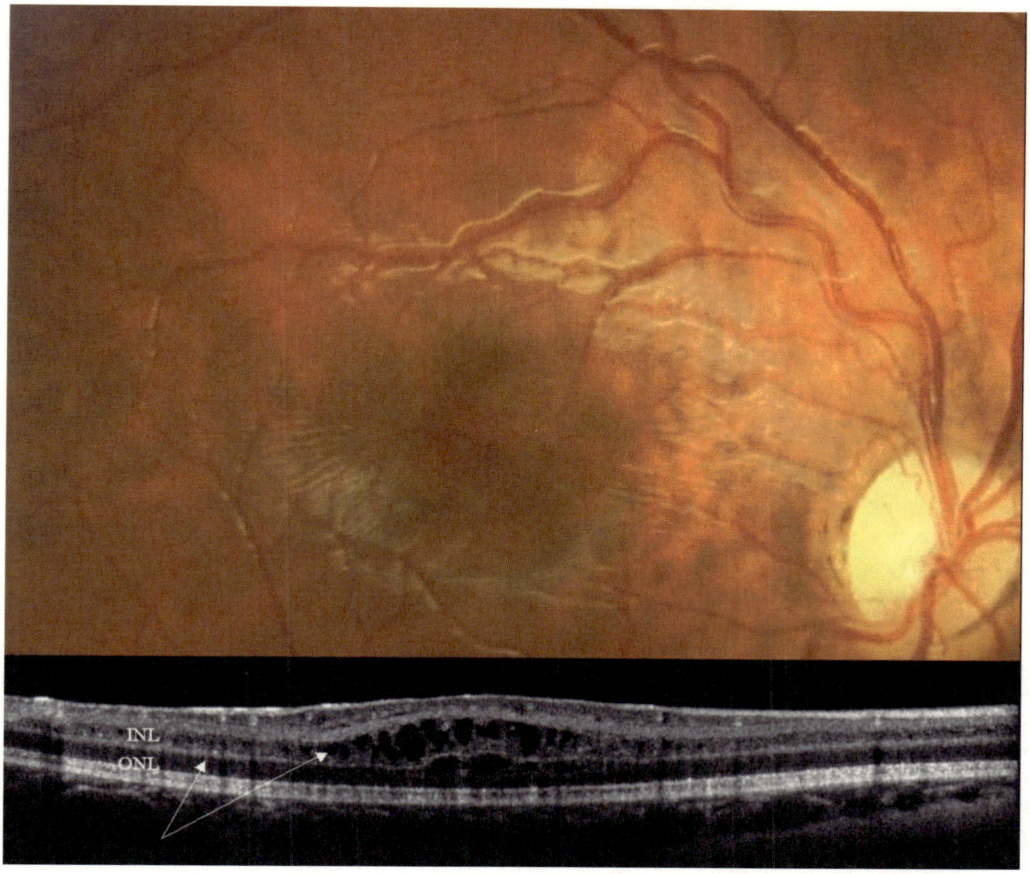

Fig. 31. Spectral OCT pattern of an X-linked retinoschisis in a young boy. The entire retina is affected, and cysts (arrows) have developed within the inner (INL) and outer nuclear layers (ONL).

4.4 Malattia Leventinese

Malattia Leventinese was described by Vogt in 1925 (in families in the Leventine valley in Switzerland). However, the first cases were reported by Doyne in 1899 (Doyne's honeycomb retinal dystrophy). In addition to the autosomal dominant transmission of the disorder, drusen in Malattia Leventinese have specific features depending on the age of onset (child or young adult), their localization, their radial arrangement in the periphery, and their confluency (fig 32).

This maculopathy is rare, and linked to a mutation in the EFEMP1 gene (EGF containing fibulin-like extracellular matrix protein 1). Visual acuity decreases after 40 years of age, with blindness at around the 7th decade, related to atrophy or to choroidal neovessels [5].

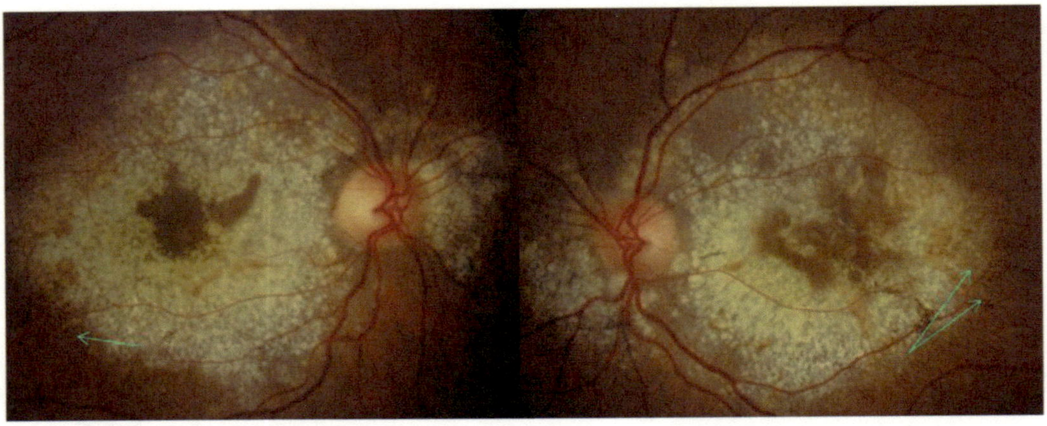

Fig. 32. Typical Malattia Leventinese with a honeycomb-like appearance in a 46-year-old woman with a visual acuity of 20/200 in both eyes. The drusen are dense, with a specific macular and peripapillary topography. Note the radial distribution of the fine peripheral drusen (arrows).

Its appearance in OCT is very specific, with a thick, continuous, homogenous, hyperreflective material between the Bruch membrane and the pigment epithelium (Gerth et al, 2009). These deposits push back and lift the entire retina, which does not show much morphological modification but which becomes wavy (fig 33). The dark cones correspond to alterations of the pigment epithelium. The photoreceptor layer is not altered until later.

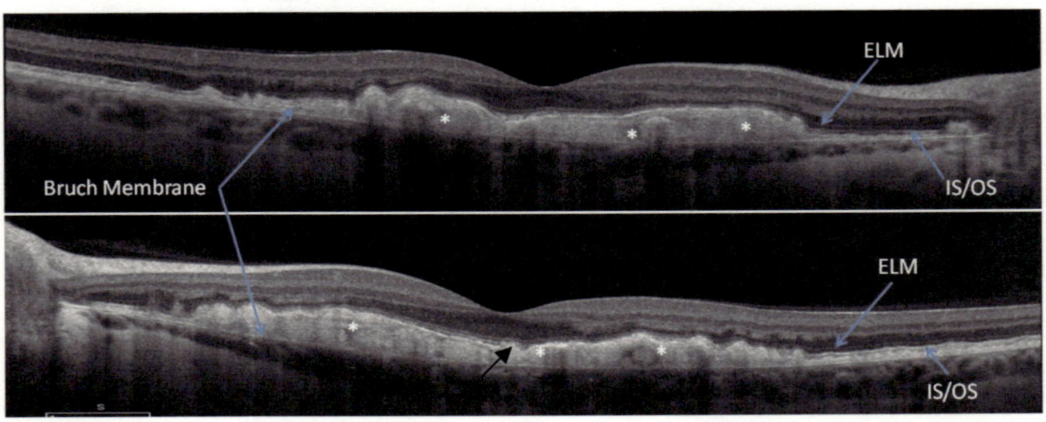

Fig. 33. Malattia Leventinese. OCT scans of a 36-year-old woman. Visual acuity is 20/20 in the right eye, 20/30 in the left eye. The material lies above the Bruch Membrane, and a part of the subfoveal IS/OS line is interrupted in the left eye (bottom, black arrow).

4.5 Sorsby's fundus dystrophy

Initially described by Sorsby in 1949, this hereditary autosomal dominant dystrophy is characterized by great clinical heterogeneity. The initial clinical profile can be limited to unilateral choroidal neovascularization, unusual for the age of onset (non-myopic young adults), and associated with a family history of retinal disease. This dystrophy is not limited to maculopathy: multiple non-specific lesions appear in varying combinations at the posterior pole and later in the periphery, progressing centrifugally. At a more evolved stage, the damage is bilateral and polymorphic, including diverse lesions at the posterior pole: yellowish-white drusen-like lesions, yellowish plaque-like subretinal deposits, streaks, patches of fibrotic scarring, and in the periphery, abnormal pigmentation and patches of depigmentation or atrophy. This rare dystrophy is linked to a mutation of the *TIMP3* gene (tissue inhibitor of metalloprotease 3), expressed by the cells of the pigment epithelium. Choroidal neovessels are the first cause of the reduction in visual acuity in this dystrophy (fig 34). The mean age at which the first eye is affected is 46 years, and 50 years for the second eye. This complication is very frequent (60% of cases) with a bilateral involvement in 50% of cases. The second factor for the severe loss of visual acuity (less than 20/200) is macular atrophy, which occurs at a mean age of 50 years for the first eye and 52 years for the second.

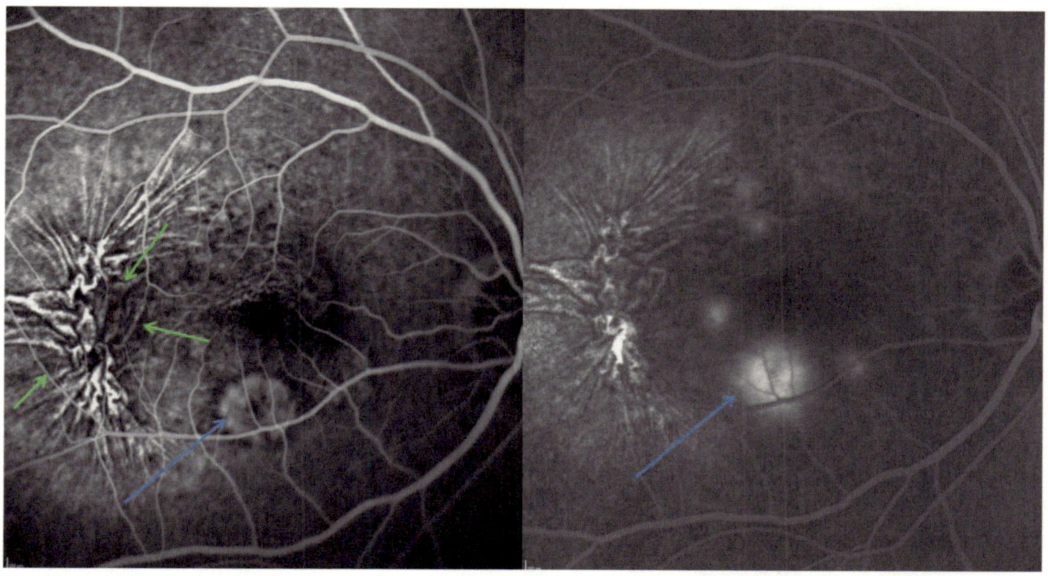

Fig. 34. A 40-year-old man referred for acute visual loss in the right eye due to choroidal neovascularization. The sea-fan-shaped complex is hyperfluorescent in an early frame (left), with diffusion of the fluorescein dye at a later phase (blue arrows). The exudation extends temporally through the retinal pigment epithelium and detaches the overlying retina. There is a contraction of the neovascular net, as revealed by chorioretinal folds (green arrows).

In OCT, the retina has a very particular appearance. Independent of neovascularization (fusiform hyperreflectivity, cavities, serous detachment, detachment of the pigment epithelium), the pigment epithelium-choroid complex is abnormally hyperreflective in certain zones of the posterior pole (Saihan et al, 2009). This hyperreflectivity is characteristic, and different from the abnormal hyperreflectivity of the choroid due to atrophy of the overlying pigment epithelium (fig 35).

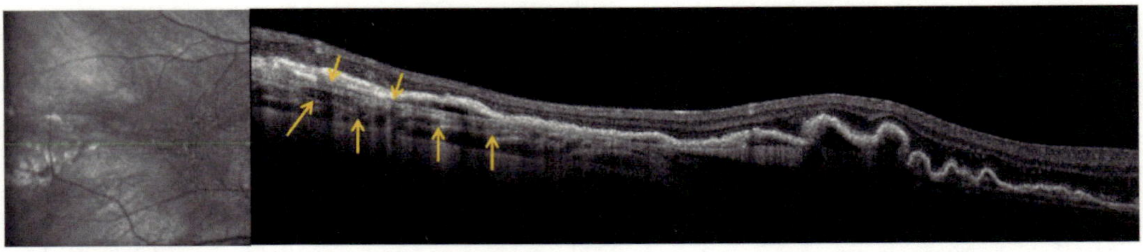

Fig. 35. OCT scan of the patient described in figure 33 demonstrates hyperreflective signals at the level of the retinal pigment epithelium-choroid complex (yellow arrows).

4.6 North Carolina dystrophy

North Carolina dystrophy, initially described by Lefler, is a maculopathy that is remarkable for its lack of evolutivity and the relative conservation of visual acuity. Each patient has a characteristic level of visual acuity and type of macular lesion (Grade 1, 2 or 3) that is invariable over time. Only grade 3 lesions are distinctive: the macula is excavated, colobomatous, and includes fibrous tissue and pigmented zones (fig 37). Grade 1 and 2 lesions (drusen) are non-specific, but their age of onset is very unusual [1-3]. This autosomal dominant dystrophy is very rare. A first identified locus, 6q14-q16.4, is thought to be involved in the approximately 5000 American cases (from an ancestral mutation carried by three Irish brothers who emigrated to North Carolina).

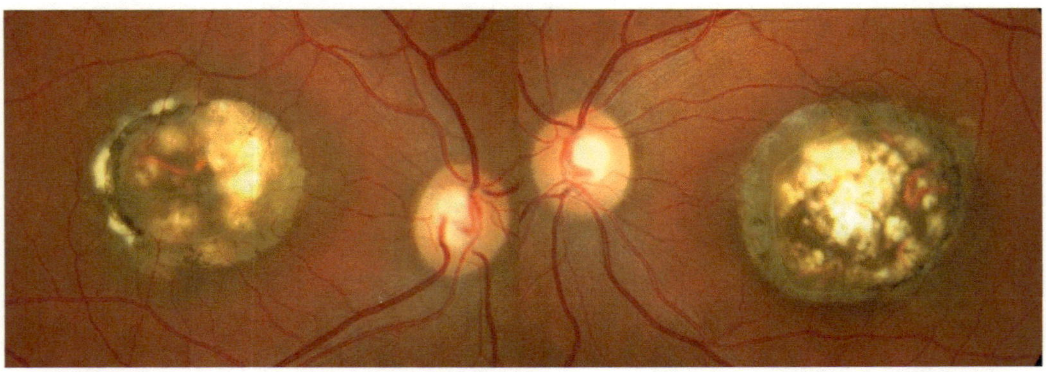

Fig. 37. A 41-year-old woman with a visual acuity of 5/10 in right eye and 3/10 in left eye. The reduced visual acuity is stable, and was already noted at the age of 12 years. There is a family history of maculopathy: the mother, the daughter and the brother of the patient are affected. In the fundus, the lesion is very large and extends over more than 6PD at the posterior pole, delimited in part by a fibrous band; the development of fibrosis can also be seen in the lesion.

The macular lesion characteristic of North Carolina dystrophy does not correspond to a coloboma or a staphyloma (Khurana et al, 2009). The term "crater" or "macular caldera" is therefore used. In this "crater" with steep edges, retinal tissue is limited to the innermost layers of the retina (fig 38). The lines representing the pigment epithelium and photoreceptors only reappear outside the lesion.

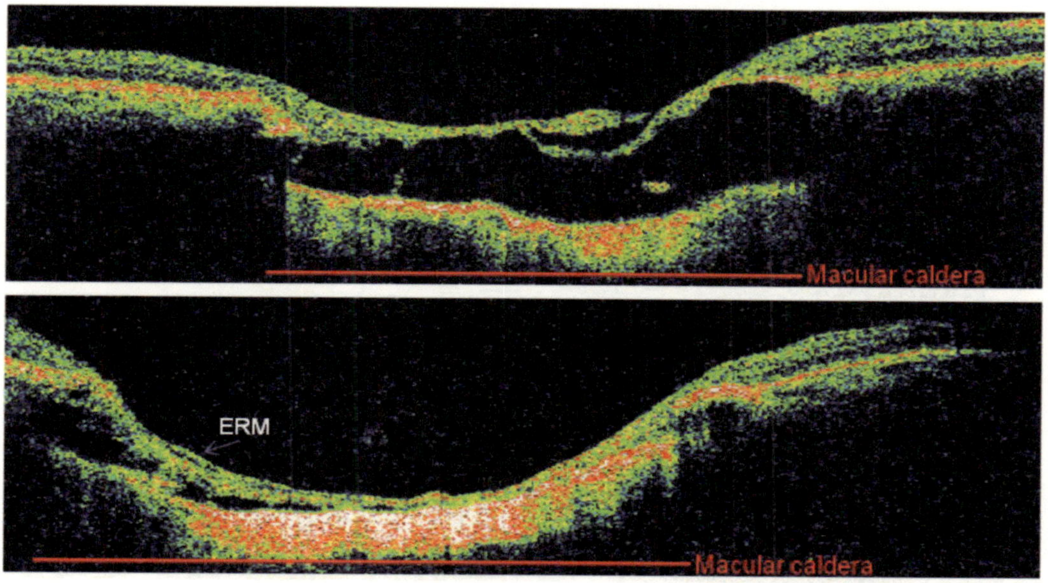

Fig. 38. With time-domain OCT (Stratus OCT, Carl Zeiss Meditec, and a resolution of 10μ), the lesion has the appearance of a crater with steep edges.

5. Conclusion

The possibility of visualizing in vivo all the retinal layers of the posterior pole, the different types of intraretinal and subretinal deposits and even choroidal abnormalities, using spectral-domain optical coherence tomography in combination with autofluorescence imaging, could lead to accurate diagnosis and phenotyping. These two imaging techniques have indisputably replaced fluorescein angiography in the study of inherited retinal dystrophies. OCT is very pertinent in revealing alterations to the neurosensory retina from very early stages, before any modification of the macula in the fundus. Nevertheless, the evaluation of disease state, disease progression and follow-up treatment are not as accurate beyond a certain degree of disorganization of the neurosensory retina.

6. References

Berger, W., Gruissem, BK., Neidhardt, J. The molecular basis of human retinal and vitreoretinal diseases. *Prog Retin Eye Research*, 2010, 29, pp. 335-375.

Ergun E, Hermann, B., & Wirtitsch, M. Assessment of central visual function in Stargardt's disease/fundus flavimaculatus with ultrahigh-resolution optical coherence tomography. *Invest Ophthalmol Vis Sci*, 2005, 46, pp. 310-316.

Ferrara, DC., Costa, RA., & Tsang, S. Multimodal fundus imaging in Best vitelliform macular dystrophy. *Graefes Arch Clin Exp Ophthalmol*, 2010, 248, pp. 1377–1386.

Gerth, C., Zawadzki, RJ., & Werner, JS. Retinal microstructure in patients with *EFEMP1* retinal dystrophy evaluated by Fourier domain OCT. *Eye*, 2009, 23, pp. 480-483.

Hyewon, C., Jong-Uk, H., & June-Gone, K. Optical coherence tomography in the diagnosis and monitoring of cystoids macular edema in patients with retinitis pigmentosa. *Retina*, 2006, 26, pp. 922-927.

Khurana, RH., Sun, X., Pearson, E. A reappraisal of the clinical spectrum of North Carolina dystrophy. *Ophthalmology* 2009, 116, pp. 1976–1983.

Querques, G., Leveziel, N., & Benhamou, N. Analysis of retinal flecks in fundus flavimaculatus using optical coherence tomography. *Br J Ophthalmol*, 2006, 90, pp. 1157-1162.

Saihan, Z., Li, Z., & Rice, J. Clinical and biochemical effects of the E139K missense mutation in the TIMP3 gene, associated with Sorsby fundus dystrophy. *Mol Vis*, 2009, 15, pp. 1218-1230.

Sandberg, MA., Brockhurst, RJ., & Gaudio, AR. Visual acuity is related to parafoveal retinal thickness in patients with retinitis pigmentosa and macular cysts. *Invest Ophthalmol Vis Sci*, 2008, 49, pp. 4568-4572.

Yu, J., Ni, Y., & Keane, PA. Foveomacular schisis in juvenile X-linked retinoschisis: an optical coherence tomography study. *Am J Ophthalmol*, 2010, 149, pp.973-978.

9

Study of the Effects of Aging, Refraction and Intraocular Pressure Levels on Retinal Nerve Fiber Layer Thickness of Normal Healthy Eyes

Maki Katai and Hiroshi Ohguro
Department of Ophthalmology, Sapporo Medical University School of Medicine
Japan

1. Introduction

Glaucomatous optic neuropathy (GON), clinically characterized by progressive visual field defects that correspond with glaucomatous optic disc changes, is known as one of the major causes of irreversible blindness worldwide (Quigley, 1999). Thus far, there is no known cure for GON. Thus, early diagnosis and treatment to slow down the disease progression is considered of most importance. To diagnose earlier stages of GON, a sensitive and reliable methodology to detect the specific glaucomatous optic disc changes required. To this point, retinal nerve fiber layer (RNFL) thickness measurements by optical coherent tomography (OCT) has been widely utilized (Bowd et al., 2000; Katai et al., 2003). However, the optic disc appearance is quite variable within even healthy populations. In fact, recent studies have revealed that its incidence exclusively varies with races, ages and others, and therefore, these factors should be taken into account to perform better analyses through OCT (Katai et al., 2006). The purpose of the present study is to investigate the effects of aging, refraction, and intraocular pressure levels on RNFL thickness. To do so, the eyes of healthy Japanese individuals were evaluated and compared with those of Europeans.

1.1 Subjects and methods

1.1.1 Subjects

246 eyes of 126 healthy Japanese subjects (53 men, 73 women) over 18 years of age were recruited from 2002 to 2009 at Sapporo Medical University Hospital. The present study protocol was approved by the Ethics Committee of the Sapporo Medical University School of Medicine and conducted in accordance with the Declaration of Helsinki. After an explanation of the study's purpose and its protocol were provided, written informed consent was obtained from all participants before inclusion. To ensure that they had no systemic and ocular diseases including ocular surface diseases, uveitis, and retinal vascular diseases other than, early cataract, all subjects were asked to provide their past medical histories. Next, their eyes were examined by a slit-lamp biomicroscope, and they also underwent a fundus examination. The mean age, spherical equivalent (SE), and intraocular pressure (IOP) of the subjects were 45.5 ± 16.5 years (22 – 87 years), +2.2 ± 3.1 D (-12.8 - +2.9 D), and 14.2 ± 2.9 mmHg (7.0 - 20.0 mmHg), respectively. The best corrected visual acuity

ranged between 16/20 to 30/20. IOP of the subjects was measured by non-contact tonometer or Goldmann applanation tonometry.

When examining the effects of aging on the RNLF thickness, 152 eyes of 80 healthy subjects were further divided in-to 6 groups: 20 to 29 years (20 eyes), 30 to 39 years (35), 40 to 49 years (25), 50 to 59 years (29), 60 to 69 years (18), and 70 to 79 years (25).

For evaluation of the effects of myopia, subjects were initially divided into two groups according to their SE values: a myopic eyes group (SE ≤-3.0 D) and a non-myopic eyes group (-3.0 D < SE) (Mitchell et al., 1999). Myopic eyes consisted of 88 eyes of 47 subjects (mean age 37.1 ± 10.3 years (22 – 63 years)) and non-myopic eyes comprised 158 eyes of- 83 subjects (mean age 50.1 ± 17.6 years (22 - 87 years)). To study the effects of refractive errors on RNFL thickness, 47 myopic eyes and 83 non-myopic eyes from subjects over 40 years old were selected and included in the analysis. No significant difference was found in average age distribution and IOP levels between the two groups.

To investigate the ocular hypertension on RNFL thickness, other subjects with ocular hypertensive eyes with more than 21 mmHg IOP were also recruited at the Sapporo Medical University Hospital. Before inclusion in the present study, in addition to ocular examinations described above, a visual field test by a Humphrey Field Analyzer (HFA: HFA 30-2 SITA fast; Humphrey-Zeiss, San Leandro, CA) was performed to make sure that the subjects' eyes had no glaucomatous visual field changes (The Japan Glaucoma Society [JGS], 2006), thereafter (JGS, 2006). 45 ocular hypertensive eyes of 25 subjects (7 men, 18 women, mean age 59.9 ± 12.1 (36 - 83 years), mean SE -1.2 ± 2.5 D (-6.8 - +4.1 D), mean IOP 23.5 ± 2.0 mmHg (21.0 - 30.0 mmHg)) were included in the current study. As a control, 147 eyes of 75 healthy subjects (30 men, 45 women, mean age 55.9 ± 13.2 years (38 - 87 years), mean SE -1.6 ± 3.2 D (-11.6 - +3.0 D), mean IOP 14.1 ± 2.7 mmHg (7.0 - 20.0 mmHg)) were randomly selected and employed among the healthy eyes described above.

1.1.2 OCT (Optical Coherence Tomography) measurement

To measure RNFL thickness, OCT3 (Optical Coherence Tomography 3000; Zeiss-Humphrey, Dublin, CA) was used for. This contained an interferometer that resolved retinal structures by measuring the echo delay time of light that was reflected and backscattered from different microstructural features in the retina. The OCT3 projected a broad bandwidth near-infrared light beam (820 nm) onto the retina from a super luminescent diode. The light reflected from the retina consisted of multiple echoes and the distance traveled by various echoes was determined by varying the distance to the reference mirror. This produced a range of time delays of the reference light for comparison.

The OCT3 software package included 18 scan acquisition protocols and 19 analysis protocols. The fast RNFL thickness scan mode was used, and this protocol acquired three 3.4 mm diameter circle scans in 1.92 seconds of scanning. The RNFL thickness average analysis protocol calculated peripapillary RNFL thickness as the distance between vitreoretinal interface and the anterior surface of the retinal pigment epithelium/choriocapillaris region. These values were then averaged to yield 12 clock-hour thickness, four quadrant thickness, and a global average RNFL thickness measurement (360° measure) (Figure 1).

These values were then compared against a normative database of age-matched controls to derive percentile values. Statistical determinations of confidence bands at 1 %, 5 %, 95 %, and 99 % were then calculated. The OD and OS graphics displayed red, yellow, green, and white colored bands, corresponding to the Normal Distribution Percentiles as estimated by the RNFL Normative Database. The subject ethnicity of this normative database is comprised of 95 % whites, blacks, and Hispanic, classified as European, with the remaining 5 % classified as other races. Asians comprise only 3 % (Patella, 2003) (Figure 2).

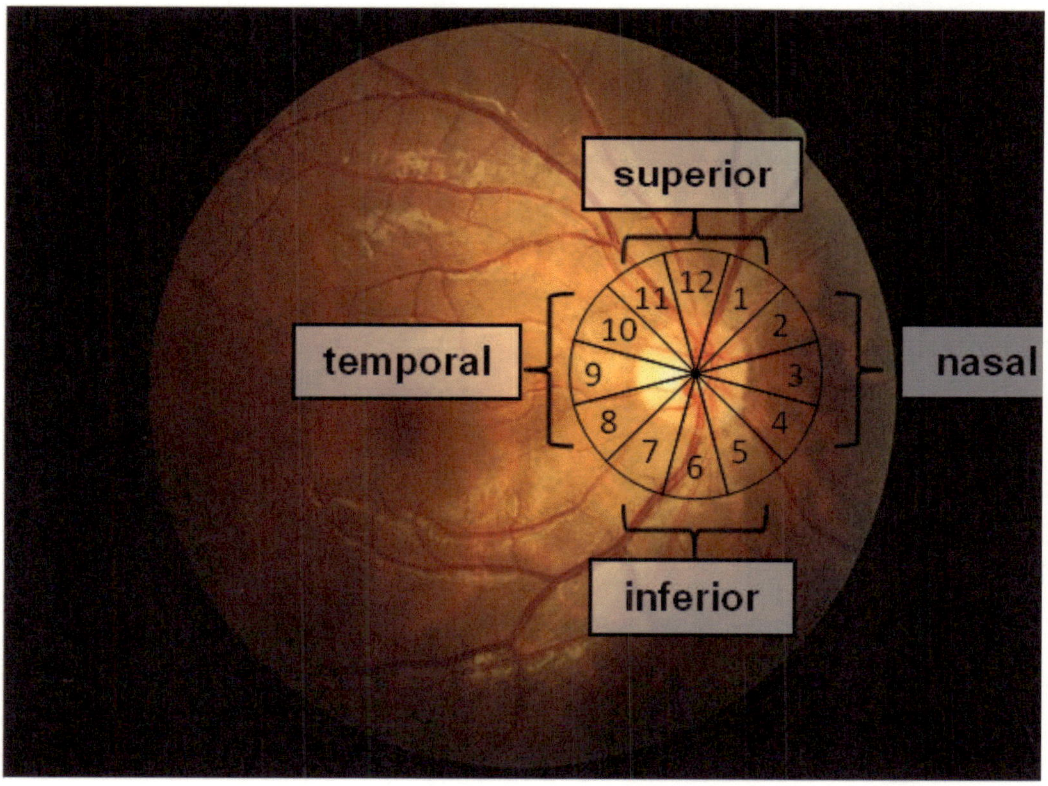

Fig. 1. Twelve 30-degree clock-hour sector of peripapillary RNFL (Right eye). Using OCT3, average RNFL thickness and each of the twelve 30-degree clock-hour sector averages were measured. Superior quadrant: 11, 12, 1 o'clock, Temporal quadrant: 8, 9, 10 o'clock, Inferior quadrant: 5, 6, 7 o'clock, Nasal quadrant: 2, 3, 4 o'clock.

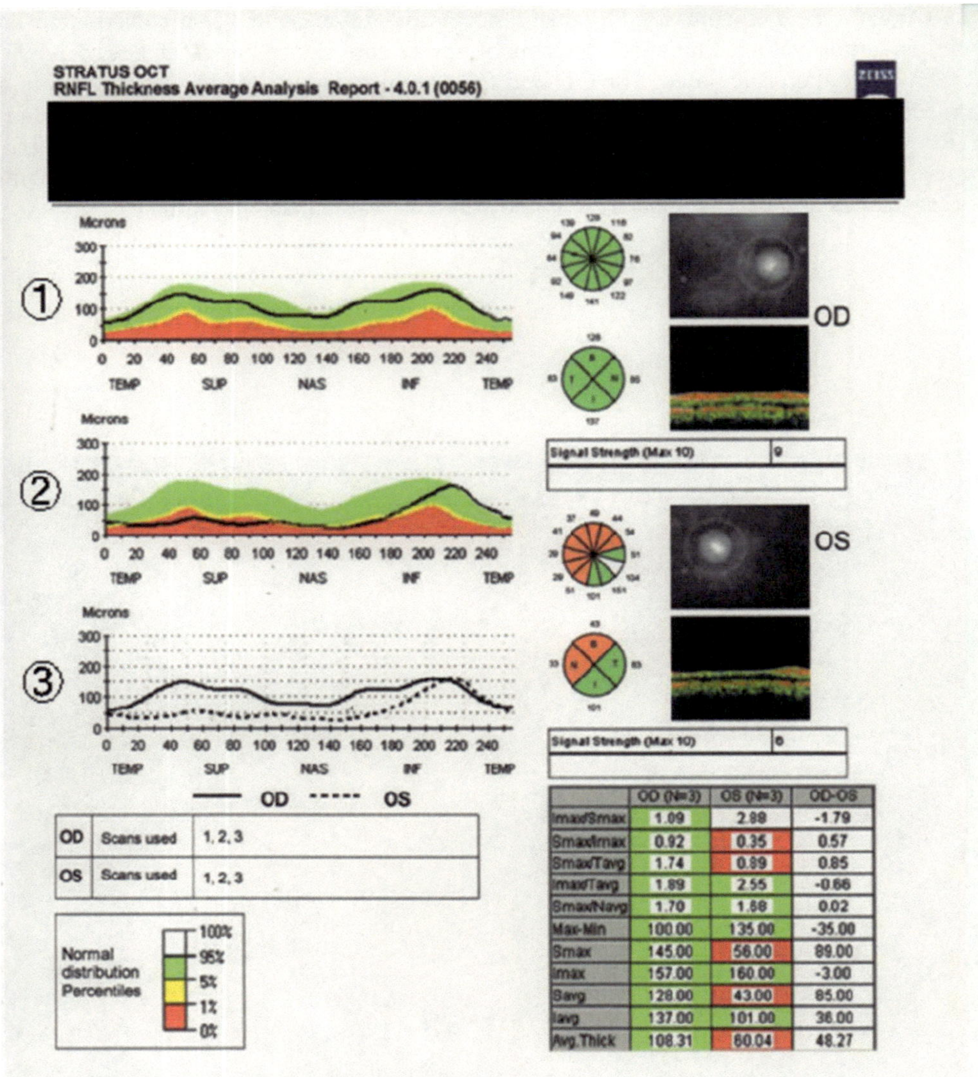

Fig. 2. Representative a sample OCT3 display data. RNFL was measured and analyzed using normative database of OCT3. (1) Right eye, (2) Left eye, (3) Comparison of both eyes (a solid line represented right eye, a dotted line represented left eye). X axis of these graphs indicated superior-temporal segment, superior segment, inferior segment, and inferior-temporal segment from the left. Y axis of these graphs indicated RNFL thickness (micrometer). Green, yellow and red colors indicated normal distribution percentiles of 5-95%, 1-5%, and 0-1%, respectively using normative database installed.

1.1.3 Statistical analysis

Statistical comparisons were performed using Mann-Whitney's U test. Mann-Whitney's U test was also known as Wilcoxon Rank sum test, and basically a non-parametric version of t test. Multiple comparisons between groups were conducted using analysis of variance (ANOVA). ANOVA was a method to compare multiple linear models, a very common way to use an ANOVA test was to test the difference in means among more than two groups. So, the intuition was a t test which accommodated more than two groups to compare. Where any significant change was identified by ANOVA, post hoc analysis using Tukey, Scheffe, and Bonferroni multiple comparisons was utilized to confirm any significant differences among the groups (Field, 2005). P<0.05 was considered statistically significant.

1.2 Mean RNFL thickness in normal Japanese eyes

The 3rd generation of OCT3 installed a normative database in which Caucasians and Hispanics composed of 95 % of the samples, with the remaining 5 % comprised of other races. In our previous preliminarily studies, we evaluated RNFL thickness of patients with glaucoma using OCT3 and found that that of some of the patients were within the normal distribution percentiles of 5-95 %. We therefore suggested that the normal distribution percentiles of 5-95 % of RNFL thickness of normal Japanese population may differ from the normative database installed with the OCT3.

In the current study, we measured the optic nerve head appearance by OCT3 of 246 eyes (158 non-myopic and 88 myopic eyes) from 126 normal healthy Japanese volunteers whose ages ranged from 22 to 87 years. As shown in Figure 3 and Table 1, mean global RNFL thickness was 106.3 ± 12.0 μm and thus mean RNFL thickness in normal Japanese eyes was thicker than that in European eyes. Furthermore, 12 clock-hour thickness showed double apical shapes which were thicker within upper and lower segments and thinner within nasal and temporal segments.

	Clock-hour	Total n=246	Non-myopic n=158	Myopic n=88	OH n=45
superior	11 o'clock	140.0 ± 24.7	137.9 ± 24.1	143.8 ± 25.4	128.3 ± 25.7
	12 o'clock	128.3 ± 25.1	131.7 ± 25.3	122.0 ± 23.7	119.5 ± 32.2
	1 o'clock	109.1 ± 27.2	113.7 ± 27.8	100.9 ± 24.4	107.6 ± 31.5
nasal	2 o'clock	84.2 ± 26.3	88.4 ± 26.9	76.6 ± 23.7	80.0 ± 22.0
	3 o'clock	68.9 ± 16.1	71.9 ± 16.8	63.4 ± 13.3	60.1 ± 12.8
	4 o'clock	84.2 ± 23.1	90.4 ± 23.9	73.1 ± 16.7	69.6 ± 17.0
inferior	5 o'clock	117.3 ± 26.8	125.0 ± 25.2	103.5 ± 24.1	93.9 ± 19.6
	6 o'clock	142.4 ± 27.1	146.8 ± 25.8	134.5 ± 27.7	126.7 ± 27.0
	7 o'clock	131.8 ± 39.1	124.4 ± 40.4	145.0 ± 33.1	135.3 ± 23.5
temporal	8 o'clock	82.1 ± 25.5	74.6 ± 19.9	95.4 ± 28.8	80.5 ± 22.3
	9 o'clock	76.2 ± 20.3	73.0 ± 19.4	82.0 ± 20.5	61.8 ± 15.6
	10 o'clock	110.8 ± 28.4	107.9 ± 28.0	116.1 ± 28.4	92.2 ± 25.8

OH: Ocular hypertensive eyes

Table 1. RNFL thickness (mean ± SD μm) of normal eyes and ocular hypertensive eyes.

This observation suggested that some of the glaucoma patients could be excluded from the glaucoma screening of Japanese people by the OCT3 and that a revised normative database composed of Japanese for more precise glaucoma screening (Katai et al., 2006).

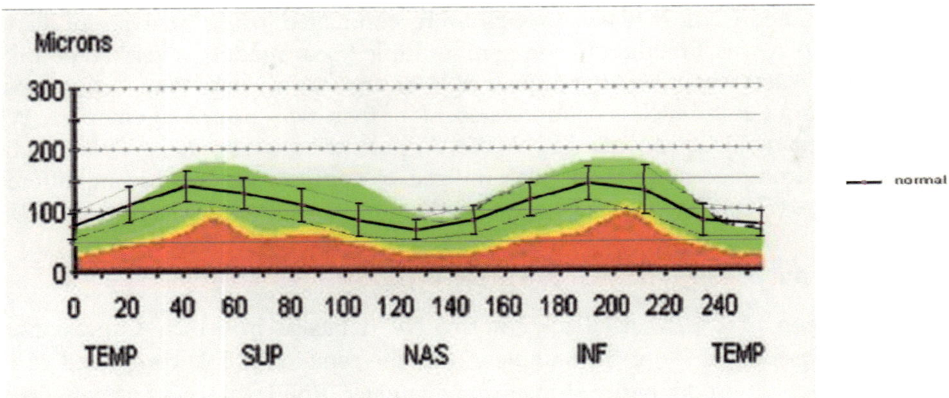

Fig. 3. Normal Japanese mean RNFL thickness and the RNFL normative database of OCT3. In most of the segments, (mean – SD) RNFL thickness of normal Japanese eyes was thicker than the RNFL normative database of OCT3, especially in temporal and nasal quadrants.

1.3 Effect of Aging on the mean RNFL thickness in normal non-myopic Japanese eyes

In the previous pilot studies, through an analysis of age-related change in the 4 quadrants of RNFL thickness, we observed a significant decrease in RNFL thickness within the temporal region in healthy Japanese eyes (Katai et al., 2004a). Therefore, it is of great interest to pursue a more detailed analysis of the effects of aging by 12 clock-hour thickness of RNFL.

To investigate the effects of aging on RNFL thickness in normal non-myopic Japanese eyes, its global and 12 clock-hour thickness was compared among the subjects with different ages, ranging from 40 years through 79 years. As shown in Figure 4-7, there was significant decrease in superior (11, 12 and 1 o'clock) and inferior-temporal (6, 7, 8 o'clock) quadrants with the advancement of age (ANOVA, $P < 0.05$).

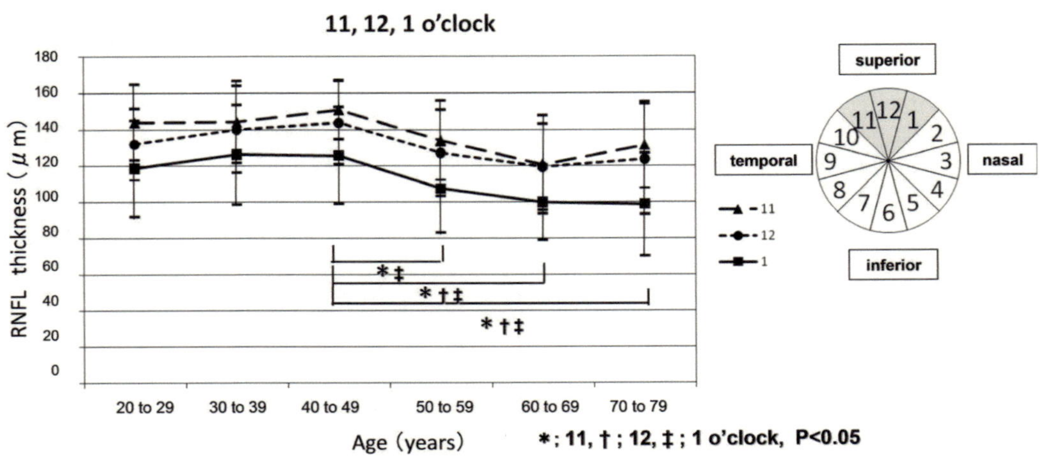

Fig. 4. RNFL thickness in the superior (11, 12, 1 o'clock) of normal non-myopic eyes stratified by age category.

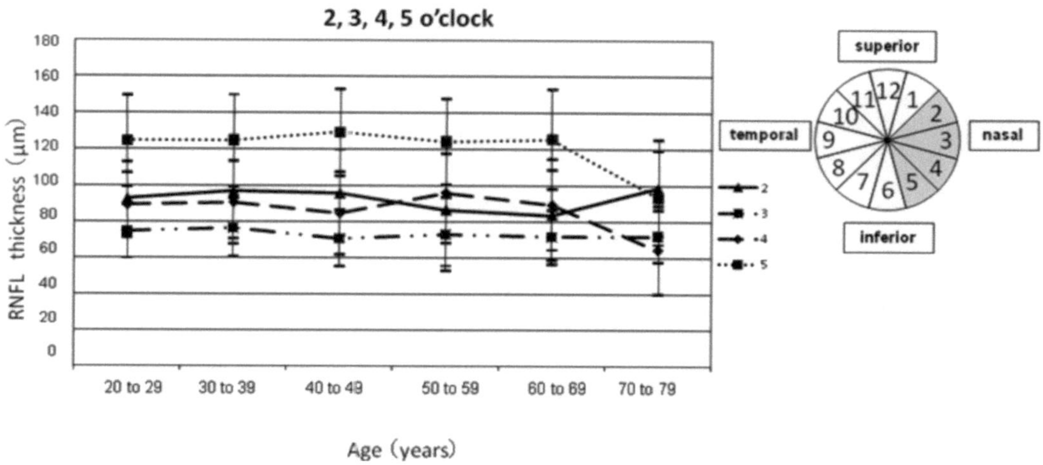

Fig. 5. RNFL thickness in the nasal (2, 3, 4, 5 o'clock) of normal non-myopic eyes stratified by age category.

In terms of effects of aging on the RNFL thickness, we found significant decreases within the superior (11, 12, 1 o'clock) (Figure 4) and inferior-temporal segments (6, 7, 8 o'clock) (Figure 6), which are known to be the most susceptible to glaucomatous optic nerve damage, in older subjects (JGS, 2006). In contrast, RNFL thickness in the other segments, nasal (2, 3, 4, 5 o'clock) (Figure 5), and temporal (9, 10 o'clock) (Figure 7) were not affected by aging.

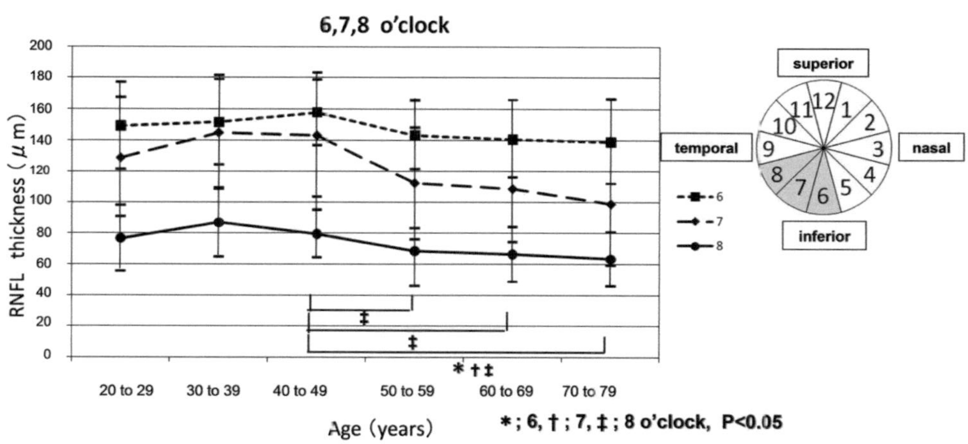

Fig. 6. RNFL thickness in the inferior-temporal (6, 7, 8 o'clock) of normal non-myopic eyes stratified by age category.

As mentioned in several previous glaucoma surveys, such as the Tajimi study (Table 2), the prevalence of glaucoma increases as people age (Suzuki et al.,2008). Thus, our present observation indicates that an age dependent natural decrease in RNFL thickness of normal Japanese may correlate with the age dependent increase in the prevalence of glaucoma.

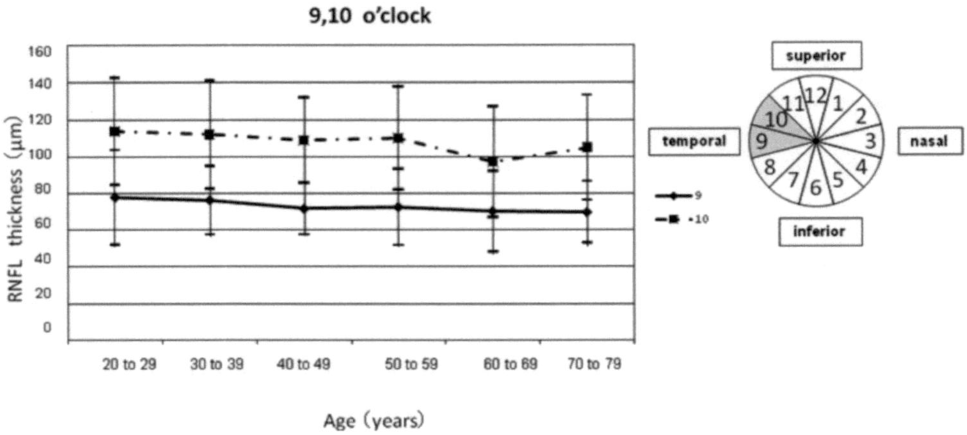

Fig. 7. RNFL thickness in the temporal (9, 10 o'clock) of normal non-myopic eyes stratified by age category.

Study	race	Glaucoma prevalence (%)	NTG prevalence (%)	Glaucoma prevalence of elderly more than 70 years (%)
Tajimi study[1)]	Japanese	5.0	3.6	10.8
Zulus[2)]	Black people	4.5	1.54	11.9
Ponza[3)]	Italian	3.8	—	—
Andhra Pradesh[4)5)]	Indian	2.8	0.7	9.5
Northern Mongolia[6)]	Mongolian	2.2	0.3	—
Proyecto VER[7)]	Latin American	2.1	1.58	—
Melbourne[8)]	Australian	2.0	—	—
Wroclaw[9)]	Caucasian	1.6	—	—
Northwest Alaska[10)]	Alaskan	0.65	—	11.7

NTG: Normal tension glaucoma —: not described

Table 2. Prevalence of glaucoma 1) Suzuki et al., 2008, 2) Rotchford & Johnson, 2002, 3) Cedrone et al., 1997, 4) Dandona et al., 2000a, 5) Dandona et al., 2000b, 6) Foster et al., 1996, 7) Quigley et al., 2001, 8) Wensor et al., 1998, 9) Nizankowska & Kaczmarek, 2005, 10) Arkell et al., 1987.

1.4 Effect of myopia on the mean RNFL thickness in normal Japanese eyes

Myopia has been reported as being a risk factor for glaucoma, and myopic fundus changes may complicate glaucomatous optic disk changes (Mitchell et al., 1999). Thus, this factor should be taken into account when evaluating RNFL changes of glaucoma in myopic eyes. Nevertheless, the normal population database for RFNL measurements, which was developed by the manufacturer and packaged within OCT3 software, did not include individuals with moderate or high degrees of myopia. Therefore, in the present study to investigate the effects of myopia on RNFL thickness in normal Japanese eyes, its global and 12 clock-hour thickness was compared in myopic and non-myopic eyes. Mean global mean RNFL thickness of non-myopic eyes (111.6 ± 10.1 µm) was significantly greater than that of myopic eyes (104.9 ± 10.6 µm) (P<0.01). In the 2 clock-hour thickness analysis, mean RNLF thickness of the segment from 12 o'clock through 6 o'clock of myopic eyes was significantly greater than that in non-myopic eyes, and conversely that of the other segment from 7 o'clock through 11 o'clock was smaller in myopic eyes than in non-myopic eyes (P<0.01) (Figure 8). Both average RNFL thickness and RNFL thickness of nasal half-quadrants in myopic eyes were thinner than those in non-myopic eyes (P < 0.01). Conversely, but with the exception of the 7, 10 and 11 o'clock positions, RNFL thickness of temporal half-quadrants in whole segments of myopic eyes was thicker than that in non-myopic eyes (P < 0.01).

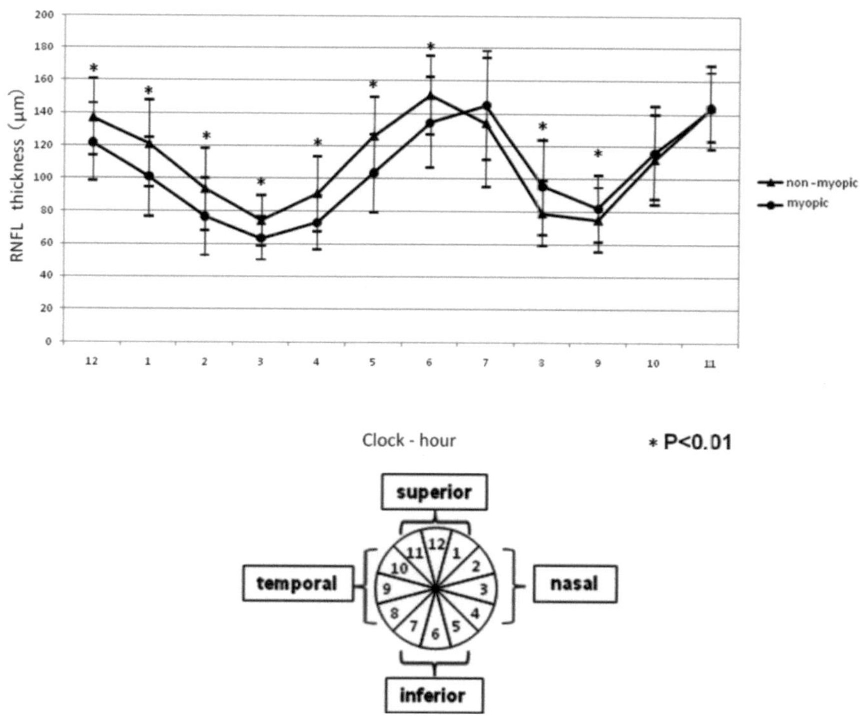

Fig. 8. RNFL thickness of myopic and non-myopic eyes. Mean RNLF thickness of the segment from 12 o'clock through 6 o'clock of myopic eyes was significantly greater than that in non-myopic eyes, and conversely that of the other segment from 7 o'clock through 11 o'clock was smaller in myopic eyes than in non-myopic eyes (Mann-Whitney's U test, P<0.01).

Several previous studies have suggested that no significant correlation is associated between myopia and RNFL thickness (Bowd et al., 2002). However, these studies may have been limited by the poorer resolution of earlier generation OCT and confocal laser devices which had lower sensitivity. Using 3rd generation OCT3, it has been reported that RNFL thickness increased with increasing hyperopia (1.7 microns per diopter) in children (91 % Hispanic, mean age 10 years, range 4-17) (Salchow et al., 2006). Alternatively, significant decrease in RNFL thickness with increasing axial length in myopia has been reported. However, its decreasing ratios varied (2-7 microns per mm) in reports; as such, its changes of RNFL thickness may depend exclusively on different races and age distributions (Hoh et al., 2006).

We demonstrated that RNFL thickness in myopic eyes appeared thicker in the temporal segments and thinner in the nasal segments in comparison to that of non-myopic eyes. It is generally known that tilted disc is more prevalent in myopic eyes, and thus this distortion of the optic nerve fibers at the myopic disc may cause a mechanical stress toward the optic nerve fibers, eventually leading to the glaucomatous optic neuropathy (Nakazawa et al., 2008). Therefore, our present data may support this mechanical theory in myopic eyes.

1.5 Comparison of mean RNFL thickness between ocular hypertensive and normal eyes in Japanese subjects

Bowd et al. has reported that global RNFL thickness of ocular hypertensive eyes is significantly thinner than it is in normal healthy eyes, especially within its inferior and nasal segments (Bowd et al., 2000). Similarly, Kamal et al. has reported significant thinning of the superior and inferior optic disc rims of ocular hypertensive eyes (Kamal et al., 2000).

To explore the effects of elevated IOPs on RNFL thickness, mean RNFL thickness was compared between ocular hypertensive and normal eyes in Japanese subjects. Global mean RNFL thickness of ocular hypertensive eyes (96.3 ± 14.1 μm) was significantly smaller than that of normal eyes (104.3 ± 12.0 μm) ($P < 0.01$), and average RNFL thickness, inferior-nasal segments, and superior-temporal segments were significantly thinner in ocular hypertensive eyes than in normal eyes ($P < 0.05$) (Figure 9).

RNFL thickness is well known to be different within the part of the ONH in a normal disc's so called "ISN'T rule". Specifically, the inferior is the thickest, followed by the superior, nasal and temporal. Since the RNFL is thickest in the inferior and superior portions of the optic nerve head, the relative blood perfusion within these portions is lower among the optic nerve head, and thus, these portions are known to be the most susceptible to glaucomatous optic nerve damage (Harris et al., 2003). It has been shown that the upper and lower visual field defects are more commonly involved in open angle glaucoma (Katai et al., 2004b). If blood perfusion is the lowest in these portions of optic nerve head as has been suggested, elevated intraocular pressure may suppress ocular blood circulation, thereby causing glaucomatous changes within the inferior and superior portions of the optic nerve head.

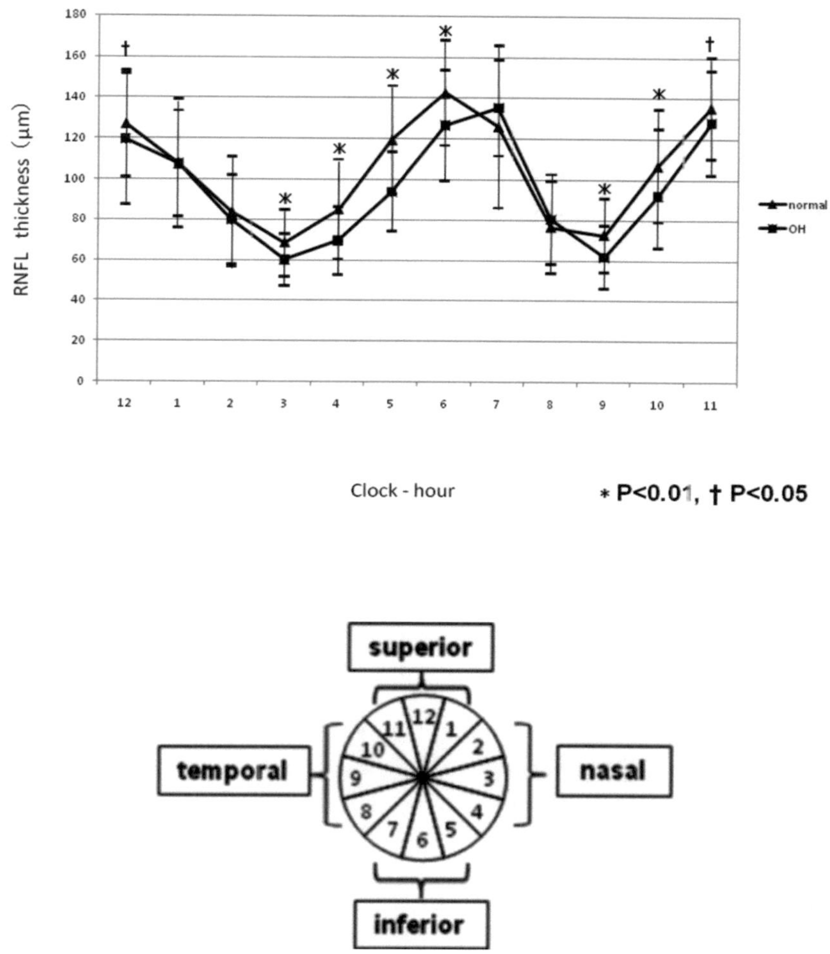

Fig. 9. RNFL thickness of normal eyes and ocular hypertensive eyes. Mean RNFL thickness, inferior-nasal segments, and superior-temporal segments were significantly thinner in ocular hypertensive eyes than in normal eyes (Mann-Whitney's U test, $P < 0.05$)

2. Conclusions

The present study demonstrates that RNFL thickness of normal Japanese eye is thicker than that of normal European eyes, and is significantly affected by aging, refraction and IOP levels. As a result, specific control data of normal Japanese eyes should be utilized in order to detect glaucoma in its early stage.

3. Acknowledgement

We especially thank Dr. Ikuyo Ohguro, Dr. Sachie Tanaka, Dr. Midori Kondo, Dr. Shuichiro Inatomi, and other members of Department of Ophthalmology, Sapporo Medical University School of Medicine, for their constructive advice for conducting this project and for their help in collecting data. We also thank Dr. Yasuo Suzuki, Teine Keijinkai Hospital, for his excellent advice regarding statistical analysis.

4. References

Arkell, SM., Lightman, DA., Sommer, A., Taylor, HR., Korshin, OM., & Tielsch, JM. (1987). The prevalence of glaucoma among Eskimos of north-west Alaska. *Arch Ophthalmol,* Vol.105, No.4, (April 1987), p.p. 482-485, ISSN 0003-9950

Bowd, C., Weinreb, RN., Williams, JM., & Zangwill LM. (2000). The retinal nerve fiber layer thickness in ocular hypertensive, normal, and glaucomatous eyes with optical coherence tomography. *Arch Ophthalmol,* Vol.118, No.1, (Janualy 2000), pp. 22-26, ISSN 0003-9950

Bowd, C., Zangwill, LM., Blumenthal, EZ., Vasile, C., Boehn, AG., Gokhale, PA., Mohammadi, K., Amini, P., Sankary, TM., & Weinreb, RN. (2002). Imaging of the optic disc and retinal nerve fiber layer: the effects of age, optic disc area, refractive error, and gender. *J Opt Soc Am A Opt Image Sci Vis,* (January 2002), Vol.19, No.1, p.p. 197-207, ISSN 1084-7529

Cedrone, C., Culasso, F., Cesareo, M., Zapelloni, A., Cedrone, P., & Cerulli, L. (1997). Prevalence of glaucoma in Ponza, Italy: a comparison with other studies. *Ophthalmic Epidemiol,* Vol.4, No.2, (Jun 1997), p.p. 59-72, ISSN 0928-65861. Quigley, HA. (1999). Neuronal death in glaucoma. *Prog Retin Eye Res,* Vol.18, No. 1, (January 1999), pp. 39-57, ISSN 1350-9462

Dandona, L., Dandona, R., Srinivas, M., Mandal, P., John, RK., McCarty, CA., & Rao, GN. (2000a). Open-angle glaucoma in an urban population in southern India. the Andhra Pradesh eye disease study. *Ophthalmology,*Vol.107, No.9, (September 2000), p.p. 1702-1709, ISSN 0161-6420

Dandona, L., Dandona, R., Mandal, P., Srinivas, M., John, RK., McCarty, & CA., Rao, GN. (2000b). Angle-closure glaucoma in an urban population in southern India. The Andhra Pradesh eye disease study. *Ophthalmology,*Vol.107, No.9, (September 2000), p.p. 1710-1716, ISSN 0161-6420

Field, A. (2005). *Discovering statistics using SPSS. (2nd edition),* SAGE Publications Ltd, ISBN 0-7619-4451-6, London, England

Foster, PJ., Baasanhu, J., Alsbirk, PH., Munkhbayar, D., Uranchimeg, D., & Johnson, GJ. (1996). Glaucoma in Mongolia. A population-based survey in Hövsgöl province, northern Mongolia. *Arch Ophthalmol,* Vol.114, No.10, (October 1996), p.p. 1235-1241, ISSN 0003-9950

Harris, A., Ishii, Y., Chung, HS., Jonescu - Cuypers, CP., McCranor, LJ., Kagemann, L., & Garzozi, HJ. (2003). Blood flow per unit retinal nerve fibre tissue volume is lower in the human inferior retina. *Br J Ophthalmol,* Vol.87, No.2, (February 2003), pp. 184-188, ISSN 0007-1161

Hoh, ST., Lim, MC., Seah SK., Lim, AT., Chew SJ., Foster PJ., &Aung T. (2006).

Peripapillary retinal nerve fiber layer thickness variations with myopia. *Ophthalmology,* Vol.113, No.5, (May 2006), pp. 773-777, ISSN 0161-6420

Kamal, DS., Garway-Heath, DF., Hitchings, RA., & Fitzke, FW. (2000). Use of sequential Heidelberg retina tomography images to identify changes at the optic disc in ocular hypertensive patients at risk of developing glaucoma. *Br J Cphthalmol,*Vol.84, No.9, (September 2000), pp. 993-998, ISSN 0007-1161

Katai, M,. Konno, S., Suzuki, Y., & Ohtsuka, K. (2003). Application of optical coherence tomography, OCT3000 to glaucoma medical examination. *J Eye,* Vol.20, No.11, (November 2003), pp. 1587-1589, ISSN 0910-1810

Katai, M., Konno, S., Suzuki, Y., & Ohtsuka, K. (2004a). Retinal nerve fiber layer thickness in normal eyes as measured with optical coherence tomography 3000. *J Eye,* Vol.21, No.2, (February 2004), pp. 275-277, ISSN 0910-1810

Katai, M., Konno, S., Maeda, S., & Ohtsuka, K. (2004b). Correlation between glaucomatous visual field loss and retinal nerve fiber layer thickness as measured by optical coherence tomography 3000. *J Eye,* Vol.21, No.12, (December 2004), pp. 1707-1709, ISSN 0910-1810

Katai, M., Konno, S., Tsunekage, H., & Ohtsuka, K. (2006). Correlation between glaucomatous visual field loss and expected retinal nerve fiber layer thickness index as calculated by optical coherence tomography, OCT3000. *J Eye,* Vol.23, No.7, (July 2006), pp. 961-965, ISSN 0910-1810

Mitchell, P., Hourihan, F., Sandbach, J., & Wang, JJ. (1999). The relationship between glaucoma and myopia: the Blue Mountains Eye Study. *Ophthalmology,* Vol.106, No.10,*(October* 1999), p.p. 2010-2015, ISSN 0161-6420

Nakazawa, M., Kurotaki, J., & Ruike, H. (2008). Longterm findings in peripaillary crescent formation in eyes with mild or moderate myopia. *Acta Ophthalmol,*Vol.86, No.6, (September 2008), pp. 626-629, ISSN 1755-3768

Nizankowska, MH. & Kaczmarek, R. (2005). The prevalence of glaucoma in the wroclaw population. The wroclaw epidemiological study. *Ophthalmic Epidemiol,* Vol. 12, No.6, (December 2005), p.p. 363-371, ISSN 0928-6586

Patella, VM.(2003). *STRATUSoct™ : Establishment of normative reference values for retinal nerve fiber layer thickness measurements,* Carl Zeiss Meditec, Inc. Dublin, CA, USA

Quigley, HA. (1999). Neuronal death in glaucoma. *Prog Retin Eye Res,* Vol.18, No. 1, (January 1999), pp. 39-57, ISSN 1350-9462

Quigley, HA., West, SK., Rodriguez, J., Munoz, B., Klein, R., & Snyder, R. (2001). The prevalence of glaucoma in a population-based study of Hispanic subjects. Proyecto VER. *Arch Ophthalmol,* Vol.119, No.12, (December 2001), p.p. 1819-1826, ISSN 0003-9950

Rotchford, AP. & Johnson GJ. (2002). Glaucoma in Zulus. A population-based cross-sectional survey in a rural district in South Africa. *Arch Ophthalmol,*Vol.120, No.4, (April 2002), pp. 471-478, ISSN 0003-9950

Salchow, DJ., Oleynikov, YS., Chiang, MF., Kennedy - Salvhow, SE., Langton, K, tsai, JC., & AI - Aswad, LA. (2006). Retinal nerve fiver layer thickness in normal children measured with optical coherence tomography. *Ophthalmology*, Vol.113, No.5, (May 2006), pp. 786-791, ISSN 0161-6420

Suzuki, Y., Yamamoto, T., Araie, M., Iwase, A., Tomidokoro, A., Abe, H., Shirato, S., Kuwayama, Y., Mishima, H., Shimizu, H., Tomita, G., Inoue, Y., & Kitazawa, Y. (2008). The Tajimi study review. *J Jpn Ophthalmol Soc,* Vol.112, No. 12, (December 2008), pp. 1039-1058, ISSN 0029-0203

Wensor, MD., McCarty, CA., Stanislavsky, YL., Livingston, PM., & Taylor, HR. (1998). The prevalence of glaucoma in the Melbourne visual impairment project. *Ophthalmology,*Vol.105, No.4, (April 1998), p.p. 733-739, ISSN 0161-6420

10

Morphological Changes of Retinal Pigment Epithelial Detachment in Central Serous Chorioretinopathy

Ari Shinojima and Mitsuko Yuzawa
Department of Ophthalmology, Surugadai Hospital of Nihon University
Japan

1. Introduction

Normal retinal tissue consists of the nine-layer sensory retina on the vitreous side and one-layer retinal pigment epithelium on the choroidal side. Serous retinal detachment is a detachment of the sensory retina from the retinal pigment epithelium. Central serous chorioretinopathy (CSC) is a condition causing local serous neurosensory detachment in the macular region. CSC causes circular or oval serous retinal detachment. Spectral domain-optical coherence tomography (SD-OCT) is a useful tool for detecting morphological changes. Spectralis® HRA+OCT (Spectralis Heidelberg retina angiograph optical coherence tomography) uses a super-luminescent diode as the light source, which has a central wavelength of 870 nm. Scanning an object with two different wavelengths allows simultaneous display of the confocal scanning laser ophthalmoscopy (cSLO) image and the OCT image of a chosen plane. Therefore, it is possible to visualize the OCT image of a lesion depicted on angiography (fluorescein angiography or indocyanine green angiography) in the same location. The angiographic image of the structure or the lesion depicted on the OCT image can both be observed. Using Spectralis® HRA+OCT, we performed fluorescein angiography, indocyanine green angiography and OCT during the clinical course of acute central serous chorioretinopathy. We studied in detail the state of the retinal pigment epithelium at the leakage point, and the relations of the leakage point to both pigment epithelial detachment and moderately to highly reflective substances.

2. Central serous chorioretinopathy

In 1866, von Graefe described some of the clinical features of "relapsing idiopathic detachment of the macula", since many reports of CSC were reported. There were a couple of reports about the pathological features of CSC, but they were reported in the era before the development of OCT. The characteristic finding in CSC is the formation of a localized neurosensory retinal detachment caused by leakage of fluid at the level of the retinal pigment epithelium. Although resolution of the serous exudation and restoration of central vision frequently takes place, some patients tend to relapse and develop permanent loss of vision. The age group affected most commonly is young adults between 30 to 50 years of age and particularly middle-aged men unilaterally; however, it can occur at 60 years of age or older. The pathogenesis of CSC remains incompletely understood, although a variety of risk factors are associated with the development of the disorder. Psychopharmacologic medication use, corticosteroid use, and hypertension are reported to be associated with central serous chorioretinopathy (Tittl et al, 1999), but Kitzmann et al reported that there were no significant risk factors identified for CSC (Kitzmann, 2008). They found that the mean annual age-adjusted incidence per 100 000 was 9.9 (95% confidence interval (CI), 7.4-12.4) for men and 1.7 (95% CI, 0.7-2.7) for women. The incidence of CSC was approximately 6 times higher in men than in women ($P<0.001$). Median time from diagnosis to recurrence was 1.3 years (range, 0.4-18.2) (Kitzmann, 2008). The chief complaints of CSC patients are image distortion or a small central scotoma, visual disturbance or impaired color vision. In the acute stage, fluorescein angiography shows a focal leak at the level of the retinal pigment epithelium, and this focal leak gradually expands into the shape of a smokestack or an inkblot pattern. In CSC, the presence of damage to the retinal pigment epithelium blood-retinal barrier, with metabolic impairment of retinal pigment epithelium transport causes focal leakage. Indocyanine green angiography shows choroidal vascular abnormalities in CSC. In active CSC, indocyanine green angiography shows choroidal filling delay, venous dilation, and focal choroidal hyperfluorescence surrounding leakage from the retinal pigment epithelium. In CSC, the grayish white lesion seems to be fibrinous exudate that accumulates in the subretinal space on OCT. The fibrinous exudate sometimes appears as a ring-shaped area (Shinojima et al, 2010) (Fig. 1).

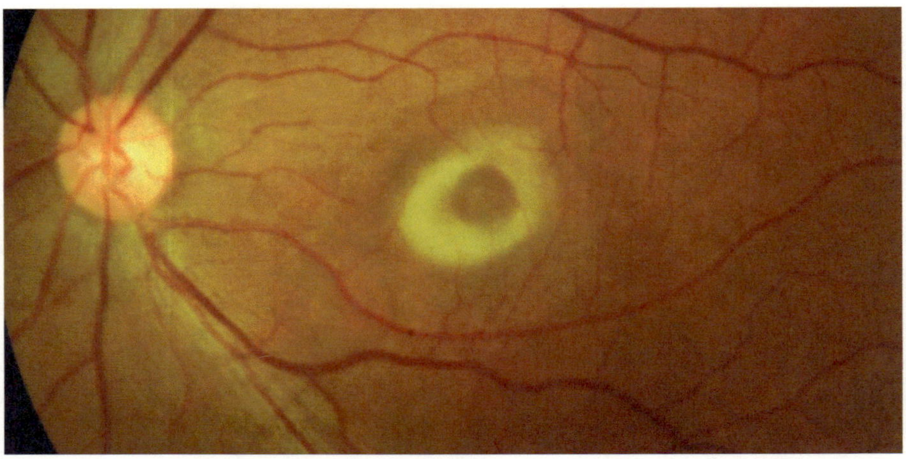

Fig. 1. Citation; Shinojima A, Hirose T, Mori R, Kawamura A, Yuzawa M. (2010). Morphologic findings in acute central serous chorioretinopathy using spectral domain-optical coherence tomography with simultaneous angiography. *Retina, Figure 4.*

2.1 Serous retinal detachment and pigment epithelial detachment in CSC

Retinal pigment epithelial detachment (PED) appears ophthalmoscopically as single or multiple, circumscribed, round or oval lesions within the posterior fundus.

There are various types of PED; serous PED, hemorrhagic PED, drusenoid PED and fibrovascular PED. Serous PED is often observed in CSC. A leakage point is often observed at PED in CSC, but some PED is not related to leakage. Recent reports describe many cases of PED in CSC (Shinojima et al, 2010). A leakage point is often observed at PED in CSC. SD-OCT has allowed the detection of small or shallow PED, which was not previously possible (Fig. 2).

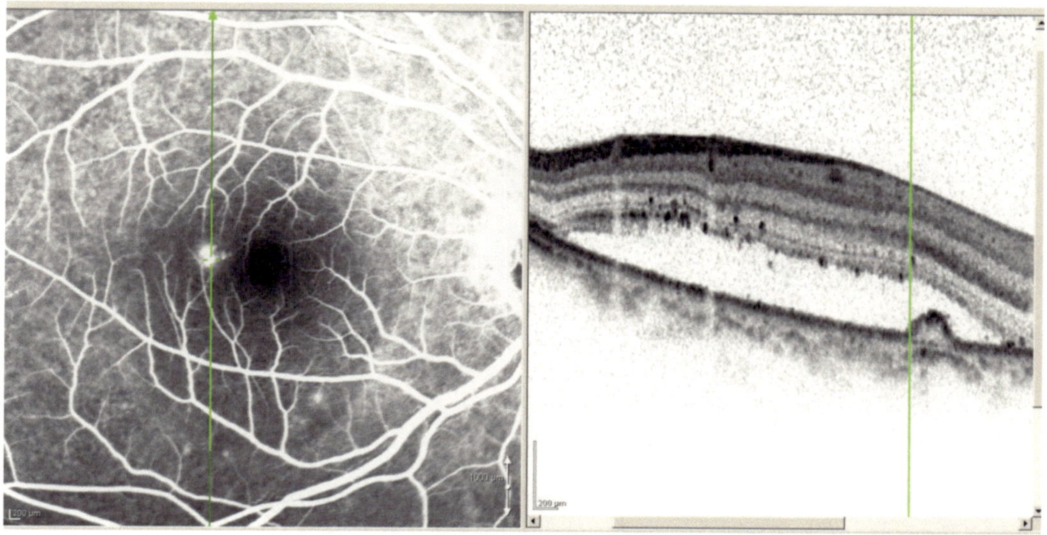

Fig. 2. Citation; Shinojima A, Hirose T, Mori R, Kawamura A, Yuzawa M. (2010). Morphologic findings in acute central serous chorioretinopathy using spectral domain-optical coherence tomography with simultaneous angiography. *Retina, Figure 3.* Simultaneous fluorescein angiography (left) and OCT photographs (right) were obtained in the early phase.

2.1.1 Morphological changes in PED

PED are often detected at leakage point in CSC. Fujimoto et al reported that among 23 leakage sites in 21 eyes, Fourier-domain OCT showed retinal pigment epithelium abnormalities in 22 (96%) sites (14 sites [61%] with a PED and 8 [35%] with a protruding or irregular retinal pigment epithelium layer). (Fujimoto et al, 2008). Shinojima et al reported that PED was recognized at 71% of leakage points in acute CSC (Shinojima et al, 2010), but sometimes PED is detected at other sites than the leakage point. In addition, SD-OCT with simultaneous cSLO enabled us to detect tiny PED by examining the area in proximity to the leakage point. We followed the changes in the PED for approximately one year.

2.1.2 Morphological changes in PED for approximately one year

Simultaneous photograph of fluorescein angiography and OCT in early phase (Fig. 3). Seven weeks after the onset of subjective symptoms, there is no serous retinal detachment at the PED in the supra-temporal region (white arrow). This PED was confirmed by fluorescein angiography, indocyanine green angiography and OCT findings. Fluorescein angiography showed pooling in the area (Figure 3). Yellow arrow indicates a smokestack pattern of leakage (left). Blue arrowheads indicate highly reflective substances just below the retinal pigment epithelium (right).

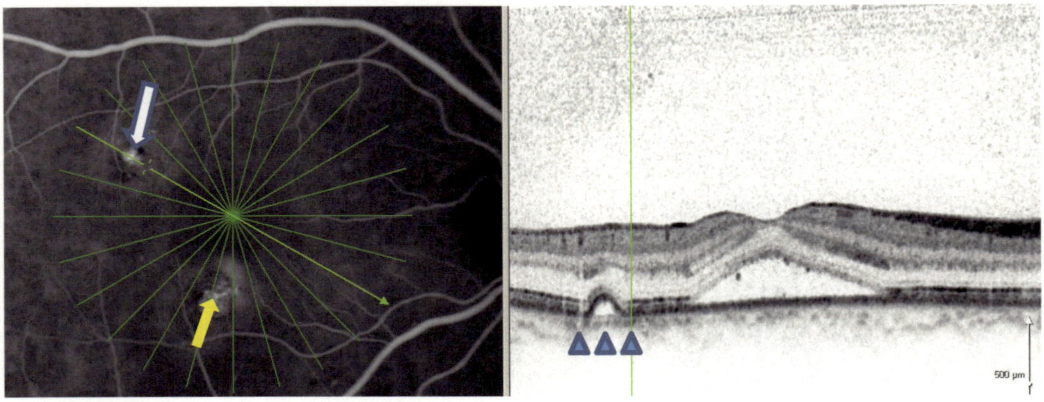

Fig. 3. PED without serous retinal detachment. Simultaneous fluorescein angiography (left) and OCT photographs (right) were obtained in the early phase.

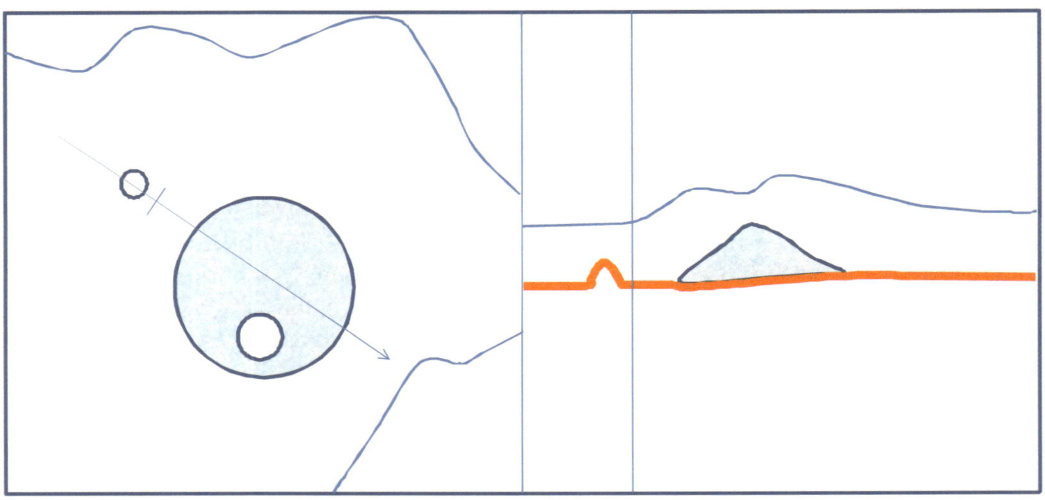

Fig. 4. Schema of Fig. 3. PED in the supra-temporal region without serous retinal detachment. Serous retinal detachment (light blue) and retinal pigment epithelium layer (orange line). There is no serous retinal detachment at the PED in the supra-temporal region.

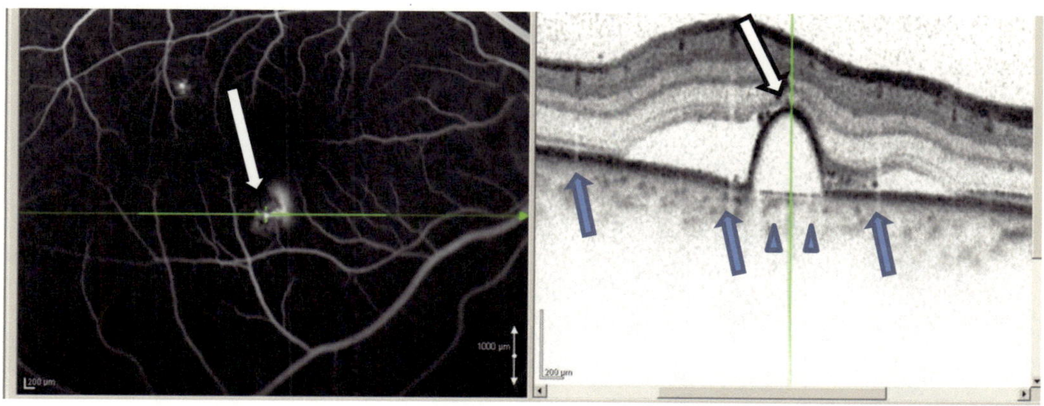

Fig. 5. Citation; Shinojima A, Hirose T, Mori R, Kawamura A, Yuzawa M. (2010). Morphologic findings in acute central serous chorioretinopathy using spectral domain-optical coherence tomography with simultaneous angiography. *Retina, Figure 2.* Seven weeks after the onset of subjective symptoms, i.e., at the same time as in Fig. 3. Simultaneous fluorescein angiography (left) and OCT photographs (right) were obtained in the early phase.The PED at the leakage point is below the sensory retina. White arrow indicates leakage point from pigment epithelial detachment. A smokestack pattern in the early phase and gradual, but increasingly marked, leakage are seen (left). The leakage point corresponds to the central part of the PED on OCT (right). Blue arrows indicate retinal vessel artifacts (right). Other OCT sections show focal serous separation, indicating one serous detachment. Blue arrowheads indicate highly reflective substances just below the retinal pigment epithelium.

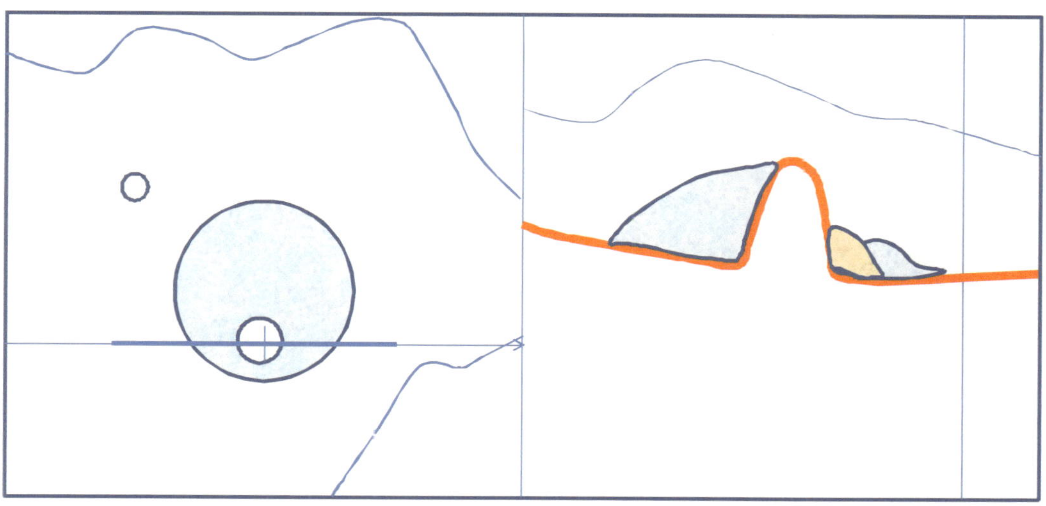

Fig. 6. Schema of Fig. 5. Serous retinal detachment (light blue), substances like fibrin (light brown) and retinal pigment epithelium layer (orange line). Retinal pigment epithelium layer (orange line) is continuous.

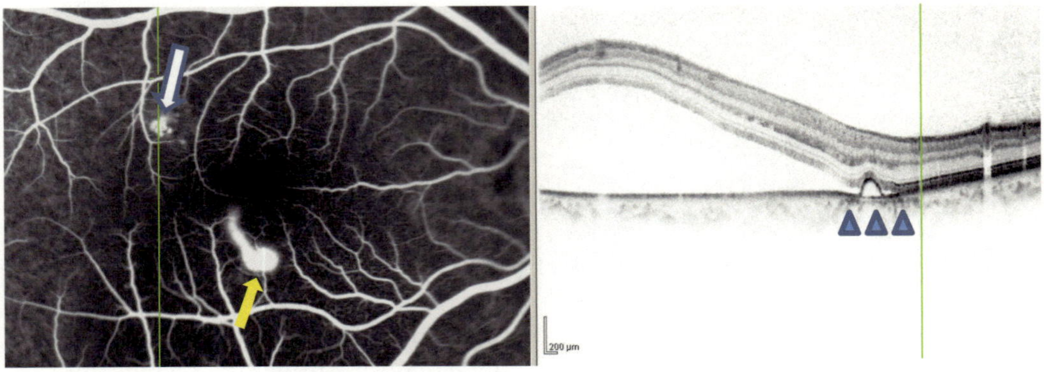

Fig. 7. PED under serous retinal detachment three months after onset. Simultaneous fluorescein angiography (left) and OCT photographs (right) were obtained in the early phase. Although SRD was not detected above PED in the supra-temporal region at seven weeks after the onset of subjective symptoms, as in Fig. 3, SRD slightly reached the PED in the supra-temporal region three months after the onset of subjective symptoms. Fluorescein angiography shows pooling (white arrow). Yellow arrow indicates a marked smokestack pattern of leakage. Blue arrowheads indicate highly reflective substances just below the retinal pigment epithelium.

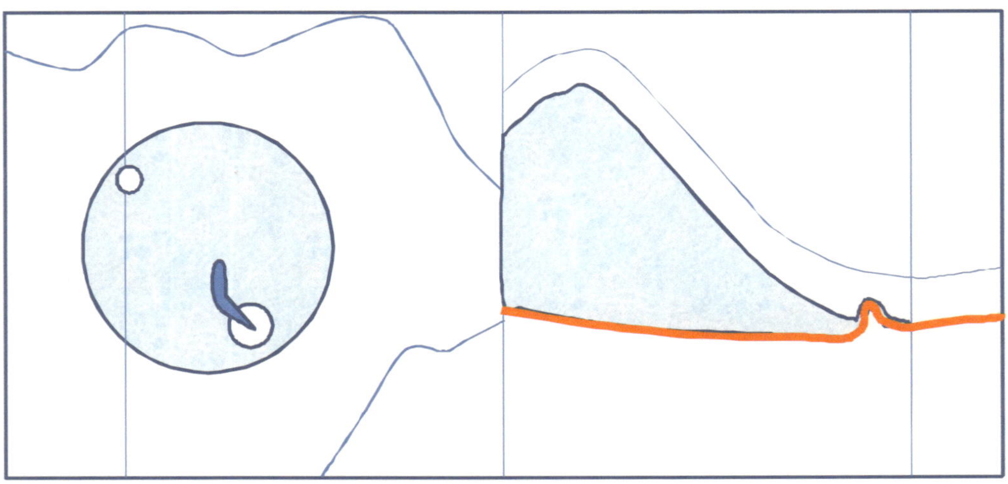

Fig. 8. Schema of Fig. 7. Serous retinal detachment (light blue), smoke-stack leakage (blue) and retinal pigment epithelium layer (orange line). Retinal pigment epithelium layer (orange line) is continuous.

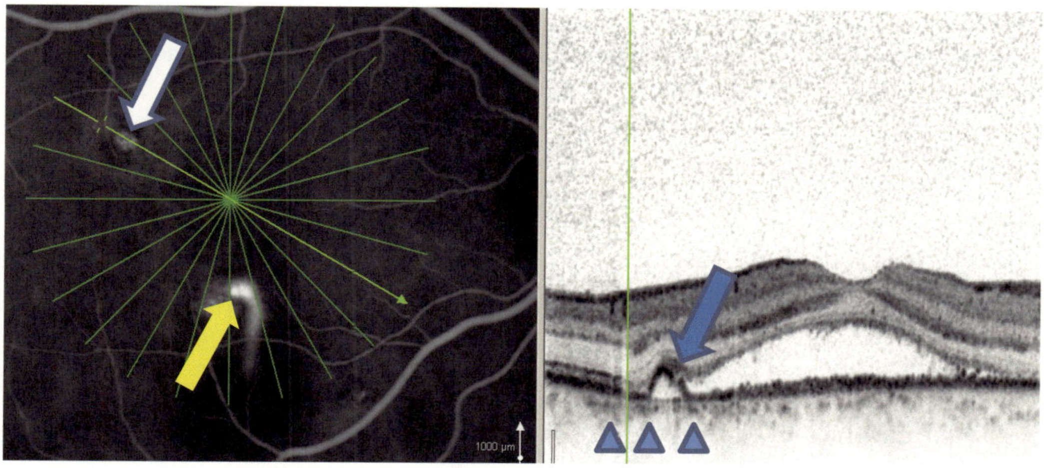

Fig. 9. Retinal pigment epithelium defect in PED. Five and a half months after the onset of subjective symptoms before photocoagulation. Simultaneous fluorescein angiography (left) and OCT photographs (right) were obtained in the early phase. Yellow arrow indicates leakage point. White arrow indicates PED (left). Blue arrow indicates a retinal pigment epithelium layer defect at PED. Blue arrowheads indicate highly reflective substances just below the retinal pigment epithelium (right). Other OCT sections show focal serous separation, indicating a serous detachment.

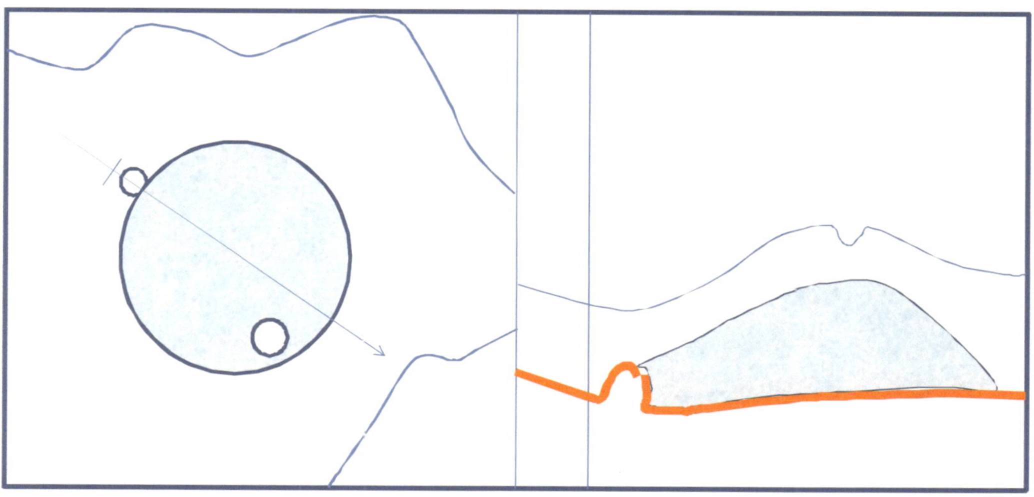

Fig. 10. Schema of Fig.9. Retinal pigment epithelium defect in PED. Serous retinal detachment (light blue) and retinal pigment epithelium layer (orange line). A retinal pigment epithelium defect (right) was detected at the PED in the supra-temporal region without leakage.

In the presence of damage to the retinal pigment epithelium blood-retinal barrier, subretinal fluid is rapidly cleared by passive forces. Thus, it is apparent that retinal pigment epithelium defects do not by themselves cause serous retinal detachment (Marmor, 1988). This description by Marmor may explain our present findings. A retinal pigment epithelium defect was not detected at the prominent leakage point, as shown in Fig. 5.

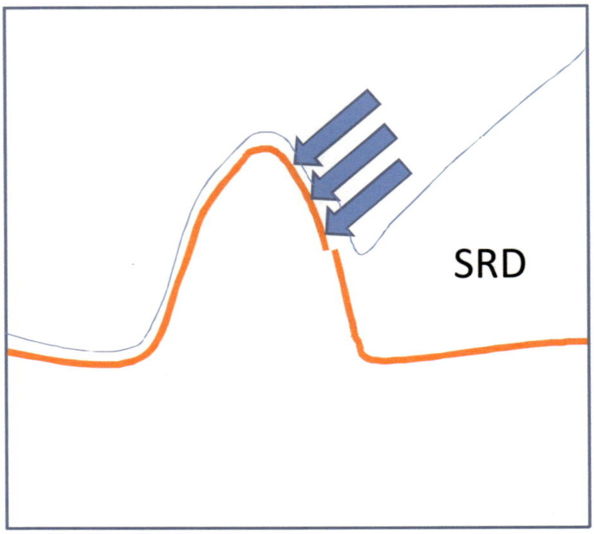

Fig. 11. Schema of Fig.9 about the PED in the supra-temporal region (Fig. 9 left, and Fig. 10 right). Retinal pigment epithelium layer (orange line) defect was detected at the PED in the supra-temporal region without leakage. It appears that PED is pushed by the neurosensory retina (blue arrow).

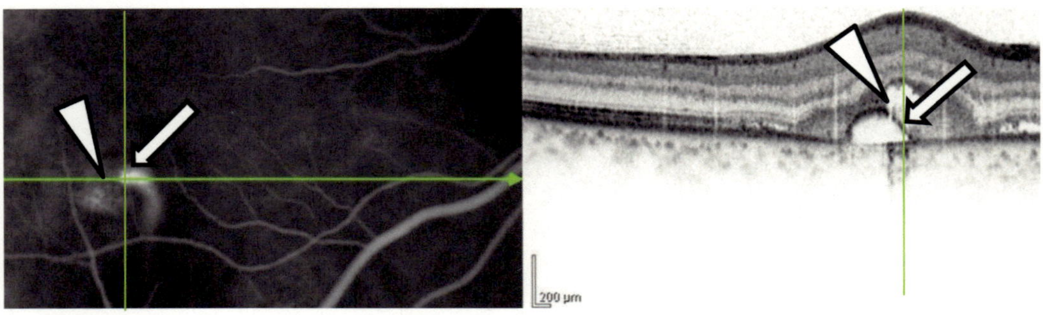

Fig. 12. Citation; Shinojima A, Hirose T, Mori R, Kawamura A, Yuzawa M. (2010). Morphologic findings in acute central serous chorioretinopathy using spectral domain-optical coherence tomography with simultaneous angiography. *Retina, Figure 2.* Five and a half months after the onset of subjective symptoms before photocoagulation. Simultaneous fluorescein angiography (left) and OCT photographs (right) were obtained in the early phase. This figure is the same part in Fig. 5. White arrow indicates leakage point from pigment epithelial detachment. A smoke stack pattern in the early phase and gradual leakage are seen. Highly reflective substances in the subretinal space and a retinal pigment epithelium defect (white arrowhead) can be seen at a point 50 µm from the leakage point at 5.5 months after the onset of subjective symptoms. The RPE layer defect does not involve the inner/outer segment.

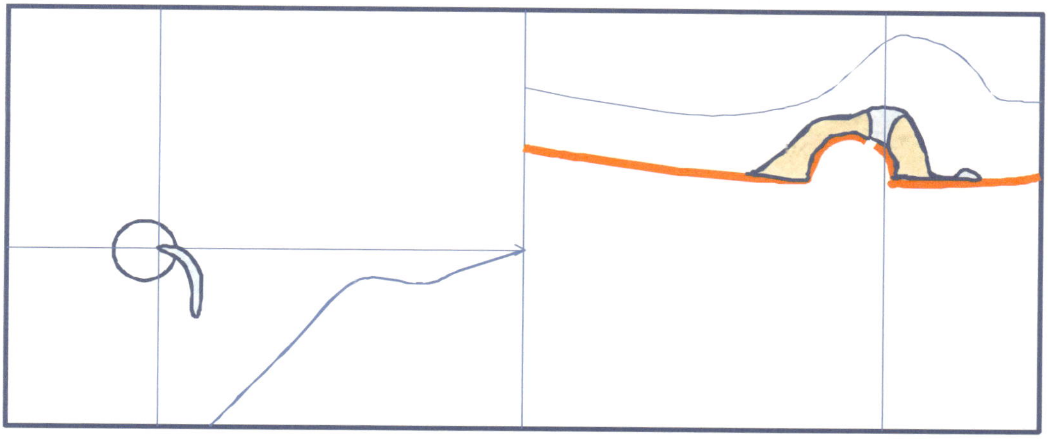

Fig. 13. Schema of Fig. 12. Serous retinal detachment (light blue), substances like fibrin (light brown) and retinal pigment epithelium layer (orange line). Highly reflective substances in the subretinal space (light brown) and a retinal pigment epithelium (orange line) defect can be seen at a point 50 µm from the leakage point at 5.5 months after the onset of subjective symptoms.

The transverse resolution of Spectralis® HRA+OCT is 14 µm, while the retinal pigment epithelium diameter in the macular region is 16 µm. Therefore, it may not always be possible to discern a one-cell defect among a row of retinal pigment epithelium cells with this device. Most retinal pigment epithelium defects in CSC patients may be too small to be detected even by SD-OCT analysis. We also speculate that these minute defects cause minute focal leakage.

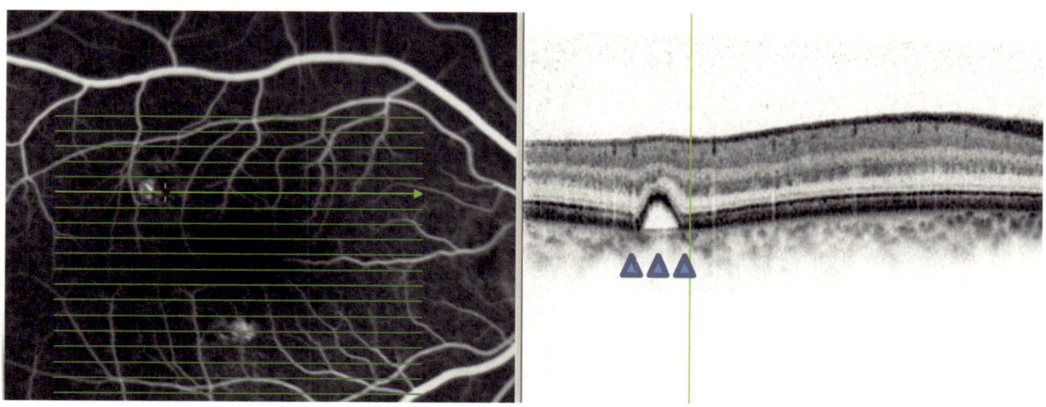

Fig. 14. PED after about 6 months after the photocoagulation. Simultaneous fluorescein angiography (left) and OCT photographs (right) were obtained in the early phase. The retinal pigment epithelium layer is continuous. Blue arrowheads indicate highly reflective substances just below the retinal pigment epithelium.

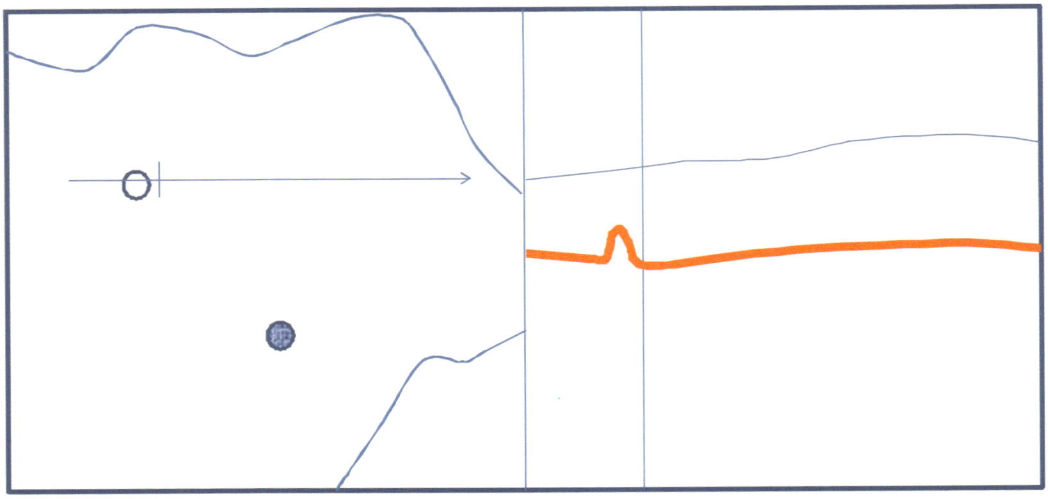

Fig. 15. Schema of Figure 14. about retinal pigment epithelium defect in PED. Retinal pigment epithelium layer (orange line) is continuous. No retinal pigment epithelial defect was detected at the PED in the supra-temporal region. Blue spot indicates the place after photocoagulation

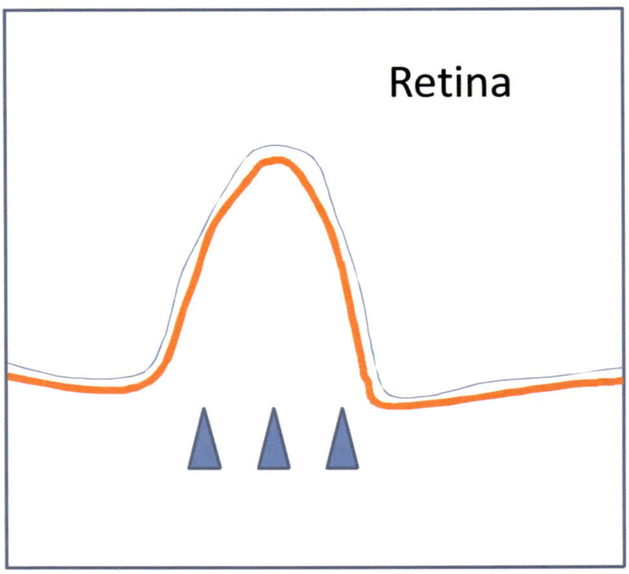

Fig. 16. Schema of Fig. 14 (right) about highly reflective substances below retinal pigment epithelium. The retinal pigment epithelium layer (orange line) is continuous. Blue arrowheads indicate highly reflective substances just below the retinal pigment epithelium.

The form of PED was maintained after reattachment. Highly reflective substances beneath the retinal pigment epithelium (blue arrowhead) undergo serous exudation secondary to congestion of choroidal venules, which may the reason for maintenance of the formation of PED.

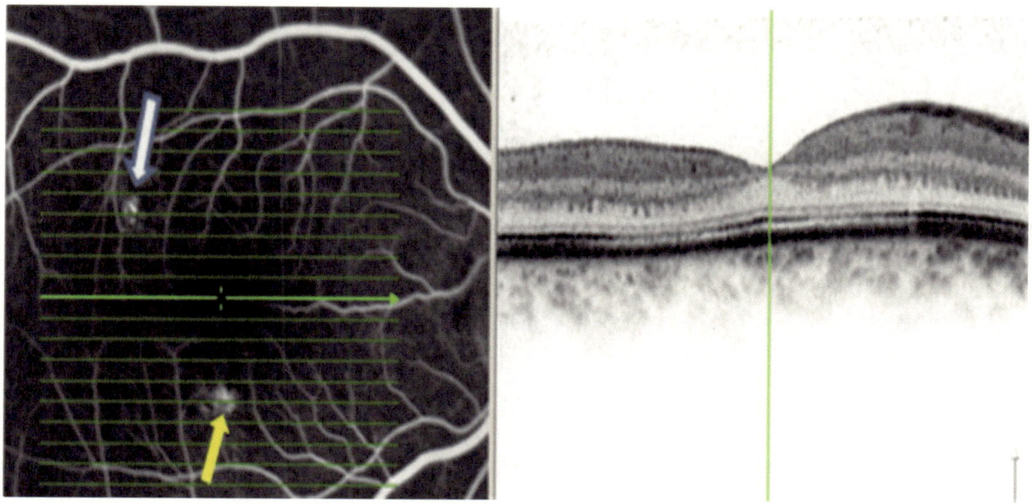

Fig. 17. Reattached serous retinal detachment about 6 months after photocoagulation. Simultaneous fluorescein angiography (left) and OCT photographs (right) were obtained in the early phase. The same time (6 months after photocoagulation) as in Fig. 14, serous retinal detachment has reattached through the fovea (fluorescein angiography +OCT). White arrow indicates PED. Yellow arrow indicates the place after photocoagulation where retinal pigment epithelium irregularities exist. A window defect was confirmed.

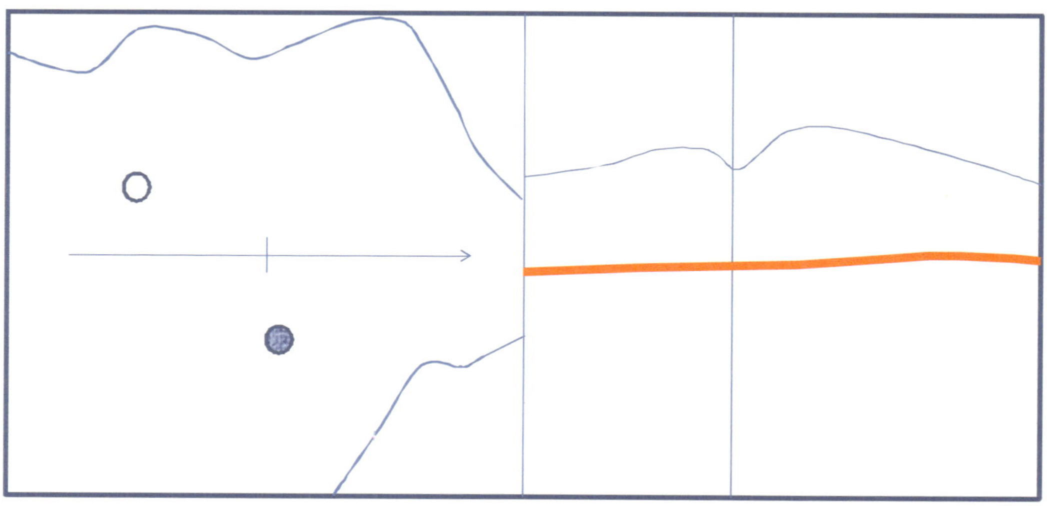

Fig. 18. Schema of Fig. 17. There is no serous retinal detachment through the fovea. The retinal pigment epithelium layer (orange line) is continuous. White spot in the supra-temporal region indicates PED and blue spot indicates the place after photocoagulation.

2.1.3 Laser photocoagulation in CSC

Photocoagulation of a leaking point can facilitate resolution of the fluid, but as long as the underlying metabolic dysfunction of the retinal pigment epithelium or choroidal hyperpermeability persists, recurrence is possible.

3. Conclusion

A retinal pigment epithelium defect at PED was detected 5.5 months after the onset of subjective symptoms. PED without leakage was restored after photocoagulation. On the other hand, PED with leakage lost its shape and changed into an RPE irregularity by local photocoagulation. Highly reflective substances may be related to PED formation. Even if a retinal pigment epithelium layer defect exists, leakage may not result. The sensory retina may compress damaged retinal pigment epithelium forming a PED, when a serous retinal detachment is reattached, and the PED may collapse morphologically.

4. References

Fujimoto H, Gomi F, Wakabayashi T, Sawa M, Tsujikawa M, Tano Y. (2009). Morphologic changes in acute central serous chorioretinopathy evaluated by Fourier-domain optical coherence tomography. *Ophthalmology,*Vol. 115. No. 9, September 2009, pp. 1494-500, 1500.e1-2.

Iida T, Hagimura N, Sato T, et al. (2000). Evaluation of central serous chorioretinopathy with optical coherence tomography. *Am J Ophthalmol,* Vol. 129. No.1 , pp. 16-20.

Kitzmann AS, Pulido JS, Diehl NN, et al. (2008). The incidence of central serous chorioretinopathy. *Br J Ophthalmol,* Vol. 115. No.1, pp. 169-73.

Marmor MF. New hypothesis on the pathogenesis and treatment of serous retinal detachment. (1988). *Graefes Arch Clin Exp Ophthalmol,*Vol. 226. No. 6. 1988, pp.548-52.

Shinojima A, Hirose T, Mori R, Kawamura A, Yuzawa M. (2010). Morphologic Findings in Acute Central Serous Chorioretinopathy Using Spectral Domain-Optical Coherence Tomography With Simultaneous Angiography. *Retina,* Vol. 30. No. 2, 2010, pp. 193-202. ISSN:0275-004X

Tittle MK, Spaide RF, Wong D, et al. (1999). Systemic findings associated with central serous chorioretinopathy. *Am J Ophthalmol,* Vol. 128. No.1 , pp. 63-8.

11

Clinical Applications of Optical Coherence Tomography in Ophthalmology

Upender K. Wali and Nadia Al Kharousi
College of Medicine and Health Sciences, Sultan Qaboos University
Oman

"In Ophthalmology, one who relies on Optical Coherence Tomography (OCT) alone is little wise, one who relies on OCT and Fluorescein angiography is wiser, and one who relies on OCT, angiography and clinical examination is the wisest."

1. Introduction

Optical coherence tomography (OCT) was first reported in 1991 as a non-invasive ocular imaging technology (Huang et al, 1991; Hrynchak & Simpson, 2007). It generates a false-color representation of the tissue structures, based on the intensity of the returned light. Over years, the clinical applications of OCT have improved dramatically in precision and specificity. It has been compared to an in vivo optical biopsy. As the resolution of OCT has been getting more and more refined, the identification, detection, localization and quantification of the tissues has accordingly, become more superior and reliable (Ryan SJ, 2006). There are several non-ophthalmic applications of OCT as well, but this chapter shall focus on its clinical applications in ocular diseases alone (Aguirre et al., 2003; Fujimoto, 2003).

2. Basic applications of optical coherence tomography in eye disorders:

Before we proceed with the clinical part of this chapter, let us have the basic information about the OCT scan and the tissues, which would permit comprehensive interpretation of the text and the abnormal images from pathologic tissues. Different models of OCT machines are in use ranging from Stratus (resolution 10 microns) to Cirrus-HD (resolution 5 microns) to ultrahigh-resolution models (resolution 2-3 microns, Drexler et al., 1999, 2001). To refresh our knowledge, we mention about the normal values first; these values help to interpret OCT scans in a better way:

- Distance between vitreoretinal interface and anterior surface of retinal pigment epithelium (RPE): 200 - 275 microns.
- Mean thickness in the foveal region: 170 – 190 microns.
- Mean thickness in peripheral retina: 220 – 280 microns.
- Mean thickness of retinal nerve fiber layer (RNFL): 270 microns (1000 microns from fovea where nerve fibers form a slight arcuate thickening).
- Normal retinal volume: 6-7 cubic mm.

The OCT scan printouts bear pseudocolor imaging and retinal mapping is based on different color codes (white, red, orange, yellow, green, blue, and black in order), White being the thickest scanned retina (>470 microns) and black the thinnest scanned retina (<150 microns) [Hee et al., 2004]. However, such color imaging or color maps may vary for different models of OCT equipment. The macular thickness stock and color code distribution depicted here is for Cirrus 3D HD-OCT (Figure 1).

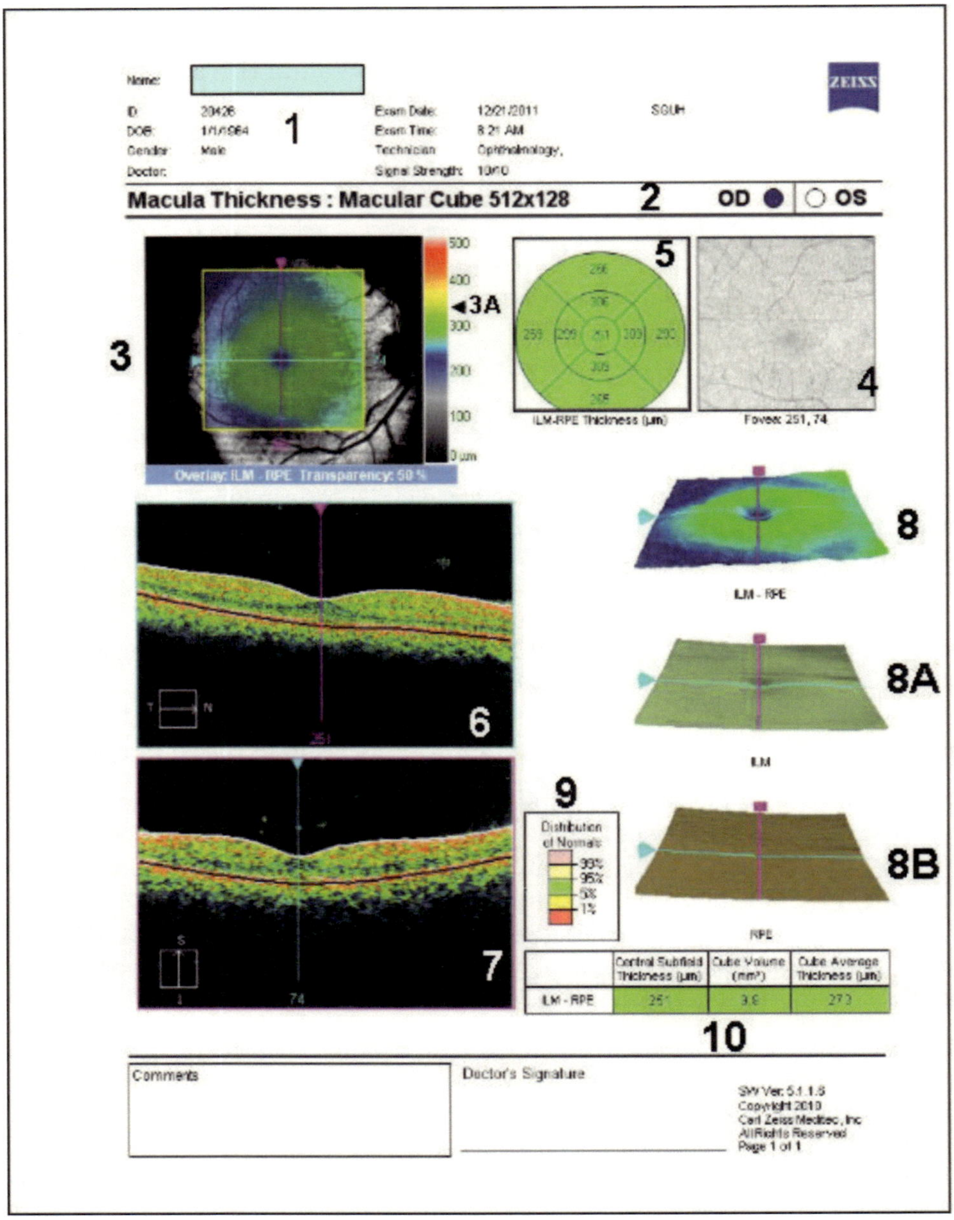

Fig. 1. OCT macular thickness stock printout.

Section 1: Patient related data, examination date, list and signal strength. It is ideal to have minimum signal strength of 5. If it is less, look for media opacities, dry cornea or a very small pupil.

Section 2: Indicates whether the scan is related to macula with its pixel strength (as in this picture) or optic disc cube (see figures 30, 31). (It also displays the laterality of the eye: OD (right eye), OS (left eye).

Section 3: Fundus image with scan cube overlay. 3A: Color code for thickness overlays.

Section 4: OCT fundus image in grey shade. It shows the surface of the area over which the measurements were made.

Section 5: The circular map shows overall average thickness in nine sectors. It has three concentric circles representing diameters of 1 mm, 3 mm and 6 mm, and except for the central circle, is divided into superior, nasal, inferior and temporal quadrants. The central circle has a radius of 500 micrometers.

Section 6: Slice through cube front. Temporal – nasal (left to right).

Section 7: Slice through cube side. Inferior – superior (left to right).

Section 8: Thickness between Internal limiting membrane (ILM) to retinal pigment epithelium (RPE) thickness map. 8A: Anterior layer (ILM). 8B: Posterior layer (RPE). All these are 3-D surface maps.

Section 9: Normative database uses color code to indicate normal distribution percentiles.

Section 10: Numerical average thickness and volume measurements. The central subfield thickness refers to the central circle of the circular map (section 5). The total volume and average thickness refer to the ILM-RPE tissue layer over the entire 6 x 6 mm square scanned area.

Red and white - High reflectivity (long white arrow); black and blue – low reflectivity (yellow arrow); green - intermediate reflectivity (small white arrow). Normal retinal structures are labeled as: red for RNFL and junction of inner and outer segments of photoreceptors (PR); green for plexiform layers, and blue/black for nuclear layers. Both PR junctions and RPE are represented by red lines, former is thinner, later is thicker. An OCT scan should be read from left to right which ensures reading from temporal field to the nasal field for right eye and nasal to temporal in the left eye. It is not possible to identify the laterality of the eye from the macular scans. This should always be checked with fundus video image of the scan.

Light rays from OCT can remarkably penetrate ocular media opacities like mild cataract, mild posterior capsular opacification, mild vitreous hemorrhage, asteroid hyalosis and mild vitritis. In such cases, OCT can give gross macular details, though, a bit compromised in quality. One can go through beautiful OCT text and atlas for images with elaborate description in recommended books (Schuman et al., 2004).

The images in this chapter are from Cirrus 3D HD-OCT (except figure 17) which provides in-vivo viewing, axial cross-sectional 3-D images and measurement of posterior ocular structures. Cirrus HD has incorporated >20% Asian individuals in its normative data base (unlike stratus OCT which has only 3%). This is important as differences in RNFL thickness have been reported between various races (Poinooswamy et al., 1997).

2.1 A word to the OCT technicians

- Miotic pupil, though not a deterrent to macular imaging, induces pupillary block of the incident light and hence affects two ends of the scan (Fujimoto et al., 2004). Mydriasis permits artifact free and a happy OCT procedure. A 3mm pupil would leave both you and your patient smiling.
- Wheel less chair adds to the stability of the patient.
- Encourage patient to blink frequently during the procedure. Wet the cornea if required.
- Instruct the patient to look at the center of the green target, not at the moving red light of the scanning beam.
- Attempt to start with fast, low resolution, and then switch to high resolution scans quickly through areas of interest.
- Remind the ophthalmologist to have prior digital fundus photos and fluorescein angiography (FA) images for correlation with OCT scans later on.
- It is possible to image retina in a silicone oil filled eye, however, in gas filled eyes, it is possible to scan only after gas bubble has receded to 45% of the fill, when inferior meniscus has reached above the foveal level (Jumper et al., 2000; Sato et al., 2003).
- Ensure that the signal strength is five and above.

Optical coherence tomography provides both qualitative (morphology and reflectivity) and quantitative (thickness, mapping and volume) analyses of the examined tissues in-situ and in real time. The indications of OCT include posterior segment lesions like detection of fluid within the retinal layers or under the retina which may not be visible clinically (Kang et al., 2004; Margherio et al., 1989; McDonald et al., 1994; Smiddy et al., 1988), macular holes (Hikichi et al., 1995; Mavrofrides et al., 2005; Wilkins et al., 1996), pseudoholes (Hikichi et al., 1995), epiretinal membranes (ERMs) [Hikichi et al., 1995; Mori et al., 2004], vitreo-macular traction (VMT) [Kang et al., 2004; McDonald et al., 1994], retinoschisis (Eriksson et al., 2004), retinal detachment (Ip et al.,1999), diabetic retinopathy (DR) [Cruz-Villegas et al., 2004; Hee et al., 1998; Schaudig et al., 2000], age-related macular degeneration (ARMD) [Mavro frides et al. 2004], retinal nerve fiber layer thickness (RNFLT), optic disc parameters, and assessment and analysis of anterior segment structures like anterior chamber area, volume and iris thickness. OCT cannot be and should not be interpreted independently vis-à-vis any ocular disease. Also, it should never be taken as the only criteria for the diagnosis or treatment of any ocular disease. The ophthalmologist must have other information available such as valid perspectives of patient's systemic and ocular disease, fluorescein angiography (FA), indocyanine green angiography (ICGA), biomicroscopy, and above all, the relevant history of the disease process. For anterior segment surgeons, especially those involved in phacoemulsification, preoperative assessment of retinal integrity with OCT may be assuring to explain about conditions like ARMD, VMT, macular holes, and ERMs, in case patient's vision does not improve after uneventful cataract surgery. Changes in the reflectivity of tissue are important elements of OCT analysis. When pathology is present, this reflectivity may be increased (hyperreflectivity) or decreased (hyporeflectivity), or a shadow zone may be observed on the scan. The strength of the signal reflected by a specific tissue depends on properties like tissue reflectivity, the amount of light absorbed by the overlying tissues, and the amount of reflected light that reaches the sensor after it has been further attenuated by the interposed tissue. So when the strength of the reflected signal is strong, the scanned tissue has high reflectivity and vice-versa. The shadow effect represents an area of dense, highly refractile tissue that produces a screening effect, which may be complete or incomplete, thereby casting a shadow on an OCT scan that hides the elements behind it. The retinal structures can be hidden at various levels in the preretinal, intraretinal, and/or subretinal regions. Tables 1 and 2 give an elaborate description for these.

Hyperreflective scans	Hyporeflective scans
Drusen	Retinal atrophy
ARMD	Intraretinal/subretinal fluid
CNVM lesions	
RNFL	
ILM	
RPE	
RPE-choriocapillaries complex	
PED	
Anterior face of hemorrhage	
Disciform scars	
Hard Exudates	
Epiretinal membrane	

Table 1. Reflectivity (signal strength) of OCT scans. (ARMD-age related macular degeneration; CNVM-choroidal neovascular membrane; RNFL-retinal nerve fiber layer; ILM-internal limiting membrane; RPE-retinal pigment epithelium; PED-pigment epithelial detachment).

Yes shadows (cone effect): *Superficial layers*	No shadows.
Normal retinal blood vessels	Serous collections
Dense collection of blood	Scanty hemorrhage
Cotton wool exudates	
Deep layers	
Hard exudates (lipoproteins)	
RPE hyperplasia	
Intraocular foreign body	
Dense pigmented scars	
Choroidal nevi	
Thick subretinal neovascular membranes	

Table 2. Shadow effects in Optical coherence tomography. (RPE-retinal pigment epithelium).

Vertical structures like PRs are less reflective than horizontal structures like RNFL or RPE layer. Other axially aligned cellular structures which show low tissue signals or reflectivity (represented by blue, green, yellow colors on OCT scans and printouts) are inner nuclear layer, outer nuclear layer and ganglion cell layers. This is due to reduced back-scattering and reduced back-reflection.

Normal ocular tissues which show high reflectivity are:

- Retinal nerve fiber layer.
- Internal limiting membrane.
- Junction between inner and outer segments of PRs, probably due to densely stacked disc membranes in outer segments (Hoang et al., 2002).
- Retinal pigment epithelium-Bruch's membrane-choriocapillaries complex.

High reflectivity is a feature of reduced retinal thickness (as in retinal atrophy) and pigmentation of the scar tissue, example, a disciform scar. Lesions showing high reflectivity may be superficial, intraretinal or deep retinal.

2.2 Superficial lesions

- Epiretinal and vitreal membranes (Figure 2).
- Exudates and hemorrhages which produce an underlying shadow effect, if dense (Figure 3).
- Cotton wool spots which are exudates at the margin of recent ischemic areas (Figure 4).

2.3 Intraretinal lesions

- Hemorrhages. OCT should be set to a maximum resolution to elicit good scans (Figure 5).
- Hard exudates: these are lipoproteins located at the margin between healthy and edematous retina (Figure 6).
- Retinal fibrosis and disciform degenerative scars (Figure 7).

2.4 Deep lesions

- Drusen (Figure 8).
- Retinal pigment epithelial hyperplasia (Figure 9).
- Intraretinal and subretinal neovascular membranes (Figure 10)
- Scarring following choroiditis, trauma or laser treatment (Figure 11).
- Hyperpigmented choroidal nevi.

2.5 Lesions causing hypo or low reflectivity

- Atrophic RPE (loss of pigment).
- Cystic or pseudocystic areas containing serous fluid (Figure 12).
- Cystoid edema, serous neural retinal detachment (Figure 13) and RPE detachment. Such lesions appear as black, optically empty spaces.

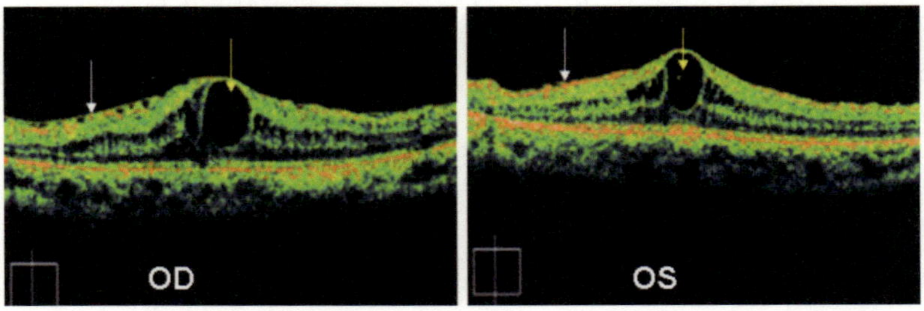

Fig. 2. Epiretinal membrane and cystoid macular edema in a patient with retinitis pigmentosa (Usher's syndrome). OCT in both eyes clearly defines hyperrefective epiretinal membranes (white arrows) which are attached to the internal limiting membranes (hyperreflective signal associated with white arrows). There is associated cystoid macular edema (yellow arrows).

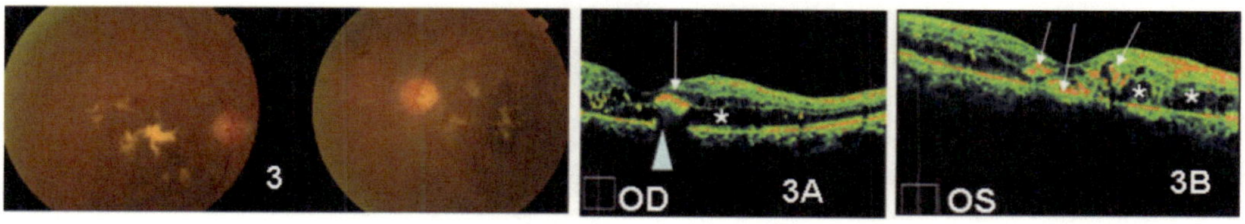

Fig. 3 Nonproliferative diabetic retinopathy. Fundus photo shows hard exudates in macular area in both eyes. 3A: OCT image of right eye: shows retinal edema (asterisk) and hard exudates in deeper retinal layers (white arrows). Note that what appears to be a missing chunk of RPE (arrowhead) is in fact shadow cast by overlying hard exudates (white arrow). 3B: OCT image of left eye showing multiple highly refractile intraretinal hard exudates (white arrows) and intraretinal edema as dark spaces (asterisks).

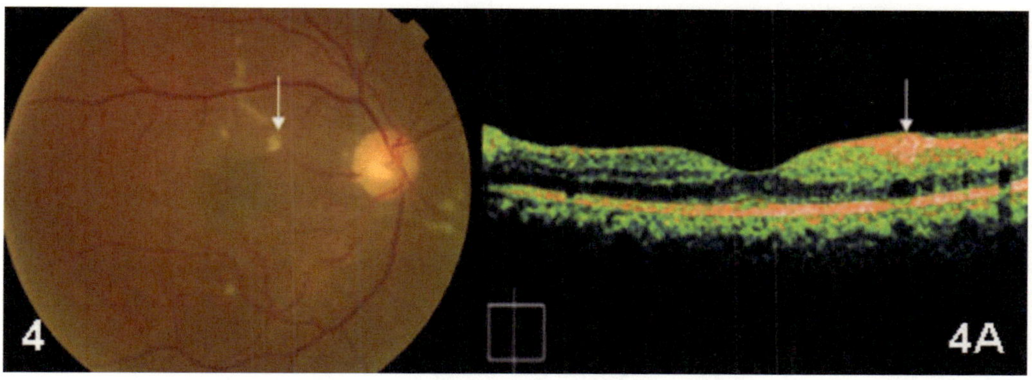

Fig. 4. Cotton wool exudates in a female diabetic patient. Fundus photo of right eye shows multiple yellowish-white soft cotton wool exudates (white arrow). 4A: OCT image has a hyperreflective signal from the exudate located nasal to the macula (white arrow).

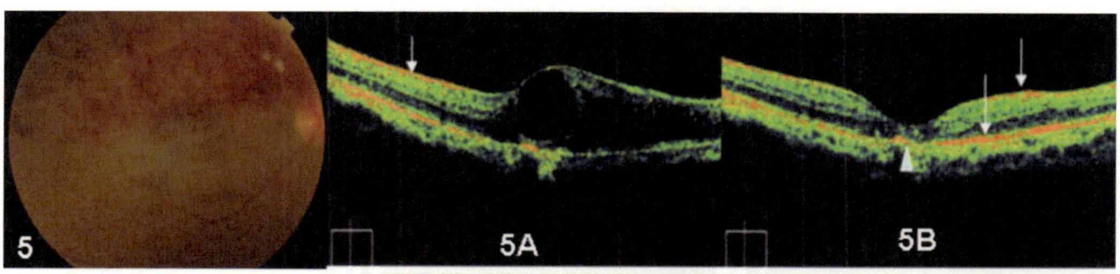

Fig. 5. Superior hemi-central venous occlusion (OD) in a 56 year old female. Fundus photo shows classical superficial and deep retinal hemorrhages. 5A: OCT image shows hyperreflective superficial hemorrhage (white arrow) and a large cystic swelling of the retina. 5B: OCT image of the same eye, six weeks after two intravitreal injections of bevacizumab shows completely resolved edema with residual subfoveal scarring (white arrow head). The hyperreflective signals (white arrows) from hemorrhages are still persisting.

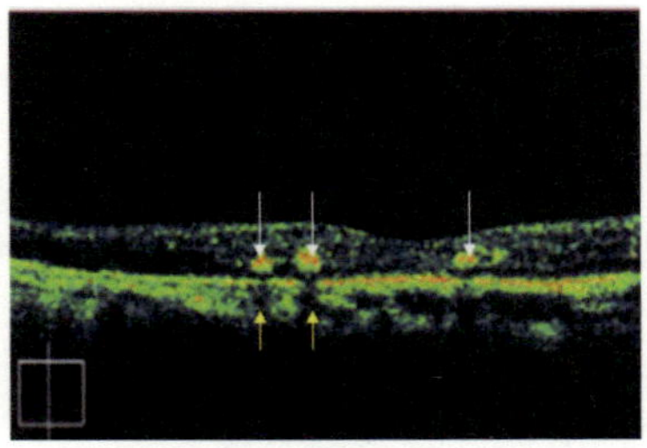

Fig. 6. Macular OCT scan of a female with diabetic retinopathy. The image (vertical scan) shows presence of hyperreflective hard exudates (white arrows) in deeper layers of retina casting underlying shadows (yellow arrows).

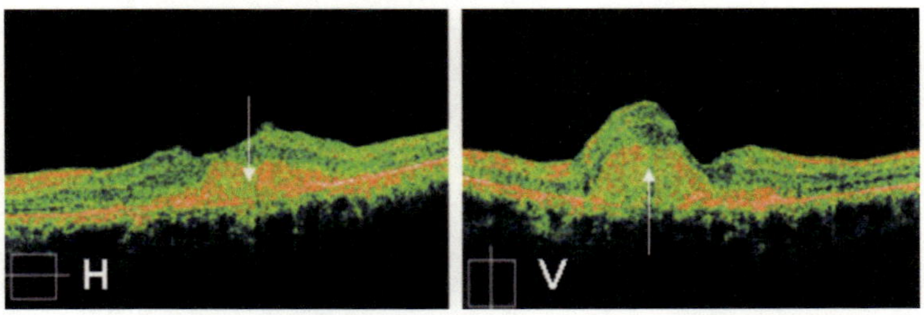

Fig. 7. Horizontal (H) and vertical (V) OCT scans showing hyperreflective subretinal scarring (Arrows) sequel to age related macular degeneration. Note the marked distortion of the macular surface.

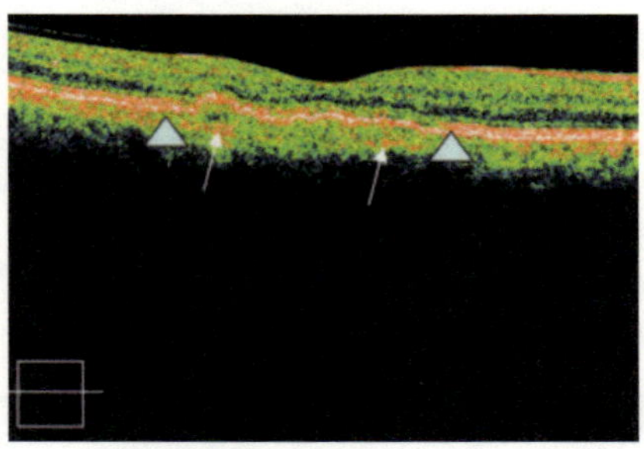

Fig. 8. Drusen. OCT image reveals hyperreflective signals from drusen under the RPE (white arrows). Note irregularity of the RPE contour in OCT (between arrowheads).

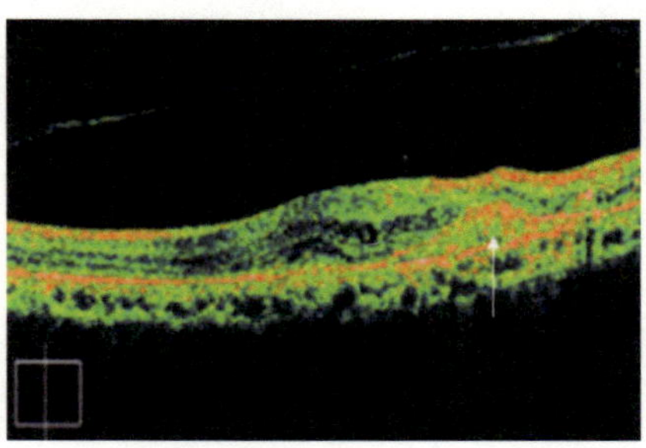

Fig. 9. Retinal pigment epithelial hyperplasia with hyperreflective signal (white arrow) in a case of ARMD.

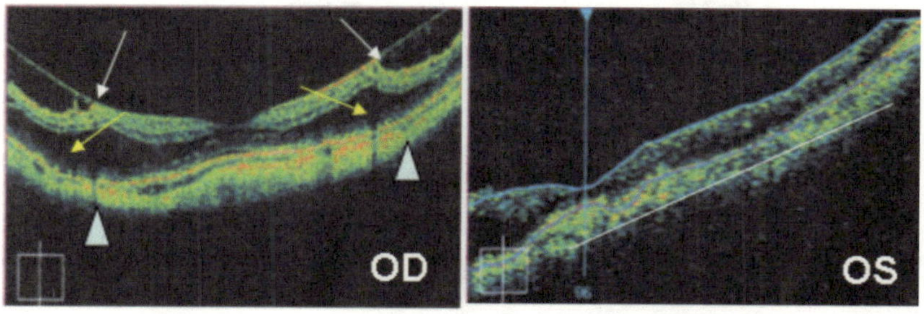

Fig. 10. Retinal vascular membranes (CNVM) with vitreo-macular traction and retinoschisis: OCT image of right eye (OD) shows residual CNVM (between arrowheads). There is VMT (white arrows) and retino-macular schisis (yellow arrows). Left eye (OS) OCT image depicts scarred CNVM (along line). There is VMT (white arrows) and retino-macular schisis (yellow arrows).

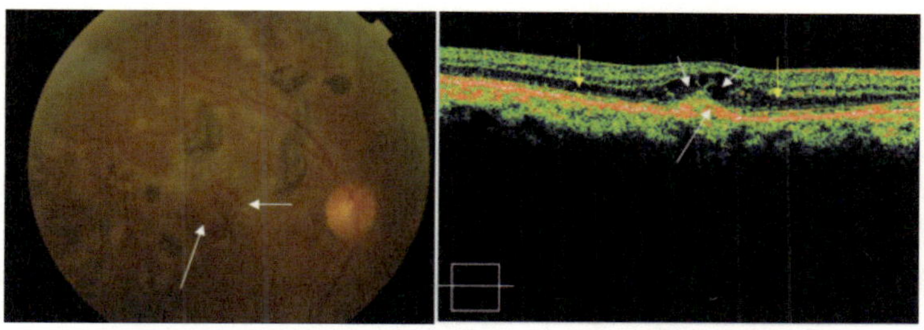

Fig. 11. Post-inflammatory CNVM (multifocal choroiditis) in right eye. Color fundus photo show subretinal exudates predominantly in macular area (small arrow), subfoveal grayish membrane (long arrow), and multiple hyperpigmented chorioretinal scars sequel to old inflammation. OCT shows hyperreflective CNVM scar (long white arrow) after PDT and four injections of ranibizumab. Note associated cystoid retinal fluid with septa (small white arrows), and a shallow neurosensory detachment (yellow arrows).

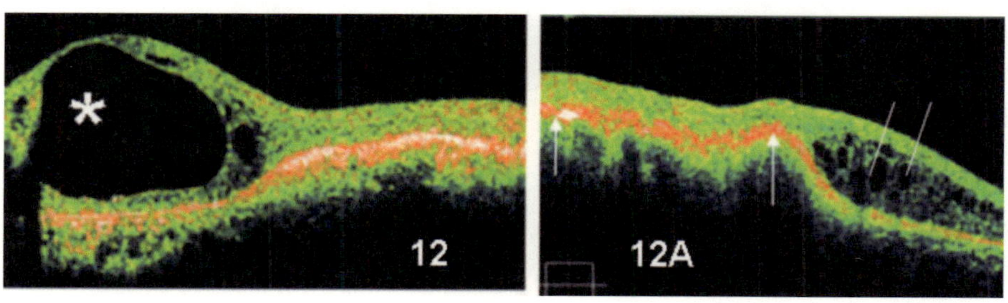

Fig. 12. OCT image showing a large cystic elevation of retina (asterisk). 12A: multiple intraretinal cystoid spaces (straight lines) with altered contour of the hyperreflective thickened retinal pigment epithelium (between arrows).

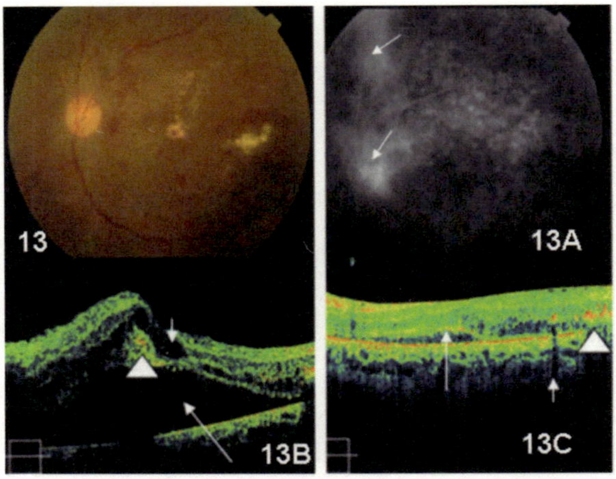

Fig. 13. Diabetic retinopathy in a 31 year old type 1 diabetes patient. Color fundus photo of left eye shows hemorrhages, exudates and retinal edema, mainly within temporal arcades. 13A: FA shows leakage (white arrows) suggestive of active proliferative diabetic retinopathy. 13B: OCT scan shows intraretinal edema (short arrow), subretinal fluid (long arrow) and hard exudates (arrowhead). Central retinal thickness (CRT) measured 470 microns). Fluid is represented by dark, optically empty spaces. Patient received intravitreal injection triamcinolone and laser. 13C: Right side OCT image: Eight weeks later there was improvement in macular edema (CRT 375 microns), with minimal residual edema and a small collection of subfoveal fluid (arrow). Hyperreflective exudates can be seen on right side of the scan (arrowhead). Also note the shadow effect of hard exudate (short arrow).

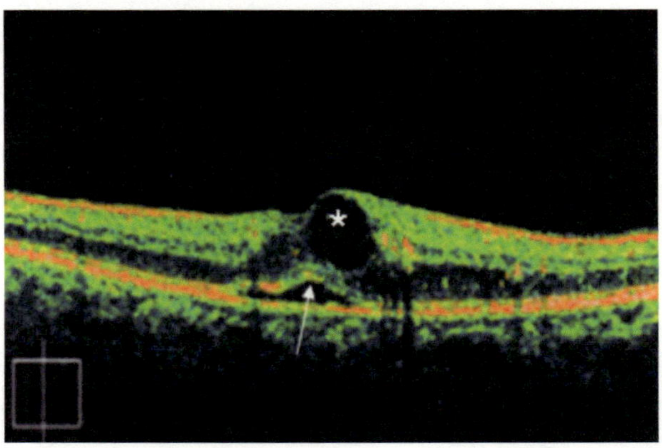

Fig. 14. A 56 year old male with type 1 diabetes mellitus. OCT shows retinal edema with an intra retinal cyst (asterisk). There is a small collection of subfoveal fluid (white arrow).

2.6 OCT deformations of the retina: common causes

- Concavity (myopia).
- Convexity (RPE detachment, subretinal cysts, subretinal tumors). It is not possible to image the entire tumor due to limitations on scanning depth (maximum 2mm).
- Disappearance of foveal depression, example clinically significant macular edema.

3. Clinical applications of optical coherence tomography in vitreo-retinal disorders (Gallemore et al., 2000; Stalmans et al., 1999)

3.1 Intraretinal fluid collections

These include focal or diffuse edema, cystoid edema, cysts, microcysts and impending macular holes. OCT provides "analytical technique" serial scans which are helpful in quantifying the amount of intraretinal and or subretinal fluid.

Retinal edema Figure 14.

The primary cause of retinal thickening is edema. One of the major achievements of OCT has been quantitative assessment of this edema in terms of measuring retinal thickness and volume, evaluate progression of the pathologic process, and monitor surgical or non-surgical intervention (Kang et al., 2004; McDonald et al., 1994). Retinal edema may present in following forms, individually or in combination.

Focal or diffuse edema: Common causes of diffuse macular edema include diabetic retinopathy, central retinal venous occlusion, branch retinal venous occlusion, arterial occlusion, hypertensive retinopathy, pre-eclampsia, eclampsia, uveitis, retinitis pigmentosa and retraction of internal limiting membrane. Initially there may be no or few visible changes. OCT may show reduced reflectivity and increased retinal thickness. As the edema progresses, OCT scan reveals spongy retina.

Cystoid macular edema (CME): Figure 15

There is intraretinal fluid collection in well defined retinal spaces (outer plexiform layer). The rosette or petalloid appearance is due to anatomical layout of the outer plexiform layer and the vertical Müller fibers. Common causes of CME include diabetic retinopathy, ARMD, venous occlusions, pars planitis, Uveitis, pseudophakos, Irvine-Gass syndrome, Birdshot retinopathy and retinitis pigmentosa. OCT usually shows diffuse cystic spaces in the outer nuclear layer of central macula, and increased retinal thickness which is maximally concentric on the fovea (Mavrofrides et al., 2004).

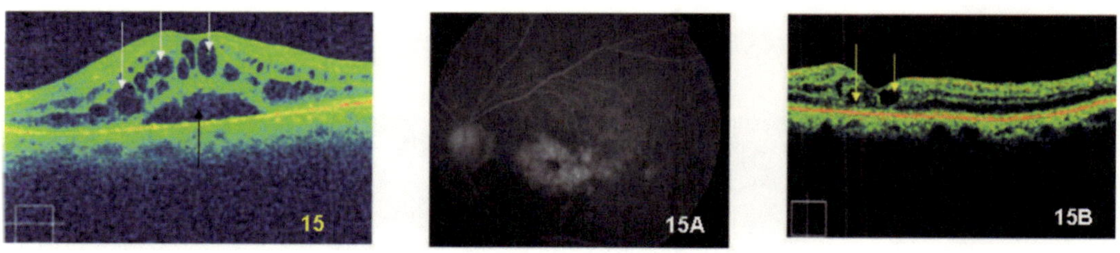

Fig. 15. Post-operative chronic cystoid macular edema. Left (15): OCT image shows multiple; optically empty cystoid spaces (white arrows) with intact septa and subfoveal fluid (black arrow). Pre-treatment central retinal thickness measured 738 microns. Note there are no underlying shadows. Middle (15A): FA shows classical cystoid macular edema. Right (15B): She received intravitreal triamcinolone, and one year later her retinal thickness measured 339 microns with few persisting cystoid spaces (yellow arrows). The subfoveal fluid has disappeared.

Serous retinal detachment: It occurs sequel to chronic edema. The cysts loose their walls and merge together forming single or multiple pools of fluid within retinal layers (Figure 16) or between retinal pigment epithelium (RPE) and the sensory retina (Villate et al., 2004).

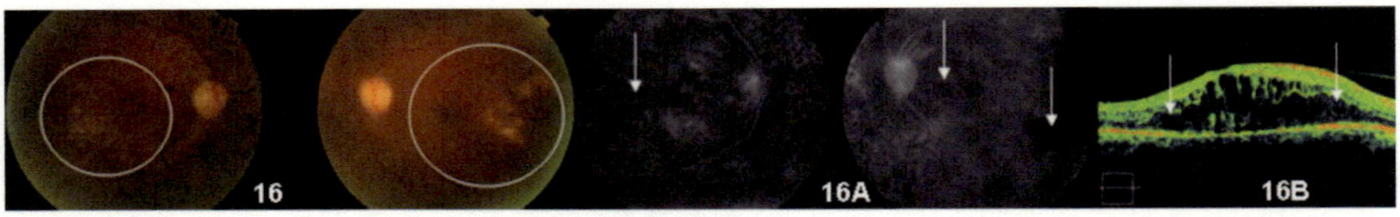

Fig. 16. Bilateral proliferative diabetic retinopathy in a 43 year old male. Color fundus photos have been taken during resolving vitreous hemorrhage, showing exudates and macular edema (encircled areas). 16A: FA shows prior laser marks and bilateral non-perfusion areas (white arrows). 16B: OCT scan highlighted merging of intraretinal fluid cysts (arrows) with some of the septa in the process of breaking down (between arrows) causing localized detachment of the neurosensory retina. OCT findings were much more informative than could be seen biomicroscopically.

3.2 Subretinal fluid collections

Serous retinal detachment: It's classical example is central serous chorioretinopathy (CSCR). Serous fluid with or without subretinal precipitates causes elevation of the sensory retina. Biomicroscopically it resembles a transparent bubble, FA shows slow filling of the dye while OCT reveals an optically empty space with or without cells or exudates (Al-Mujaini et al., 2008). Common causes of CSCR include pregnancy (Figure 17), subretinal neovascularization, optic disc colobomas, diabetic retinopathy, venous occlusions and choroiditis.

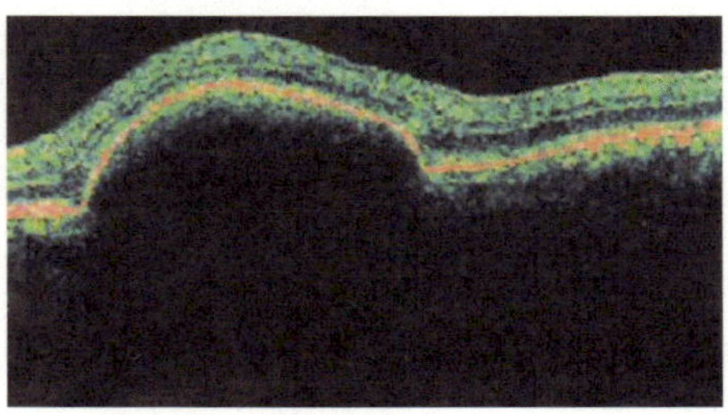

Fig. 17. Central serous chorioretinopathy with sub-retinal pigment epithelial fluid in a pregnant patient.

Retinal pigment epithelial detachment

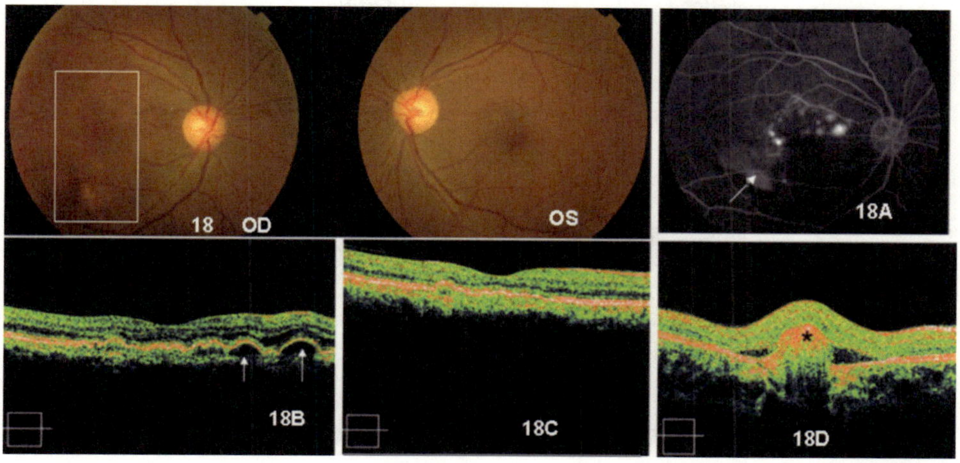

Fig. 18. Color fundus photos: OD: Retinal pigment epithelial detachment following PDT for ICG proved polypoidal choroidal vasculopathy (box). OS: Normal for comparison. 18A: FA shows multiple hyperfluorescent spots in late phase corresponding to RPE detachments/ polypoidal choroidal vasculopathy, and a well defined stained scar (arrow) infero-temporal to the fovea. 18B: OCT reveals dome shaped RPE detachments with collection of fluid under them (arrows). Patient was treated with intravitreal anti-VEGF therapy. 18C: Same patient as in 18B. OCT image shows resolution of the pathology after anti-VEGF treatment. 18D: OCT of an another 19 year old female with idiopathic CNVM scar and Pigment epithelial detachment (black asterisk).

It occurs due to leaking serous fluid from the choriocapillaries in the sub-RPE space or collection of blood under RPE causing its separation and elevation from the Bruchs membrane. OCT scans show a classical dome-shaped detachment of the RPE with intact contour in early stages (Figure 18). Differentiating features of OCT in various types of RPE detachments facilitate the clinical diagnosis (Table 3).

Serous RPED	Inflammatory RPED	Hemorrhagic RPED
Optically clear space with reflective choriocapillaries	Sub-RPE cells or precipitates like fibrin. Subdued choriocapillaries	Shadow effect that prevents choriocapillaries from being seen.

Table 3. Differentiating features of pigment epithelial detachments. (RPED-retinal pigment epithelial detachment).

Common causes of RPE detachment include CSCR, ARMD with or without sub-retinal neovascularization, melanomas and other choroidal tumors (Hee et al., 1996).

Role of OCT in CSCR

- Presence and extent of subretinal fluid and PED.
- Quantitative monitoring of subretinal fluid.

- Differentiation between CSCR and occult CNVM.
- Localization of leakage points which usually appear as PEDs (Robertson et al., 1986; Cardillo et al., 2003).

OCT in serous retinal detachment with RPE detachment: (Mavrofrides et al., 2004; Ting et al., 2002). Such detachments usually follow chronic diffuse retinal pigment epitheliopathy with optically empty contents. The detached neural retina forms shallow angle with the RPE while RPE detachment itself forms steep angles. (Figure 19).

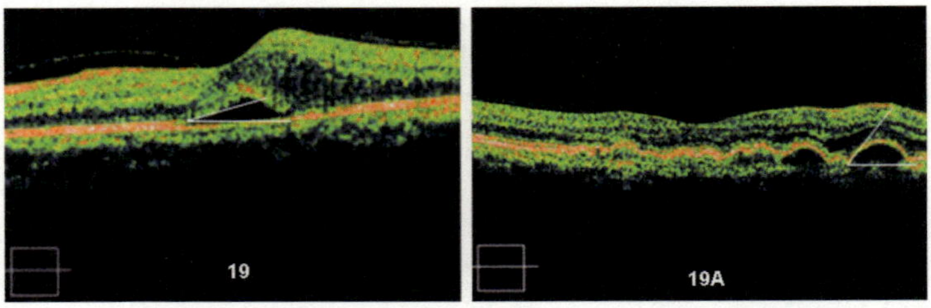

Fig. 19. The detached neurosensory retina forms shallow angle with the RPE. 19A: RPE detachment itself forms a steeper angle.

The RPE may be thickened and disrupted due to CNV. The small serous retinal detachments indicate that CNVM is active.

3.3 Epiretinal membrane (ERM) / Macular pucker (cellophane maculopathy)

Epiretinal membranes are glial proliferations on the vitreo-retinal interface. OCT does not have an impressive record of detecting ERMs; only 42% of eyes with such membranes were detected with this technique (Mavrofrides et al., 2005; Mori et al., 2004). However, other studies label OCT as an ideal instrument for detecting such membranes (Suzuki et al., 2003; Massin et al., 2000). This is due to the fact that both nerve fiber layer and epiretinal membrane are hypereflective, and the blending may sometimes make it difficult to differentiate the two. However, newer high-resolution OCT scans may show much improvement over this deficiency.

Clinical features / associations of ERMs include:

- Altered vascular architecture.
- Macular edema.
- May evolve into macular pseudoholes.
- Visual distortion and decreased vision.
- FA may show macular leakage.

Common causes of ERMs are vascular, uveitis, trauma and idiopathic. OCT scans reveal irregular retinal profile with small folds of the surface and changes in the contour of the foveal depression. Strongly adherent membranes that exert traction on the retina cause increase in retinal thickness, loss of foveal depression and retinal edema. The membrane may either elevate the retina or get itself detached from the retina. OCT enables evaluation of the density, thickness and location of such membranes. In mild cases OCT may only show increase in reflectivity along the internal retinal surface with no changes in internal limiting membrane (ILM) or intra-retinal reflectivity Figure 20).

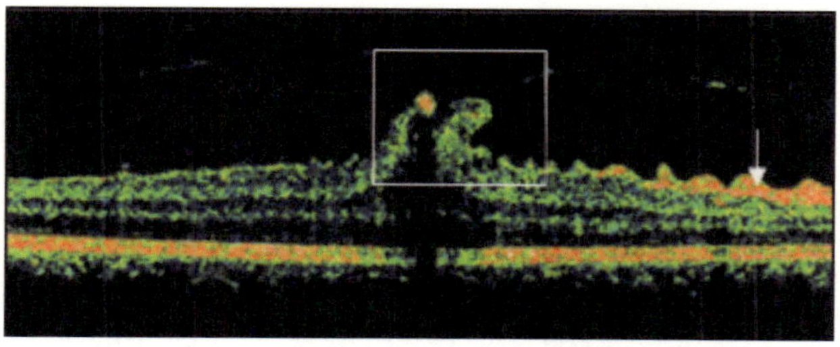

Fig. 20. Hypereflective ERM (white arrow) producing wrinkling of the retinal surface. There is associated vitreomacular traction (box). This patient had history of trauma with a football. Clinically it looked like a pseudohole which was confirmed by OCT.

Epiretinal membranes are best seen by OCT when there is some gap between the membrane and the inner retinal tissue. Conversely any epiretinal membrane that is tightly adherent to the retinal tissue may not be detected by OCT. Epiretinal membranes may induce schisis in the outer retinal layers, producing hyporeflective areas on OCT scanning. Such areas of schisis or edema may not be noticed by FA.

3.4 Vitreomacular traction (Figures 10, 20 and 21)

Clinical features of VMT: (Gallemore et al., 2000; Voo et al., 2004).

- Distortion of the macular contour.
- Antero-posterior and tangential tractional forces applied to the macula.
- Intraretinal edema with or without subretinal fluid.

Many cases of VMT are clinically undetectable; OCT is extremely valuable in such situations.

OCT features of VMT: Preretinal membranes may be thin or get thickened due to fibroglial proliferation and show hyperreflectivity. Such preretinal membranes correspond to detached posterior hyaloid membrane. The traction by the membrane to the retina induces deformations of the retinal surface (Figures 20 and 21).

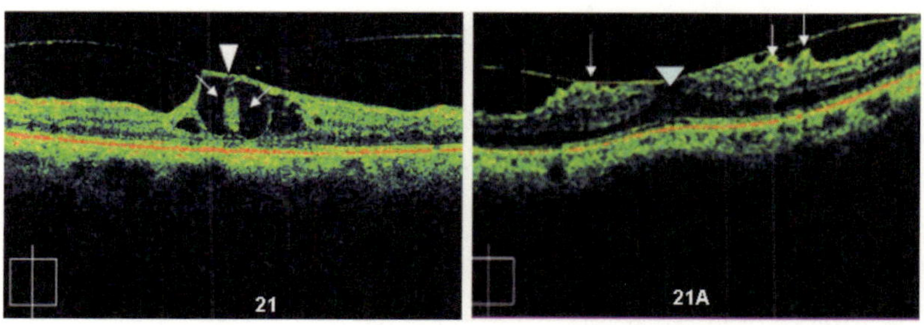

Fig. 21. An OCT image of a 51 year old diabetic and hypertensive patient having a constant vitreo-macular traction (arrowhead) causing cystoid macular edema (arrows). 21A: Vitreomacular traction: OCT of a 63 year old male shows a band in the vitreal cavity with adhesions at multiple points along the internal retinal surface (white arrows). There is increased retinal thickness, reduced intraretinal reflectivity due to edema. Note the lifted edges of the macula around the distorted foveal zone (pseudohole-arrowhead).

3.5 OCT in rhegmatogenous detachment

The scan shows elevation of neural retina with extensive subretinal fluid. (Ip et al., 1999). It also documents the status of retinal detachment at baseline, while following up retinal anatomy after surgery.

3.6 OCT in exudative retinal detachment

- To document the presence, degree and extent of subretinal fluid (Villate et al., 2004).
- More accurate assessment of the level of retinal infiltrates and sub-RPE lesions.
- Detects macular edema in patients with chronic uveitis where hazy media may prevent clinical examination to find the cause of reduced vision (Antcliff et al., 2002; Markomichelakis et al., 2004).

3.7 Macular pseudoholes and lamellar holes

Pseudoholes occur in presence of epiretinal membranes with central defects. They overlay the fovea and may be ophthalmoscopically visible as true holes.

OCT features: (Figure 22-all features may not be displayed in a single scan).

- Homogenous increase in foveal and perifoveal retinal thickness.
- Diffuse reduction in intraretinal reflectivity due to edema.
- Increased perifoveal thickness leads to increase in apparent physiological foveal depression giving a false impression of a partial thickness macular hole, so called a pseudohole. This is a common feature with ERMs.
- In partial thickness or lamellar macular hole, OCT shows presence of residual retinal tissue at the base of the hole (above the RPE).

Macular hole: A macular hole is mostly age-related, common in females in the sixth or seventh decade. It results from centrifugal displacement of the photoreceptors from a central defect in the foveola. It should be noted that it is uncommon to have subretinal fluid in macular holes, when present, it is minimal. On the other hand macular holes are more often associated with intraretinal fluid accumulation and vitreofoveal traction (usually Gass stages 2 and 3) which give a curled-up appearance to the edges of the hole. OCT gives a sequence of documentation in ascertaining such changes in the genesis of a macular hole (Hee et al., 1995; Gaudric et al., 1999). Common causes of macular holes include idiopathic, trauma, high myopia, vascular causes (DR, venous occlusions, and hypertensive retinopathy) and subretinal neovascularization.

OCT and clinical features in macular holes: Table 4 and Figure 22 (not all features may be seen in a single scan).

- Complete absence of foveal retinal reflectivity. No residual retinal tissue.
- Thickened retinal margins around the hole with reduced intraretinal reflectivity.
- Perilesional cystoid edema, appearing as small cavities.
- Increased reflectivity of the inner retinal surface around the macular hole may represent posterior vitreous detachment (PVD-Figure 23), commonly seen as perifoveal vitreous separation which may be subclinical or not clinically visible (Roth et al., 1971; Sidd et al., 1982).

- A hyperreflective band or a spot may be seen in front of the macula, which represents foveal pseudooperculum. (Pseudooperculum means separation of vitreous from fovea).
- Confirmation of successful surgical closure (Jumper et al., 2000; Sato et al., 2003).
- In partial or unsuccessful surgeries, OCT evaluates the retinal anatomy to find reason for poor visual outcome (Hee et al., 1995; Hikichi et al., 1995).

Often biomicroscopy and FA may not be conclusive in differentiating "ERMs associated pseudomacular holes" from true macular holes. OCT readily differentiates such lesions by depicting presence or absence of retinal tissue under the holes respectively.

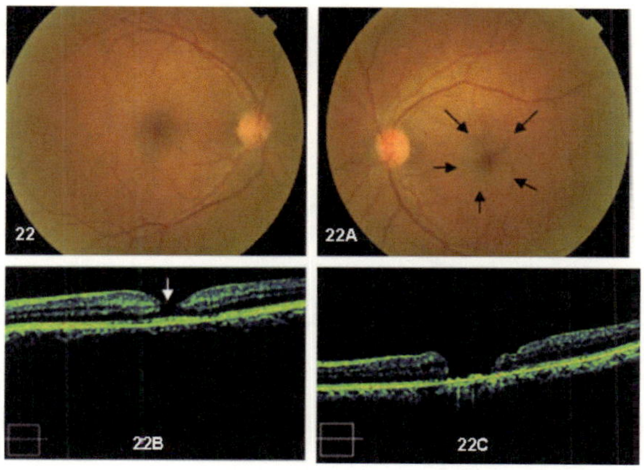

Fig. 22. Upper left: Fundus photo of normal right eye (for comparison). Upper right: (22A) Fundus photo of left eye showing a grayish white epiretinal membrane with a pseudohole appearance (within arrows). Lower left (22B): OCT image displaying an impending macular hole. A thin rim of intact tissue can be seen (white arrow). Lower right: (22C): OCT image of a non-responding full thickness macular hole of a long duration. See figure 1 for comparison with a normal macular-foveal retinal tissue morphology.

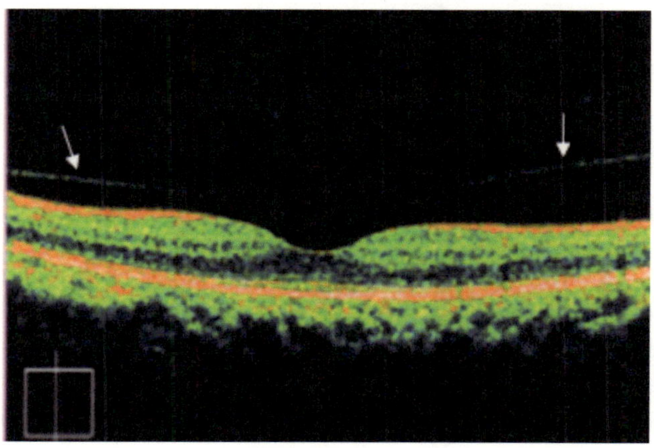

Fig. 23. Posterior vitreous detachments (arrows).

Stage-wise OCT features of genesis of macular holes: Gass classification; (Gass, 1995; Ip et al., 2002; Ullrich et al., 2002; Kasuga et al., 2000).

STAGE	CLINICAL FEATURES	OCT FEATURES
1A 1B	Foveolar detachment Foveal detachment	Perifoveal separation of the posterior hyaloid. Vitreous attached to the fovea.
2A 2B	Full thickness-Eccentric Full thickness-central	Small, full thickness retinal defect or rupture of the roof of the pseudocyst.
3A 3B	Hole with operculum Hole without operculum	Full thickness retinal defect. Adjacent neurosensory detachment. Intraretinal edema. Epiretinal membrane.
4	Hole with posterior vitreous separation	Full thickness retinal defect. Adjacent neurosensory detachment. Intraretinal edema. Epiretinal membrane.

Table 4. Oct and macular hole staging.

As a rule impending macular holes have no pseudooperculum; partial thickness macular holes with ERM do have a pseudooperculum.

Pseudooperculum	Operculum	Weiss' ring
Separation of vitreous from fovea.	Separation of roof of the pseudocyst from the foveal margin.	Separation of vitreous from the optic disc.

Table 5. Features of macular hole-related attachments.

3.8 Retinoschisis (Figure 10)

Definition: It is the separation or splitting of the neurosensory retina into an inner (vitreous) and outer (choroidal) layer with severing of neurons and complete loss of visual function in the affected area. In typical retinoschisis the split is in the outer plexiform layer, and in reticular retinoschisis, which is less common, splitting occurs at the level of nerve fiber layer. Retinoschisis may be degenerative, myopic, juvenile or idiopathic. Presence of vitreoretinal traction is an important pathogenic factor in its initiation. In X-linked retinoschisis, OCT reveals wide hyperreflective space with vertical palisades and splitting of the retina into a thinner outer layer and thicker inner layer (Eriksson et al., 2004).

3.9 OCT in diabetic retinopathy (Cruz-Villegas et al., 2004; Schaudig et al., 2000)

About three decades ago FA and laser photocoagulation improved our knowledge about pathogenesis and benefits of treatment in patients with DR. Since 2002 OCT has given a tremendous boost to the understanding of DR and its complications. This non-invasive technique has revolutionized the evaluation, treatment and prognosis of DR.

3.9.1 Nonproliferative diabetic retinopathy (NPDR) and diabetic macular edema

Though OCT retinal thickness maps can be used to direct laser therapy, and sometimes may be better than biomicroscopy alone, one must be cautious not to proceed with laser photocoagulation in diabetic macular edema (DME) based solely on OCT findings. Ischemic retina may appear thinner on OCT. It is proper to include clinical examination and FA to guide treatment line in DR. Macular traction is an important association in DME which does not respond to laser therapy or intravitreal steroids (Pendergast et al., 2000). Such eyes have taut posterior hyaloid and show diffuse leakage on FA. OCT is very useful in recognizing this condition with following findings: Figure 24

- Diffuse cystic retinal thickening.
- Flat foveal contour.
- Thickened, hyperreflective vitreoretinal surface (Kaiser et al., 2001).

OCT enables the following analysis in DR:

- As an aid in finding the cause of visual impairment.
- Location and extent of retinal edema as a whole and within retinal layers.
- Indications and extent of photocoagulation therapy.
- Monitoring the effectiveness of laser, intravitreal or surgical therapy.

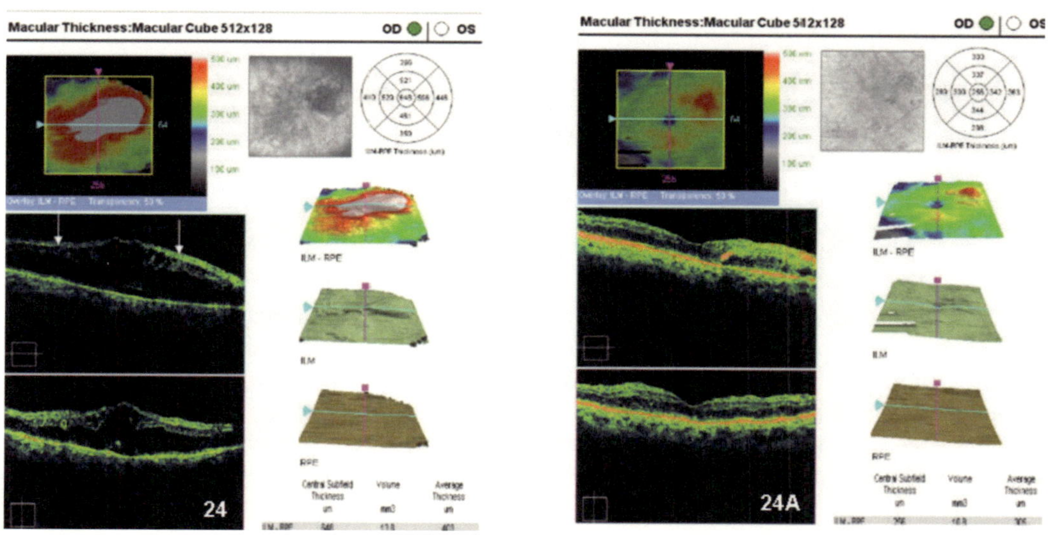

Fig. 24. Severe NPDR: Left image: Right eye of a sixty year old male with diabetic macular edema (before injection bevacizumab). Note the multiple intraretinal cystoid spaces, increasing the central retinal thickness to 648 microns. Right image (24A) belongs to same patient after intravitreal injection of bevacizumab (1.25mg) showing marked reduction in retinal edema (258 microns). Note the difference in color coded maps of retinal thickness as well. OCT has been valuable in following up this patient.

3.9.2 OCT appearance in common pathophysiologic lesions in DR

- Cotton-wool spots: as hyperreflective nodular or elongated lesions in nerve fiber layer, often casting a shadow on posterior layers. (Figure 4)
- Hard exudates: (Figures 6). Appear as hyperreflective formations in deeper retinal layers. Common causes include DR, hypertensive retinopathy, Coats disease, telangiectasias and radiation retinopathy.
- Retinal hemorrhages: hyperreflective scans with shadows on posterior layers.
- Fibrous tissue: Appears as a hyperreflective area with deformation of macular outline. (Figure 7)
- Retinal edema: (Figures 3, 12, 13, 14) seen in OCT scans as thickened and hyporeflective, spongy retina. The edema is located by retinal mapping and quantified through measurement of retinal thickness and volume. OCT permits better localization of edema than can be done with FA. The external plexiform layer displays the greatest amount of edema. The spongy retina detected by OCT is thought to represent altered Möller cells. Over years, microcavities merge to form pseudocysts which are depicted clearly in OCT scans (Figure 15). Fully developed CME can involve full thickness of the retina with disappearance of retinal tissue, coalescence of the cavities, subsequently leading to a true serous neurosensory retinal detachment. OCT in such eyes reveals an optically clear cavity between elevated retina and RPE (Figure 25). One of the real supremacy of OCT in the field of CME from different causes has been to monitor the effectiveness of intravitreal therapeutic drugs in terms of retinal thickness and retinal volume (Figures 5, 13, 15, 18, 24, and 25).

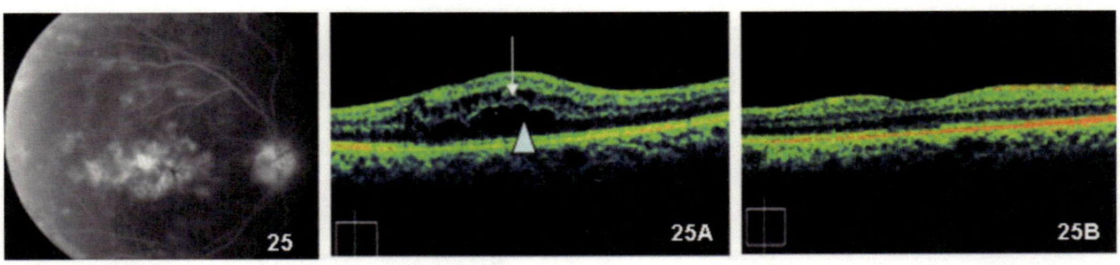

Fig. 25. Postoperative endophthalmitis: FA shows petalloid cystoid macular edema. 25A: OCT image shows persistent cystoid macular edema (white arrow) with central subfoveal thickness of 530 microns and shallow neurosensory detachment (arrowhead). She was given intravitreal triamcinolone. 25B: Repeat OCT after 2 weeks showed marked reduction in macular edema (central subfoveal thickness 230 microns). Patient continued to be free of macular edema six months after intravitreal injection.

3.9.3 OCT and proliferative diabetic retinopathy (PDR) Figure 26

Proliferative diabetic retinopathy occurs commonly in young individuals where newly formed vessels appear at the margin of the ischemic area. Common causes of retinal neovascularization include DR, CRVO, Eale's disease, vasculitis, pars planitis and sickle cell anemia. Uncommon causes include leukemias and multiple myelomas. The newly formed abnormal blood vessels are thin and fine and are picked up in OCT scans only when glial tissue is present with vessels.

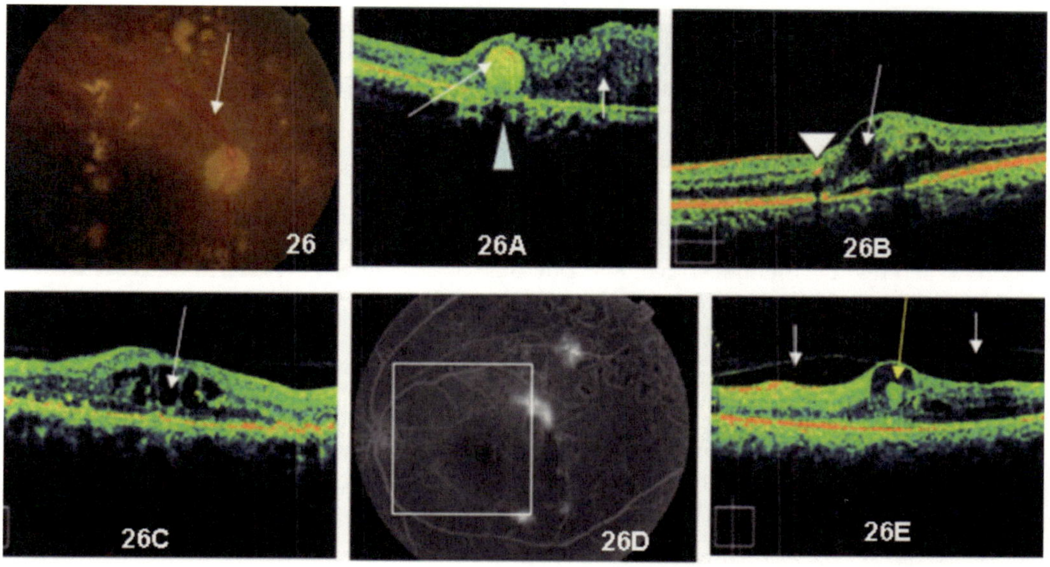

Fig. 26. Proliferative diabetic retinopathy: Color fundus photo shows extensive hard exudates and glial tissue proliferation (arrow). 26A: OCT image of the same patient depicts partially hyperreflective round exudate (long white arrow) amidst macular edema (short arrow). Note the underlying shadow cast by overlying exudate (arrowhead). 26B Another patient with cystoid macular edema (arrow) and intraretinal exudate (arrowhead).

Bottom row: A 42 year old male diabetic patient with bilateral proliferative diabetic retinopathy. 26C: OCT image shows clinically significant macular edema (Central subfoveal thickness 619 microns). Note the optically empty cysts (arrow) do not caste any underlying shadows. 26D: FA shows ischemic retinopathy (white rectangle) with areas of non-perfusion and leaking NVE. 26E: Large intraretinal cyst (yellow arrow) with vitreo-macular traction (white arrows).

3.9.4 OCT in traction with or without retinal detachment

OCT typically shows points of traction on the retina causing its elevation (FIGURES 10, 20, 21), intraretinal fluid accumulation causing retinal thickening. (Figure 21) and Subretinal fluid collection (Figure 20). If OCT rules out traction as a cause of vision loss, macular ischemia should be a strong reason then.

4. Drusen

Drusen are round, yellowish colloidal bodies associated with Bruch's membrane. They may be single (large single drusen also called vitelliform) or multiple (geographic), hard or soft, later variety being more damaging to the retinal pigment epithelium-photoreceptor layer.

OCT findings in drusen (Mavrofrides et al., 2004)

Highly refractive irregular, convex excrescences in the form of thickenings or deformities of the RPE-Bruch's membrane complex (external band), leading to its irregular or undulating outline (Figure 8). Geographic atrophy of RPE elicits increased reflectivity from underlying exposed choroid. Retinal thinning due to focal or diffuse retinal atrophy may ensue. Drusen unlike hard exudates do not cast any underlying shadows in OCT scans.

5. Age Related Macular Degeneration (ARMD)

Drusen are the earliest findings in ARMD. The disease has dry (atrophic) form in 80 percent of cases and wet (exudative) form in 20 percent of cases. OCT is particularly useful in evaluating different modes of therapies, namely photodynamic therapy (PDT), intra-vitreal anti-angiogenic therapies and surgical treatment (Giovannini et al., 1999, 2000; Rogers et al., 2002).

5.1 Dry (atrophic) ARMD

Macular region shows clusters of drusen and progressive atrophy of RPE, photoreceptors and choriocapillaries. OCT scans show reduced retinal thickness, increased RPE reflectivity due to reduced light attenuation by atrophic retinal tissue (Mavrofrides et al., 2004)

5.2 Wet (exudative) ARMD (Ting et al., 2002)

The typical components of exudative ARMD include serous elevation of RPE and neurosensory retina, hemorrhage under RPE and Subretinal hemorrhage. Figures 27, 28

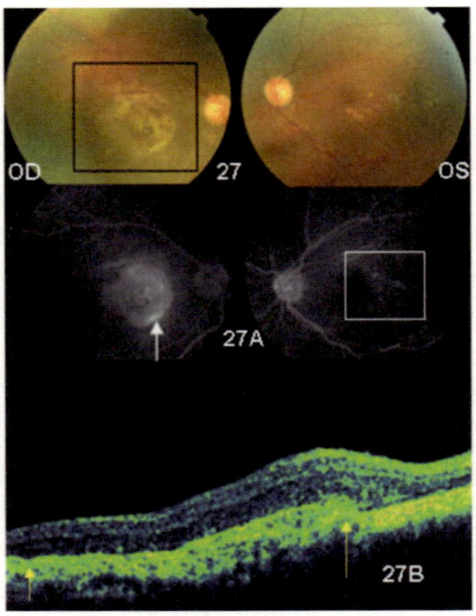

Fig. 27. Age related macular degeneration with scarred CNVM (right eye) in a 62 year old male. Color fundus photo of right eye (OD) shows a large grayish elevated macular lesion with drusen infero-temporal to the macula (square). Left eye (OS) color fundus photo shows multiple drusen inferior and temporal to macula. 27A: FA shows stained scarred CNV with doubtful activity inferiorly (arrow) in right eye and stained small drusen bodies in the left eye (white square). 27B: OCT scan right eye showed minimal reflectivity (between yellow arrows). Patient was earlier treated with intravitreal ranibizumab and bevacizumab injections. The vision remained unchanged in the treated eye.

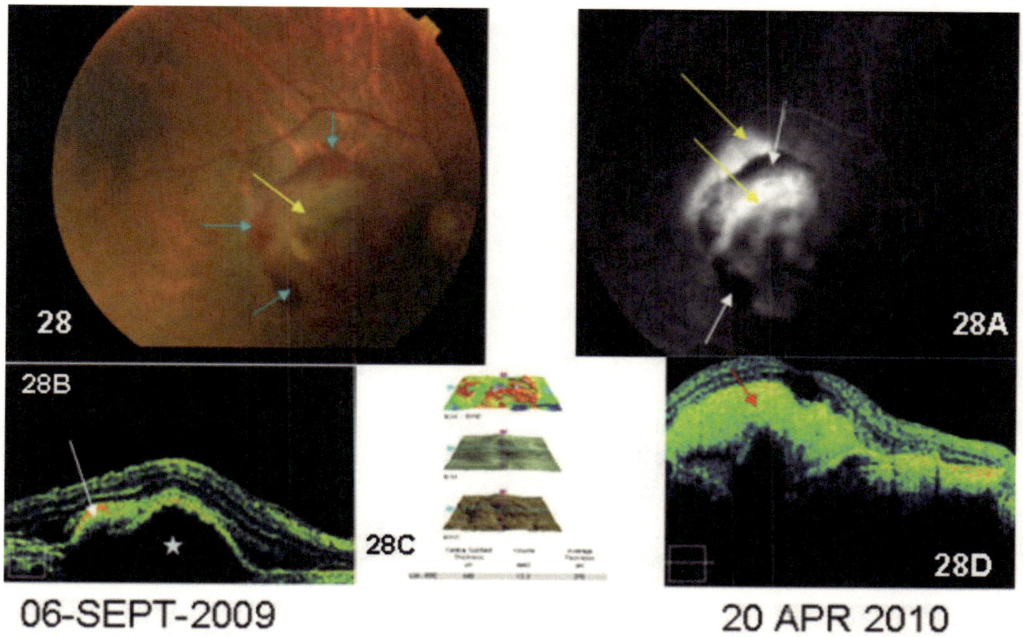

Fig. 28. Advanced age-related macular degeneration in an 89 year old male (right eye). Color fundus photo shows a large subfoveal hemorrhage (blue arrows) and a large disciform scar (yellow arrow). 28A: FA shows blocked fluorescence (white arrows) due to hemorrhage and hyperfluorescent areas (yellow arrows) defining stained fibrous tissue. 28B: OCT image shows black, optically empty area corresponding to presence of fluid (star) and hyperreflective scar (white arrow). 28C: Note the irregularity in the color maps. Patient received three injections of intravitreal bevacizumab. 28D: OCT after 8 months (April 2010): The CNVM scar remained unchanged (red arrow). Patient did not show any visual improvement. Treatment was abandoned.

5.3 OCT in ARMD Figures 27 and 28

It provides vital information about different presentations of ARMD in different stages, more common and more important being the following:

- Serous RD.
- Hemorrhagic RD.
- Retinal edema.
- Cystoid edema.
- RPE detachment.
- Neovascular membranes.
- Subretinal fibrosis.
- As an adjunct to FA/Indocyanine angiography.

Fluorescein Angiography may not be equivocal in defining intraretinal, subretinal or sub-RPE fluid; OCT scans all these components vividly and identifies location and level of such fluid, besides giving clue to the contents of the fluid (blood, serous fluid, pigment, and fibrosis). Unlike FA, OCT yields quantitative data about retinal thickness, volume and size of the CNV.

6. Classic choroidal neovascular membranes - OCT findings (Figure 10)

Neovascular lesions appear as highly refractile, fusiform areas beneath the retina. Secondary exudation may be seen as intraretinal or subretinal fluid. Intraretinal edema may be mild or diffuse and cystic. OCT is highly sensitive in picking up even small amounts of subretinal fluid (seen as non-reflective space) between outer retina and highly refractile external band (RPE-choriocapillaries complex). No technique other than OCT can monitor the quantitative response of different methods of treatment in CNV (Giovannini et al., 1999, 2000; Rogers et al., 2002).

Occult choroidal neovascular membranes: Usually located sub-RPE and may lead to fibrovascular PED. FA shows mottled hyperfluorescence. OCT reveals PED with irregular external band and variable subretinal or intraretinal fluid.

7. Pigment epithelial detachment (PED)

Usually accompanies occult CNV lesions. Other common causes include idiopathic, CSCR (Figure 17) and ocular inflammations. Classical PEDs have continuous, highly reflective bands on both sides of the lesion. Any discontinuity favors an RPE tear or presence of an overlying inflammatory exudate, blood or fibrin which block the incident OCT beam of light.

OCT and serous PED: Figure 18 The OCT findings include a dome shaped optically clear space between RPE and choriocapillaries. Detached RPE forms a steep angle with underlying choriocapillaries. The contents of the serous cavity may be clear or contain cells or fibrin. The detachments may be single or multiple. Sometimes they may merge and form a bubble; however, this does not obstruct the view of the underlying choroid.

OCT and hemorrhagic PED: The source of blood is a neovascular membrane. The RPE detachment, like serous detachment, forms a steep angle with choriocapillaries but, unlike serous detachment, obscures the underlying choriocapillaries and all other posterior layers due to inability of OCT light beam to penetrate blood. The anterior face of the hemorrhage elicits a very high optical reflectivity.

8. RPE tears

(Gelisken et al., 2001; Pece et al., 2001; Srivastava et al., 2002). RPE tear is a serious complication of ARMD and PDT.

Common causes:

- Serous and hemorrhagic PED.
- Following laser treatment like PDT.
- Long standing sub-RPE fluid collection due to active CNV.

OCT changes in RPE tear include:

- Thickening (secondary to retraction of RPE) and folding of RPE layer.
- Blood under RPE. This may induce dense shadow on posterior layers.
- An area of irregular, thick hyperreflective outer band with intense backscattering. This area corresponds to where RPE has retracted and underlying choriocapillaries have been bared.

OCT is valuable in aiding clinical diagnoses in many other RPE lesions like hamartomas and hyperplasias (Lopez & Guerrero, 2006; Shukla et al., 2005).

9. Choroidal Neovascular Membrane (CNVM-Figure 10)

FA is invaluable in detecting both classic and occult CNV. OCT reveals CNVM as a hyperreflective area in front of or in contact with, or slightly separated from an irregular RPE. When active, OCT invariably shows retinal edema or neurosensory RD. With involuntary regression of CNVM, OCT images become less evident. In Occult CNVM the new vessels predominantly lie in sub-RPE space. Such occult neovascular membranes are difficult to identify clinically or sometimes even with FA. OCT clearly depicts an irregular, thickened, disrupted and fragmented RPE in such cases. There may be associated retinal cystoid edema and neurosensory RD opposite the membrane (Figure 10). Common causes of CNVM include exudative from of ARMD, myopia (usually with axial length of more than 26mm), idiopathic neovascularization in young patients, idiopathic polypoidal vasculopathy, retinal angiomatosis, traumatic choroidal ruptures, post-photocoagulation therapy, angioid streaks, choroiditis and histoplasmosis.

10. Idiopathic polypoidal vasculopathy (IPV) or polypoidal neovascular membranes (Figure 18)

This disorder is a variant of ARMD, found in patients aged fifty years and above (Yannuzzi et al., 1997). FA / ICG reveals dilated choroidal vessels with ectasias or aneurysms, often in clusters. There may be associated serous or hemorrhagic detachment of the retina and RPE.

It may masquerade as CSCR. ICG differentiates the two conditions (Yannuzzi et al., 2000).

Laser treatment yields good results. OCT shows cup-shaped elevation of RPE and serous (no underlying shadow) or hemorrhagic (with shadow effect) detachments of the retina and or RPE.

11. Retinal angiomatous proliferans

Clinical features:

- Intraretinal neovascularization.
- Intraretinal hemorrhage with or without PED.
- Cystic retinal edema.

OCT features:

- Intraretinal cystic edema.
- PED.

- Hyperreflective intraretinal neovascular complex (Yannuzzi et al., 2001 ; Zacks & Johnson, 2004).
- Serous subretinal or sub-RPE fluid.

12. Idiopathic juxtafoveal retinal telangiectasia

Clinical features:

- Common retinal vascular disorder affecting young to middle aged males.
- Telangiectatic vessels have predilection for temporal macula.
- Macular edema as reason for reduced vision.
- Telangiectasis appears often in small, right angled venular groups which are seen better in high magnification.
- FA shows leakage mostly temporal to the macula.
- OCT shows normal foveal contour and horizontally oriented oblong, small, inner retinal cysts.

13. Disciform scars / subretinal fibrosis (Figure 7, 28, 29)

Scars develop as a sequel to regression of subretinal hemorrhages and prolonged retinal edema. They are composed of fibrovascular tissue and hyperplastic RPE. There usual location being between altered Bruch's membrane and the retina which is often elevated. They may mask the end stage of untreated CNVMs. On FA the scars may appear as areas of hyperfluorescence with late staining. This may be confused with persisting leakage from a CNVM lesion. The decision whether or not to re-treat such a lesion with PDT is facilitated by OCT imaging. In dry variety (common) there is pronounced destruction of almost all retinal layers, while in rarer exudative variant there may be serous or hemorrhagic exudation from leaking CNVM, causing retinal elevation. OCT findings include an area of nodular hyperreflectivity with deformation or irregularity of adjacent retina and RPE. In exudative type, OCT scans show diffuse or cystoid retinal edema and RPE detachments. Absence of intraretinal thickening or subretinal fluid usually indicates non-active CNV complex within the scar tissue complex. OCT greatly facilitates differentiation between active CNV complexes from subretinal fibrosis. Occasionally chronic end-stage, burnt out CNV may be associated with overlying intra-retinal cysts-this could be an associated chronic inflammation rather an active CNV.

14. Post-therapeutic assessment by OCT (Figures 5, 13, 15, 18, 24, 25)

OCT provides an accurate outcome of the effect of pharmacological or surgical interventions like PDT, transpupillary thermotherapy, vitreoretinal surgery, anti-VEGF therapy, intravitreal steroid therapy and therapeutic Intravitreal implants (Rogers et al., 2002).

15. Retinal venous occlusions: Figure 5

In Branch retinal venous occlusion, technician should be asked to arrange vertical scan through the foveal center. This shows classical vertical disparity between normal retina and thick cystic retina.

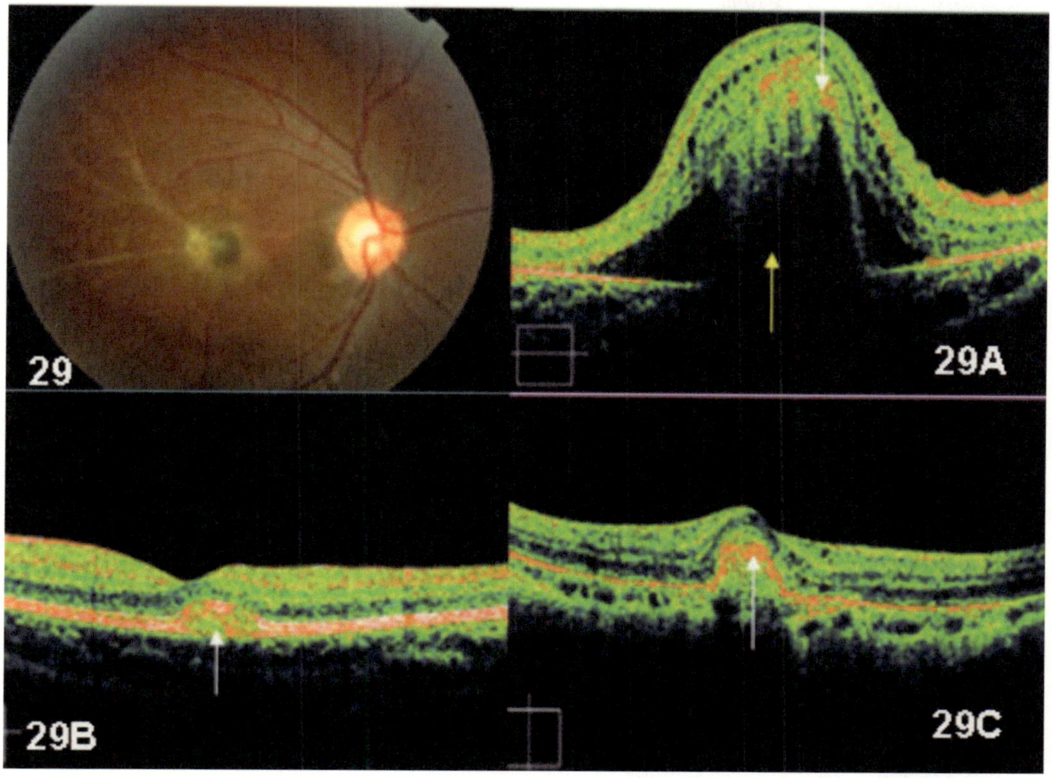

Fig. 29. A 15 year old male patient with Best disease. Color fundus photo shows central fibrosis following resolved CNVM with RPE hyperplasia. 29A: OCT right eye shows hyperreflective scar (white arrow) within markedly elevated macula with subretinal fluid (yellow arrow). 29B: OCT left eye shows a hyperreflective dome shaped lesion (white arrow) which was clinically compatible with a circumscribed scrambled egg lesion. Note the absence of subretinal fluid in left eye. 29C: (another patient): CNVM after LASIK: OCT image of a 31 year old female who developed CNVM after LASIK procedure. OCT shows a post-CNVM hyperreflective macular scar (white arrow) following three PDT therapies and intravitreal bevacizumab.

OCT findings:

- Diffuse intraretinal cystic collections causing retinal thickening. Such cysts are evenly distributed throughout the macula (Ip et al., 2003; Lerche et al., 2001; Sekiryu et al., 2000).
- Subretinal fluid.

There are certain rarer conditions that show significant intraretinal cystic spaces in OCT scans, but do not leak on FA. These include X-linked juvenile retinoschisis, Goldman-Favre-vitreoretinal degeneration, nicotinic acid maculopathy, docetaxel (anti-neoplastic drug) toxicity and few variants of vitreomacular traction (Spirn et al., 2003; Teitelbaum & Tresley 2003).

16. Optic disc pits

Recently it has been proposed that fluid from the vitrous enters through the pit and then traverses between the inner and outer layers of the retina producing a retinal schisis. OCT has confirmed such an inner retinal schisis preceding the outer retinal layer detachment (Krivoy et al., 1996; Lincoff & Kreissig, 1998). It was found from OCT scans that the RNFL thickness is reduced in the quadrant corresponding to the optic nerve pit (Myer et al., 2003).

17. Retinitis pigmentosa

OCT displays the associations of this disease like epiretinal membrane and cystoid macular edema. (Figure 2) The outer nuclear layer thickness may appear normal in the foveal region, but becomes abnormally thin in the macular periphery. UHR-OCT may show progressive thinning of the outer and inner segments of the photoreceptors outside of the foveal region (Ko et al., 2005).

18. OCT in rarer posterior segment lesions

Melanomas: OCT does not detect the internal characteristics of melanocytic tumors (Espinoza et al., 2004). It identifies the associated features like subretinal fluid (Muscat et al., 2004), intraretinal cystic changes and schisis-like splitting of the overlying neurosensory retina.

Choroidal osteomas: OCT is not of much help in assisting the diagnosis, however, may help in confirming associated clinical features like overlying CNV, subretinal fluid, retinal edema or thinning and attenuation of the overlying RPE. Osteomas induce partial shadowing of the choroids (Fukasawa & Lijima, 2002).

19. Optical coherence tomography and its applications in glaucoma

The RNFL represents a highly reflective band whose anterior limit begins at the vitreo-retinal interface, and the posterior limit is detected on the basis of signal thresholding. OCT provides both qualitative and quantitative information regarding the optic nerve and the RNFL. The images in this chapter are based on Cirrus 3D HD domain, therefore, may differ from older versions of the OCT. The measurement of the RNFL thickness marks one of the most important applications of OCT in the field of ophthalmology. The authenticity of pathological specificity of OCT RNFL measurements correlates with histological measurements in primate and human studies, and this has been correlated with visual field changes as well (Chen et al., 2006). An OCT RNFL report generated by Cirrus-3D HD OCT in a normal person reads as following: Figure 30.

Section 1 and 1A: RNFL thickness maps for right eye and left eye respectively. The maps report thickness using GDx (glaucoma diagnostics) color pattern, where warm colors (reds, yellows) represent thicker areas and cool colors (blues and greens) represent thinner areas.

Section 2 and 2A: RNFL thickness deviation maps for right and left eyes respectively. These maps report statistical comparison against normal thickness range, overlaid on the fundus OCT image. These maps apply only yellow and red colors. The green color is not applied because it may obscure the anatomical details in the underlying OCT fundus image, as most of the superpixels would be green for normal patients. Any region that is not red or yellow means it falls within normal limits. One can have a gross clue of the cup-disc ratio and position of the vessels in the cup.

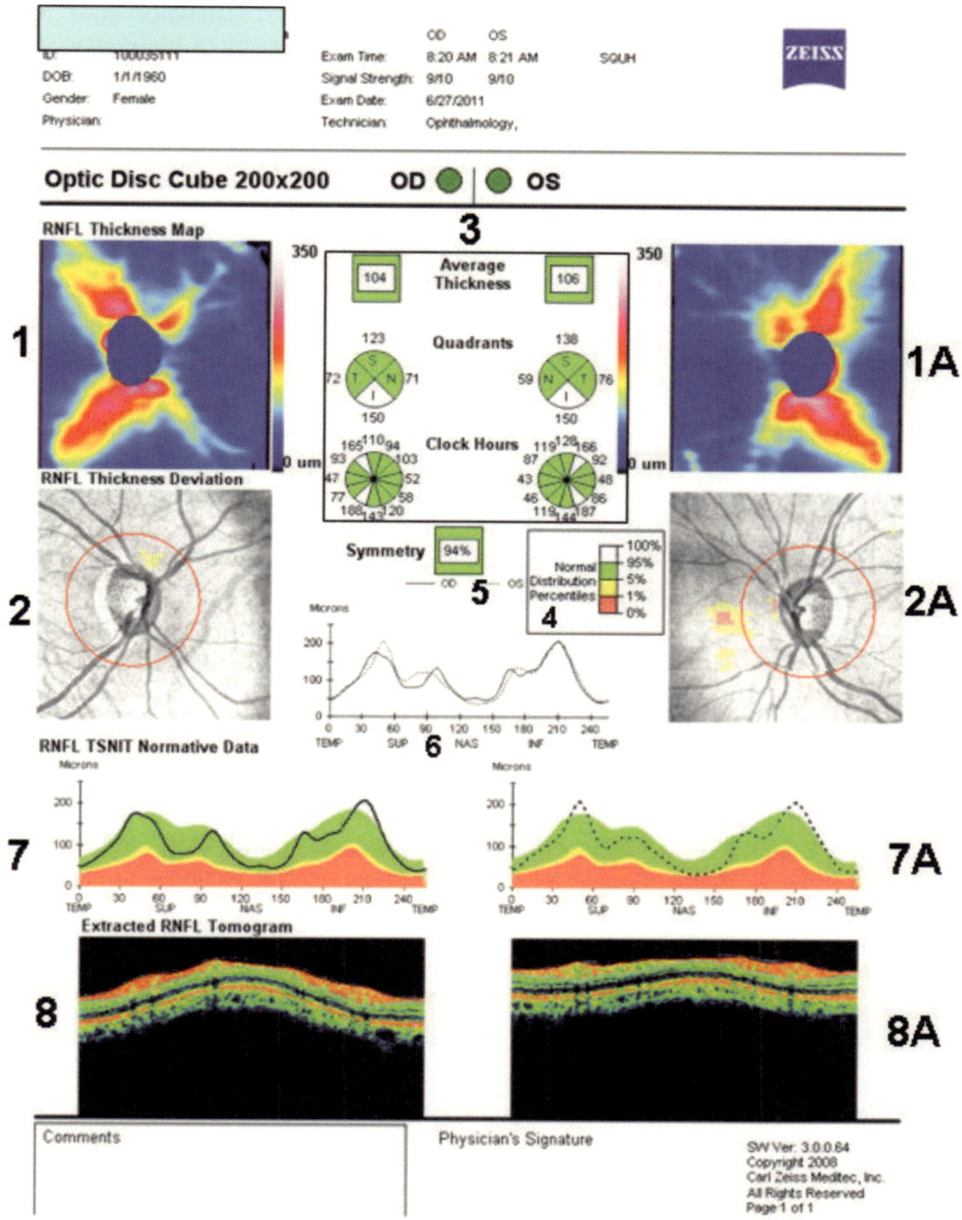

Fig. 30. See text.

Section 3: Displays average RNFL thickness along the whole calculation circle (squares in the print out, as well as quadrant and clock hour measurements). These measures are represented in pseudocolor (means these colors are not same as the RNFL in vivo) coded programs by comparing the measured RNFL thickness to age-matched data in the normative database of the OCT machine. Green and white colors indicate normal RNFLT (white color means thickest). Note that red color in the map (section 1) denotes more thickness of the RNFL contrary to red color of boxes or quadrants or clock hours in section 2 where red indicates reduced average thickness of the RNFL.

Sections 4: The RNFL normative database uses a white-green-yellow-red color code to indicate the normal distribution percentiles. The color code applies to the quadrant, clock hour, graphs, and to the right (OD) and left (OS) columns. The percentiles apply as follows (among same-age individuals in the normal population):

Red represents thinnest 1% of measurements and is considered outside normal limits.

Yellow represents thinnest 5% of measurements and is considered suspect.

Green represents 90% of measurements and is considered normal.

White area represents thickest 5% of all measurements.

Note: Ophthalmologists must exercise clinical judgment while interpreting the normative data because one out of twenty normal eyes (5%) will fall below green.

Section 5: Symmetry: Indicates the extent of symmetry of distribution of RNFL thickness in TSNIT (temporal-superior-nasal-inferior-temporal) quadrants between two eyes. The symmetry parameter is a correlation coefficient, converted to a percentage and does not have much applicability in patient management. One can ignore this parameter in clinical decisions.

Section 6: RNFL-TSNIT thickness graph: OU (Both eyes): This section plots RNFL thickness in Y axis (vertical) and retinal quadrants in X axis (horizontal). This normally has a "double hump" appearance owing to the thicker RNFL measurements in the superior and inferior quadrants compared with the nasal and temporal quadrants. This profile shows right and left eye RNFL thickness together, to enable comparison of symmetry in specific regions.

Section 7 and 7A: Separate RNFL-TSNIT normative data graph for right and left eyes respectively. The graph is superimposed against the color codes. If the graph dips into red color in any quadrant, the RNFL thickness in that quadrant is not normal (Figure 31 section 7 and 7A)

Section 8 (OD) and 8A (OS): Extracted RNFL tomograms. Display the reflectivity of the RNFL. Not of much clinical significance in taking clinical decisions. Some models of OCT can display optic disc modules including parameters like cup-disc ratio (vertical and horizontal), neuroretinal rim area, disk area, cup area, cup volume, rim volume etc.

An OCT RNFL report generated by Cirrus-3D HD OCT in a patient with glaucoma is interpreted as following: Figure 31.

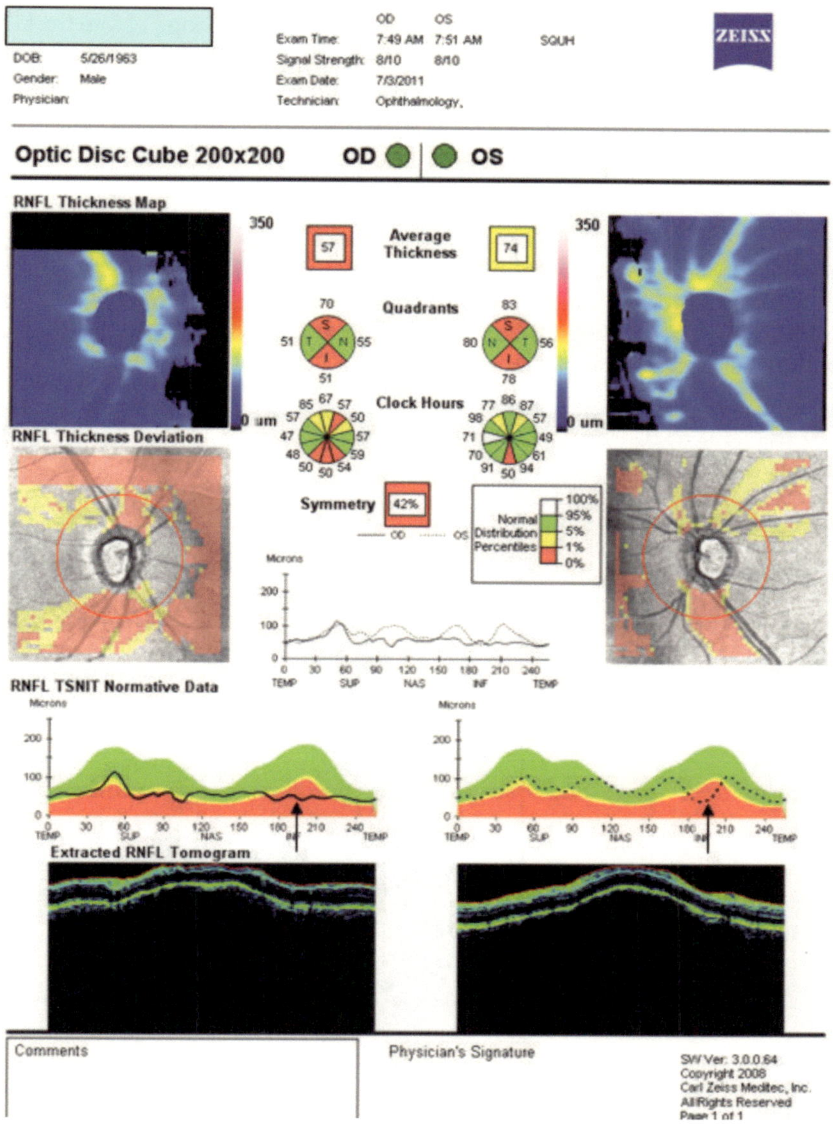

Fig. 31. Section 1: Note absence of red color code compared to normal OCT. This indicates thinning of RNFL. Section 2: There is a pink-red brush paint appearance (absent in normal OCT). This again indicates wedge shaped NFL defect. Section 3: The average RNFL thickness in the right (OD) eye is represented in red square, which indicates abnormal (reduced) NFL thickness (red denotes values ≤1% of what would be expected when compared with a reference population of the same age as the patient while the average RNFL thickness in the left (OS) eye is represented in yellow square, indicating a value which is borderline or suspect, or a subclinical involvement, or a normal variant (such patients need regular follow up). Section 4: Same interpretation as for normal scan. Section 5: An abnormal symmetry (red square) of RNFLT between two eyes. Note that symmetry square in normal OCT scan is green and healthy. Section 6: Absence of double-hump due to

marked thinning and asymmetry of NFLT between two eyes. Section 7: Note the significant dipping of graph into red zone in both eyes (black arrows). This happens when there is advanced atrophy of nerve fibers (in this case due to glaucoma). Another important cause could be MS. Section 8: same interpretation as in normal OCT.

20. OCT in systemic diseases

The application of OCT has gone beyond the borders of ophthalmology. Ocular manifestations of systemic diseases are widely accepted as important clues to the diagnosis, treatment and follow up of such disorders. OCT has added a new dimension in this field. Few examples from hematological and neurological disorders have been cited in this chapter, but the list is much more (Figure 32).

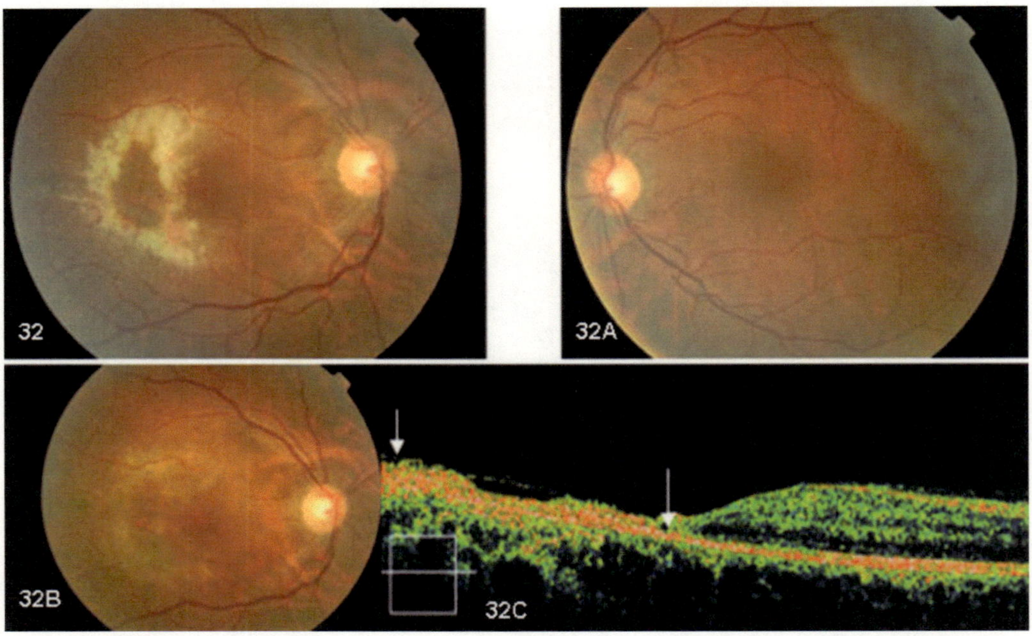

Fig. 32. OCT in systemic disease: A 45 year old male with acute lymphoid leukemia (ALL) complained of reduced vision (6/60) in right eye. His associated ocular co-morbidity included cytomegalovirus retinitis in right eye. Figure 32: Fundus photo in June 2011 revealed paramacular ring shaped retinal opacification, with hemorrhages, which were attributed to leukemic cell infiltration and possible CMV retinitis. 32A: normal left eye for comparison. Patient received chemotherapy. 32B: After 5 weeks, fundus examination revealed marked resolution of retinal opacification, replaced by scarring. 32C: OCT in July 2011 showed marked retinal atrophy and a hyperreflective scar (between arrows-central subfield thickness 38 microns). Compare it to the normal retinal thickness nasal (right side of the scan) to the fovea.

OCT in multiple sclerosis (MS): The first study to report ocular OCT findings in MS patients was published by Parisi et al in 1999. Both academic and industrial scientists have been quick to realize the potential utility of OCT as a surrogate marker of axonal integrity in

MS. As a result OCT research in MS has grown exponentially in recent years and it has become an undisputed corroborator into the design of ongoing clinical trials. The disability level in MS is best correlated with axonal damage, but axonal damage is poorly appreciated on MRI. The RNFL is composed primarily of unmyelinated axons that originate from the ganglion cells. In addition to providing an indication of axonal integrity through measurement of RNFL thickness, OCT provides evaluation of the outer macula which is felt to provide an estimate of neuronal integrity within the retina (Burkholder et al., 2009; Moura et al., 2007). OCT measurement of RNFL thickness reflects axonal integrity, while its measurement of total macular volume reflects retinal neuronal integrity. MRI does not provide insight into the process of subclinical optic neuropathy or the subsequent neurodegenerative sequelae that ensue in the retina as a result of optic neuropathy. Studies found that the thickness of RNFL was reduced in patients with MS, and it correlated with visual evoked potential P100 amplitude (a reflection of axonal integrity) than with P100 latency (a reflection of myelin integrity), supporting the notion that RNFL thinning in MS is attributed to axonal degeneration and this, in turn reflects the degree of brain atrophy (Gordon-Lipkin et al., 2007). OCT imaging following acute inflammatory optic neuritis has shown that approximately 75% of patients ultimately sustain 10-40 micron reduction in RNFL thickness in the affected eye within 3-6 months, indicating significant and rapid axonal degeneration secondary to demyelination. OCT has documented that RNFL thickness threshold of 75 microns, below which there is a reduction in visual function. This observation has been confirmed with automated perimetry testing (Costello et al., 2006).

Based on the correlating findings of OCT, it appears that individuals with progressive MS variants suffer greater RNFL thinning than those with relapsing-remitting variants (Pulicken et al., 2007). Pathological specificity of OCT RNFL measurements correlates with histological measurements in primate and human studies and yields good structure-function correlation between RNFL thickness and low-contrast visual acuity (Fisher et al., 2006; Pulicken et al., 2007).

21. Aberrant variations of OCT scan

It may be due to retinal edema, denser media opacities and ERMs which may be located at a very short distance from the retinal surface. Such measurements complicate the interpretation and may not correspond to the reality. New versions of OCT may perform better in such situations.

22. OCT in anterior segment imaging (Console et al., 2008; Devereux et al., 2000; Wang et al., 2010; Wu et al., 2011)

Anterior segment imaging is a rapidly advancing concept in ophthalmology. New technologies offering non-contact cross-sectional imaging of the cornea and the anterior segment are now commercially available. These new modalities, based on rotating Scheimpflug imaging and anterior segment OCT; supplement the already established imaging techniques like slit corneal topography and ultrasound biomicroscopy. One of such applications of anterior segment OCT is commercially available as Visante OCT. It uses the physical principle of low-coherence interferometry to generate images of the anterior segment. Anterior segment OCT uses a longer wavelength (1310nm) that permits deeper penetration through the highly reflective tissues of the sclera and is minimally affected by corneal opacifications. The system provides anterior segment images up to 6mm in depth and 16mm in width. Therefore, this technology permits morphological and morphometric plus qualitative and quantitative analysis of the anterior segment. (Fishman GR et al., 2005; Li H et al., 2007). One of the most valuable advantages of anterior segment OCT is its ability to produce a reliable representation of anterior chamber structures in presence of total loss of corneal transparency.

OCT is used in evaluating the anterior segment of the eye e.g. cornea, iris, anterior chamber and the central portion of the lens. It analyses the anterior chamber angle in patients with different angle configurations, particularly when gonioscopy is not possible due to different prevailing circumstances (Landoy-Kalev et al., 2007). This technique appears to be a promising tool in assessment of the anterior chamber angle configuration in various angle closure glaucomas as well as in glaucoma suspects, and those with ocular hypertension (Radhakrishan et al., 2007). OCT depicts changes induced by laser iridotomies, and can be used as a rapid screening tool for detection of occludable angles.

Visante OCT was approved by FDA in 2005 as a non-contact, high resolution tomographic and biomicroscopic device for in-vivo imaging and measurement of ocular structures in the anterior segment such as corneal and LASIK flap thickness. Fourier-domain OCT and Visante OCT (time-domain) have been studied in assessing corneal and trabecular-iris angle disorders, central corneal thickness, trabecular–iris angle, and angle-opening distance (Pekmezci et al.,2009; Wylegala et al., 2009). OCT devices with biomicroscopy provide images of the scleral spur, ciliary body, ciliary sulcus, anterior chamber depth, and even canal of Schlemm in some eyes. Such anatomical landmarks help in phakic intra-ocular lens implantation (Konstantopoulos et al., 2007).Though OCT has been utilized for imaging of trabeculectomy blebs (Singh et al., 2007), capsular block syndrome (Lau et al., 2007), residual Descemet's membrane after Descemet's stripping endothelial keratoplasty (Kymionis et al., 2007), as well as visualization of aqueous shunt position and patency (Sarodia et al., 2007), there is currently inadequate evidence to support its application in these indications. Anterior-segment OCT has imaged small hypopigmented tumors with complete penetration, however, cysts behind iris pigment epithelium, highly pigmented tumors, large tumors, and ciliary body could not be penetrated completely. In these situations, ultrasound biomicroscopy was undoubtedly superior to the OCT (Pavlin et al., 2009).

23. Future strategy

Adaptive optics in combination with SD-OCT is going to be a new high-definition, three-dimensional retinal microstructural imaging technology in coming years. OCT derived pachymetry to capture focal thinning in keratoconus is being developed. Coming up are OCT-guided femtosecond laser capsulotomies in cataract surgeries where accuracy of the capsulotomy size, shape, and centration has been quantified in porcine and human eyes (Freidman et al., 2011).

24. OCT in artificial vision

This innovation provides qualitative and quantitative information about the retina-implant interface. It enables to follow epiretinal implants anatomically in both animal models and human patients (Panzan et al, 2004).

25. References

Aguirre AD, Hsiung P, Ko TH, Hart I, Fujimoto JG, et al. (2003). High-resolution optical coherence microscopy for high speed, in vivo cellular imaging. *Opt Lett,* Vol. 28, No. 21, (Nov), pp. 2064-2066.

Al-Mujaini A, Wali U, Ganesh A, Montana C. (2008). Natural course of Central Serous Chrioretinopathy without subretinal exudates in Pregnanacy. *Can J Ophthalmol,* Vol. 43, No. 5, (Oct), pp. :588-90.

Antcliff RJ, Stanford MR, Chauhan DS, Graham EM, Spalton DJ, et al. (2002). Comparison between Optical coherence tomography and fundus fluorescein angiography for the detection of cystoid macular edema in patients with uveitis. *Ophthalmology,* Vol. 107, No. 3, (Mar), pp. 593-599.

Burkholder BM, Osborne B, Loguidice MJ, Bisker E, Frohman TC, et al. (2009). Macular volume determined by optical coherence tomography as a measure of neuronal loss in multiple sclerosis. *Arch Neurol,* Vol. 66, No. 11, (Nov), pp. 1366-1372.

Cardillo Piccolino F, Eandi CM, Ventre L, Longrais RC, Grignolo FM, et al. (2003). Photodynamic therapy for chronic central serous chorioretinopathy. *Retina,* Vol. 23, No. 6, (Dec), pp. 752-763.

Chen TC, Cense B, Miller JW, Rubin PA, Daschler DG, et al. (2006). Histologic correlation of in vivo optical coherence tomography images of the human retina. *Am J Ophthalmol,* Vol. 141, No. 6, (Jun), pp. 1165-1168.

Console JW, Sakata LM, Aung T, Friedman DS, He M. (2008). Quantitative analysis of anterior segment Optical coherence tomography images: the Zhongshan angle assessment program. *Br J Ophthalmol,* Vol. 92, No. 12, (Dec), pp. 1612-1616.

Costello F, Coupland S, Hodge W, Lorello GR, Koroluk J, et al. (2006). Quantifying axonal loss after optic neuritis with optical coherence tomography. *Ann Neurol,* Vol. 59, No. 6, (Jun), pp. 963-969.

Cruz-Villegas V, Flynn HW Jr. Diabetic retinopathy. In: Schuman JS, Puliafito CA,

Cruz-Villegas V, Puliafito CA, Fujimoto JG. (2004). Retinal vascular diseases. In: Schuman JS, Puliafito CA, Fujimoto JG, eds. Optical coherence tomography of ocular diseases. Thorofare, NJ: SLACK, Inc.; 103-156.

Devereux JG, Foster PJ, Baasanhu J, Uranchimeg D, Lee PS, et al. (2000). Anterior chamber depth measurement as a screening tool for primary angle closure glaucoma in the East Asian population. *Arch Ophthalmol,* Vol. 118, No. 2, (Feb), pp. 257-263.

Drexler W, Morgner U, Ghanta RK, Kärtner FX, Schuman JS, Fujimoto JG. (2001). Ultrahigh resolution ophthalmic optical coherence tomography. *Nat Med,* Vol. 7, No. 4, (Apr), pp. :502-507.

Drexler W, Morgner U, Kärtner FX, Pitris C, Boppart SA, et al. (1999). In vivo ultrahigh resolution Optical coherence tomography. *Optics Lett,* Vol. 24, No. 17, (Sep), pp. 1221-1223.

Eriksson U, Larsson E, Holmstrom G. (2004). optical coherence tomography in the diagnosis of juvenile X-linked retinoschisis. *Acta Ophthalmol Scand,* Vol. 82, No. 2, (Apr), pp. 218-23.

Espinoza G, Rosenblatt B, Harbour JW. (2004). Optical coherence tomography in the evaluation of retinal changes associated with suspicious choroidal melanocytic tumors. *Am J Ophthalmol*, Vol. 137, No. 1, (Jan), pp. 90-95.

Fisher JB, Jacobs DA, Markowitz CE, Galetta SL, Volpe NJ, et al. (2006). Relation of visual function and retinal nerve fiber layer thickness in multiple sclerosis. *Ophthalmology*, Vol. 113, No. 2, (Feb), pp. 324-332.

Fishman GR, Pons ME, Seedor JA, Liebmann JM, Ritch R. (2005). Assessemnt of central corneal thickness using Optical coherence tomography. *J Cataract Refract Surg*, Vol. 31, No. 4, (), pp. 707-711.

Friedman NJ, Planker DV, Schuele G, Anderson D, Marcellino G, et al. (2011). Femtosecond laser capsulotomy. *Journal of cataract and refractive surgery*, Vol. 37, No. 7, (Jul), pp. 1189-1198.

Fujimoto JG, eds. Optical coherence tomography of ocular diseases. Thorofare, NJ: SLACK, Inc., 2004:157-214.

Fujimoto JG, Hee MR, Duang D et al. Principles of optical coherence tomography. In: Schuman JS, Puliafito CA, Fujimoto JG, eds. Optical coherence tomography of ocular diseases. Thorofare, NJ: SLACK; 2004: 3-20.

Fujimoto JG. (2003). Optical coherence tomography for ultrahigh resolution in vivo imaging. *Nat Biotechnol*, Vol. 21, No. 11, (Nov), pp. 1361-1367.

Fukasawa A, Lijima H. (2002). Optical coherence tomography of choroidal osteoma. *Am J Ophthalmol*, Vol. 133, No. 3, (Mar), pp. 419-421.

Gallemore RP, Jumper JM, McCuen BW 2nd , Jaffe GJ, Postel EA, Toth CA (2000). Diagnosis vitreoretinal adhesions in macular disease with optical coherence tomography. *Retina*, Vol. 20, No. 2, pp. 115-120.

Gass JD. (1995). Reappraisal of biomicroscopic classification of stages of development of a macular hole. *Am J Ophthalmol*, Vol. 119, No. 6, (Jun), pp. 752-759.

Gaudric A, Haouchine B, Massin P, Pacques M, Blain P, Erginay A. (1999). Macular hole formation: new data provided by optical coherence tomography. *Arch Ophthalmol*, Vol. 117, No. 6, (Jun), pp. 744-751.

Gelisken F, Inhoffen W, Partsch M, Schneider U, Kreissig I. (2001). Retinal pigment epithelial tear after photodynamic therapy for choroidal neovascularisation. *Am J Ophthalmol*, Vol. 131, No. 4, (Apr), pp. 518-520.

Giovannini A, Amato G, Mariotti C, Scassellati-Sforzolini B. (2000). Optical coherence tomography in the assessment of retinal pigment epithelial tear. *Retina*, Vol. 20, No. 1, pp. 37-40.

Giovannini A, Amato GP, Mariotti C, Scassellati-Sforzolini B. (1999). OCT imaging of choroidal neovascularisation and its role in the determination of patients' eligibility for surgery. *Br. J Ophthalmol*, Vol. 83, No. 4, (Apr), pp. 438-442.

Gordon-Lipkin E, Chodkowski B, Reich DS, Smith SA, Pulicken M, et al. (2007). Retinal nerve fiber layer is associated with brain atrophy in multiple sclerosis. *Neurology*, Vol. 69, No. 16, (Oct), pp. 1603-1609

Hee MR, Baumal CR, Puliafito CA, Duker JS, Reichel E, et al. (1996). Optical coherence tomography of age-related macular degeneration and choroidal neovascularisation. *Ophthalmology*, Vol. 103, No. 8, (Aug), pp. 1260-1270.

Hee MR, Fujimoto JG, Ko T et al. Interpretation of the optical coherence tomography image. In: Schuman JS, Puliafito CA, Fujimoto JG, eds. Optical coherence tomography of ocular diseases. Thorofare, NJ: SLACK, Inc.; 2004:21-56.

Hee MR, Puliafito CA, Duker JS, Reichel E, Duker JS, et al. (1998). Topography of diabetic macular edema with optical coherence tomography. *Ophthalmology,* Vol. 105, No. 2, (Feb), pp. 360-370.

Hee MR, Puliafito CA, Wong C, Duker JS, Reichel E, et al. (1995). Optical coherence tomography of macular holes. *Ophthalmology,* Vol. 102, N0. 5, (May), pp. 748-756.

Hee MR, Puliafito CA, Wong C, Duker JS, Reichel E, et al. (1995). Quantitative assessment of macular edema with optical coherence tomography. *Arch Ophthalmol,* Vol. 113, No. 8, (Aug), pp. 1019-1029.

Hikichi T, Yoshida A, Trempe CL. (1995). Course of vitreomacular traction syndrome. *Am J Ophthalmol,* Vol. 119, No. 1, (Jan), pp. 55-61.

Hoang QV, Linsenmeier A, Chung CK, Curcio CA. (2002). Photoreceptor inner segments in monkey and human retina: mitochondrial density, optics, and regional variation. *Vis Neurosci,* Vol. 19, No. 4, (Jul-Aug), pp. 395-407.

Hrynchak P, Simpson T. (2007). Optical coherence tomography: an introduction to the technique and its use. *Optom Vis Sci,* Vol. 77, No. 7, (Jul), pp. 347-356.

Huang D, Swanson EA, Lin CP, Schuman JS, Stinson WG, et al. (1991). Optical coherence tomography. *Science,* Vol. 254, No.5035, (Nov), pp.1178-1181.

Ip M, Garza-Karren C, Duker JS, Reichel E, Swartz JC, et al. (1999). Differentiation of degenerative retinoschisis from retinal detachment using optical coherence tomography. *Ophthalmology,* Vol. 106, No. 3, (Mar), pp. 600-605.

Ip M, Kahana A, Altaweel M. (2003). Treatment of central retinal vein occlusion with triamcinolone acetonide: an optical coherence tomography study. *Semin Ophthalmol,* Vol. 18, No. 2, (Jun), pp. 67-73.

Ip MS, Baker BJ, Duker JS, Reichel E, Baumal CR, et al. (2002). Anatomical outcomes of surgery for idiopathic macular hole as determined by optical coherence tomography. *Arch Ophthalmol,* Vol. 120, No. 1, (Jan) pp. 29-35.

Jumper JM, Gallemore RP, McCuen BW 2nd , Toth CA. (2000). Features of macular hole closure in the early postoperative period using optical coherence tomography. *Retina,* Vol. 20, No. 3, pp. 232-237.

Kaiser PK, Riemann CD, Sears JE, Lewis H. (2001). Macular traction detachment and diabetic macular edema associated with posterior hyaloidal traction. *Am J Ophthalmol,* Vol. 131, No. 1, (Jan), pp. 44-49.

Kang SW, Park CY, Ham DI. (2004). The correlation between fluorescein angiographic and optical coherence tomographic features in clinically significant diabetic macular edema. *Am J Ophthalmol,* Vol. 137, No. 2, (Feb), pp.313-322.

Kasuga Y, Arai J, Akimoto M, Yoshimura N. (2000). Optical coherence tomography to confirm early closure of macular holes. *Am J Ophthalmol,* Vol. 130, No. 5, (Nov), pp. 675-676.

Ko TH, Fujimoto JG, Schuman JS, Paunescu LA, Kowalevicz AM, et al. (2005). Comparison of ultrahigh-and standard resolution optical coherence tomography for imaging macular pathology. *Ophthalmology*, Vol. 112, No. 11, (Nov), pp. 1922-1935.

Konstantopoulos A, Hossain P, Anderson DF. (2007). Recent advances in ophthalmic anterior segment imaging: A new era for ophthalmic diagnosis. *Br J Ophthalmol*, Vol. 91, No. 4, (Apr), pp. 551-577.

Krivoy D, Gentile R, Liebmann JM, Stegman Z, Rosen R, et al. (1996). Imaging congenital optic disc pits and associated maculopathy using optic coherence tomography. *Arch Ophthalmol*, Vol. 114, No. 2, (Feb), pp. 165-170.

Kymionis GD, Suh LH, Dubovy SR, Yoo SH. (2007). Diagnosis of residual Descemet's membrane after Descemet's stripping endothelial keratoplasty with anterior segment Optical coherence tomography. *J Cataract Refract Surg*, Vol. 33, No. 7, (Jul), pp. 1322-1324.

Landoy-Kalev M, Day AC, Cordeiro MF, Migdal C. (2007). Optical coherence tomography in anterior segment imaging. *Acta Ophthalmol Scand*, Vol. 85, No.4, (Jun), pp. 427-430.

Lau FH, Wong AL, Lam PT, Lam DS. (2007). Photographic assay. Anterior segment Optical coherence tomography findings of early capsular block syndrome. *Clin Experiment Ophthalmol*, Vol. 35, No. 8, (Nov), pp. 770-771.

Lerche RC, Schaudig U, Scholz F, Walter A, Richard G. (2001). Structural changes of the retina in retinal vein occlusion-imaging and quantification with optical coherence tomography. *Ophthalm Surg Lasers*, Vol. 32, N0. 4, (Jul-Aug), pp. 272-280.

Li H, Leung CK, Cheung CY, -----(2007). Repeatabilty and reproducibility of anterior chamber angle measurement with anterior segment Optical coherence tomography. . *Br J Ophthalmol*, Vol. 91, No. 11, ( ), pp. 1490-1492.

Lincoff H, Kreissig I. (1998). Optical coherence tomography of pneumatic displacement of optic disc pit maculopathy. *Br J Ophthalmol*, Vol. 82, No. 4, (Apr), pp. 367-372.

Lopez JM, Guerrero P. (2006). Congenital simple hamartoma of the retinal pigment epithelium: optical coherence tomography and angiography features. *Retina*, Vol. 26, No. 6, pp. 704-706.

Margherio RR, Trese MT, Margherio AR, Cartright K. (1989). Surgical management of vitreomacular traction syndromes. *Ophthalmology*, Vol. 96, No. 9, (Sept), pp. 1437-1445.

Markomichelakis NN, Halkiadakis I, Pantelia E, Peponis V, Patelis A, et al. (2004). Patterns of macular edema in patients with uveitis: qualitative and quantitative assessment using Optical coherence tomography. *Ophthalmology*, Vol. 111, No. 5, (May), pp. 946-953.

Massin P, Allouch C, Haouchine B, Metge F, Pâques M, et al. (2000). Optical coherence tomography of idiopathic macular epiretinal membranes before and after surgery. *Am J Ophthalmol*, Vol. 130, No. 6, (Dec), pp. 732-739.

Mavrofrides EC, Cruz-Villegas V, Puliafito CA. Miscellaneous retinal diseases. In: Schuman JS, Puliafito CA, Fujimoto JG, eds. Optical coherence tomography of ocular diseases. Thorofare, NJ: SLACK, Inc.; 2004:457-482.

Mavrofrides EC, Puliafito CA, Fujimoto JG. Central serous chorioretinopathy . In: Schuman JS, Puliafito CS, Fujimoto JG, eds. Optical coherence tomography of ocular diseases. Thorofare, NJ: SLACK, Inc; 2004:215-242.

Mavrofrides EC, Rogers AH, Truong S et al. Vitroretinal interface disorders. In: Schuman JS, Puliafito CA, Fujimoto JG, eds. Optical coherence tomography of ocular diseases. Thorofare, NJ: SLACK, Inc.; 2005: 57-102.

Mavrofrides EC, Villate N, Rosenfeld PJ et al.[eds]. Optical coherence tomography of ocular diseases. In: Schuman JS, Puliafito CA, Fujimoto JG [eds]. Optical coherence tomography of ocular diseases. Thorofare, NJ:SLACK, Inc.; 2004:243-343.

McDonald HR, Johnson RN, Schatz H. (1994). Surgical results in the vitreomacular traction syndrome. *Ophthalmology*, Vol. 101, No.8, (Aug), pp. 1397-1402.

Mori K, Gehlbach PL, Sano A, Deguchi T, Yoneya S. (2004). Comparison of epiretinal membranes of differing pathogenesis using optical coherence tomography. *Retina*, Vol. 24, No. 1, (Feb), pp. 57-62.

Moura FC, Medeiros FA, Monteiro ML. (2007). Evaluation of macular thickness measurements for detection of band atrophy of the optic nerve using optical coherence tomography. *Ophthalmology*, Vol. 114, No. 1, (Jan), pp. 175-181.

Muscat S, Parks S, Kemp E, Keating D. (2004). Secondary retinal changes associated with choroidal nevi and melanomas documented by optical coherence tomography. *Br J Ophthalmol*, Vol. 88, No. 1, (Jan), pp. 120-124.

Myer CH, Rodrigues EB, Schmidt JC. (2003). Congenital optic nerve head pit association with reduced retinal nerve fiber thickness at the papillomacular bundle. *Br J Ophthalmol*, Vol. 87, No. 10, (Oct), pp. 1300-1301.

Panzan CQ, Guven D, Weiland JD, Lakhanpal R, Javaheri M, et al. (2004). Retinal thickness in normal and RCD1 dogs using optical coherence tomography. *Ophthlm Surg Lasers Imaging*, Vol. 35, No. 6, (Nov-Dec), pp. 485-493.

Parisi V, Manni G, Spadaro M, Colacino G, Restuccia R, et al. (1999). Correlation between morphological and functional retinal impairment in multiple sclerosis patients. *Invest Ophthalmol Vis Sci*, Vol. 40, No. 11, (Oct), pp. 2520-2527

Pavlin CJ, Vasquez LM, Lee R, Simpson ER, Ahmed II. (2009). Anterior segment Optical coherence tomography and ultrasound biomicroscopy in the imaging of anterior segment tumors. *Am j Ophthalmol*, Vol. 147, No. 2, (Feb), pp. 214-219.

Pece A, Introini U, Bottoni F, Brancato R. (2001). Acute retinal pigment epithelial tear after photodynamic therapy. *Retina*, Vol. 21, No. 6, pp. 661-665.

Pekmezci M, Porco TC, Lin SC. (2009). Anterior segment Optical coherence tomography as a screening tool for the assessment of the anterior segment angle. *Ophthalmic Surg Lasers Imaging*, Vol. 40, No. 4, (Jul-Aug), pp. 389-398.

Pendergast SD, Hassan TS, Williams GA, Cox MS, Margherio RR, et al. (2000). Vitrectomy for diffuse diabetic macular edema associated with a taut premacular posterior hyaloid. Am J Ophthalmol, Vol. 130, No. 2, (Aug), pp. 178-186.

Poinooswamy D, Fontana L, Wu JX, Fitzke FW, Hitchings RA. (1997). Variation of nerve fibre layer thickness measurements with age and ethnicity by scanning laser polarimetry. *Br J Ophthalmol*,Vol. 81, No. 5, (May), pp. 350-354.

Pulicken M, Gordon-Lipkin E, Blacer LJ, Frohman E, Cutter G, Calabreci PA. (2007). Optical coherence tomography and disease subtype in multiple sclerosis. *Neurology* Vol. 69, No. 22, (Nov), pp. :2085-2092.

Radhakrishan S, See J, Smith SD, Nolan WP, Ce Z, et al. (2007). Reproducibility of anterior chamber angle measurements obtained with anterior segment Optical coherence tomography. *Invest Ophthalmol Vis Sci.,* Vol. 48, No. 8, (Aug), pp. 3683-3688.

Robertson DM. (1986). Argon laser photocoagulation treatment in central serous chorioretinopathy. *Ophthalmology,* Vol. 93, No. 7, (Jul), pp. 972-974.

Rogers AH, Martidis A, Greenberg PB, Puliafito CA. (2002). Optical coherence tomography findings following photodynamic therapy of choroidal neovascularisation. *Am J Ophthalmol,* Vol. 134, No. 4, (Oct), pp. 566-576.

Roth AM, Foos RY. (1971). Surface wrinkling retinopathy in eye enucleated at autopsy. *Trans Am Acad Ophthalmol Otolaryngol,* Vol. 75, No. 5, (Sep-Oct) pp. 1047-1059.

Ryan SJ. Retina, 4th edn, vol. 2. Elsevier Mosby 2006:1533-1556.

Sarodia U, Sharkawi E, Hau S, Barton K. (2007). Visualization of aqueous shunt position and patency using anterior segment Optical coherence tomography. *Am j Ophthalmol,* Vol. 143, No. 6, (Jun), pp. 1054-1056.

Sato H, Kawasaki R, Yamashita H. (2003). Observation of idiopathic full-thickness macular hole closure in early postoperative period as evaluated by optical coherence tomography. *Am J Ophthalmol,* Vol. 136, No. 1, (Jul), pp. 185-187.

Schaudig UH, Glaefke C, Scholz F, Richard G. (2000). Optical coherence tomography for retinal thickness measurement in diabetic patients without clinically significant macular edema. *Ophthalm Surg Lasers,* Vol. 31, No. 3, (May-Jun) pp. 182-186.

Schuman JS, Puliafito CA, Fujimoto JG [eds]. Optical coherence tomography of ocular diseases. Thorofare, NJ: Slack; 2004.

Sekiryu T, Yamauchi T, Enaida H, Hara Y, Furuta M. (2000). Retina tomography after vitrectomy for macular edema of central retinal vein occlusion. *Ophthalm Surg Lasers,* Vol. 31, No. 3, (May-Jun), pp. 198-202.

Shukla D, Ambatkar S, Jethani J, Kim R.(2005). Optical coherence tomography in presumed congenital simple hamartoma of retinal pigment epithelium. *Am. J. Ophthalmol,* Vol. 139, No. 5, (May), pp. 945-947.

Sidd RJ, Fine SL, Owens SL, Patz A. (1982). Idiopathic preretinal gliosis. *Am J Ophthalmol,* Vol. 94, No. 1, (Jul), pp. 44-48.

Singh M, Chew PT, Friedman DS, Nolan WP, See JL et al. (2007). Imaging of trabeculectomy blebs using anterior segment Optical coherence tomography. *Ophthalmology,* Vol. 114, No. 1, (Jan), pp. 47-53.

Smiddy WE, Michels RG, Glaser BM, deBustros S. (1988). Vitrectomy for macular traction caused by incomplete vitreous separation. *Arch Ophthalmol,* Vol. 106, No 5, (May), pp. 624-628

Spirn MJ, Warren FA, Guyer DR, Klancnik JR, Spaide RF. (2003). Optical coherence tomography findings in nicotinic acid maculopathy. *Am J Ophthalmol,* Vol. 135, No. 6, (Jun), pp. 913-914.

Srivastava SK, Sternberg P Jr. (2002). Retinal pigment epithelial tear weeks following photodynamic therapy with verteporfin for choroidal neovascularisation secondary to pathologic myopia. Retina, Vol. 22, No. 5 (Oct), pp. 669-671.

Stalmans P, Spileers W, Dralands L. (1999). The use of optical coherence tomography in macular diseases. *Bull Soc Belge Ophthalmol*, Vol. 272, pp. 15-30.

Suzuki T, Terasaki H, Niwa T. (2003). Optical coherence tomography and focal macular electroretinogram in eyes with epiretinal membrane and macular pseudohole. *Am J Ophthalmol*, Vol. 136, No. 1, (Jul), pp. 62-67

Teitelbaum BA, Tresley DJ. (2003). Cystic maculopathy with normal capillary permeability secondary to docetexel. *Optom Vis Sci*, Vol. 80, No. 4, (Apr), pp. 277-279.

Ting TD, Oh M, Cox TA, Meyer CH, Toth CA. (2002). Decreased visual acuity associated with cystoid macular edema in neovascular age-related macular degeneration. *Arch Ophthalmol*, Vol. 120, No. 6, (Jun) pp. 731-737.

Ullrich S, Haritoglou C, Gass C, Schaumberger M, Ulbig MW, Kampik A. (2002). Macular hole size as a prognostic factor in macular hole surgery. *Br J Ophthalmol*, Vol. 86, No. 4, (Apr), pp. 390-393.

Villate N, Mavrofrides EC, Davis J. Chorioretinal inflammatory diseases. In: Schuman JS, Puliafito CA, Fujimoto JG, eds. Optical coherence tomography of ocular diseases. Thorofare, NJ: SLACK, Inc.; 2004:371-412.

Voo I, Mavrofrides EC, Puliafito CA. (2004). Clinical applications of Optical coherence tomography for the diagnosis and management of macular diseases. *Ophthalmol Clin North Am*, Vol. 17, No. 1, (Mar), pp. 21-31.

Wang B, Sakata LM, Friedman DS, Chan YH, He M, et al. (2010). Quantitative iris parameters and association with narrow angles. *Ophhalmology*, Vol. 117, No. 1, (Jan), pp. 11-17.

Wilkins JR, Puliafito CA, Hee MR, Duker JS, Reichel E, et al. (1996). Characterisation of epiretinal membranes using optical coherence tomography *Ophthalmology*, Vol. 103, No. 12, (Dec), pp. 2142-2151.

Wu R, Nongpiur ME, He MG, Sakata LM, Friedman DS, et al. (2011). Association of narrow angles with anterior chamber area and volume measured with anterior segment Optical coherence tomography. *Arch Ophthalmol*, Vol. 129, No.5, (May), pp. 569-574.

Wylegala E, Teper S, Nowińska AK, Milka M, Dobrowolski D. (2009). Anterior segment imaging: Fourier-domain Optical coherence tomography versus time-domain Optical coherence tomography. Journal of cataract and refractive surgery, Vol. 35, No. 8, (Aug), pp. 1410-1414.

Yannuzzi LA, Ciardella A, Spaide RF, Rabb M, Freund KB, Orlock DA. (1997). The expanding clinical spectrum of idiopathic polypoidal choroidal vasculopathy. *Arch Ophthalmol*, Vol. 115, No. 4, (Apr), pp. 478-485.

Yannuzzi LA, Freund KB, Goldbaum M, Scassellati-Sforzolini B, Guyer DR, et al. (2000). Polypoidal choroidal vasculopathy masquerading as central serous chorioretinopathy. *Ophthalmology*, Vol. 107, No. 4, (Apr), pp. 767-777.

Yannuzzi LA, Negrão S, Iida T, Carvalho C, Rodriguez-Coleman H, et al. (2001). Retinal angiomatous proliferation in age-related macular degeneration. *Retina,* Vol. 21, No. 5, pp. 416-434.

Zacks DN, Johnson MW. (2004) Retinal angiomatus proliferation: optical coherence tomographic confirmation of an intraretinal lesion. *Arch Ophthalmol,* Vol. 122, No. 6, (Jun), pp. 932-933.

12

Optical Coherence Tomography in Dentistry

Yueli L. Chen[1], Quan Zhang[2] and Quing Zhu[1]
[1]*Biomedical Engineering Department, University of Connecticut, Storrs,*
[2]*Massachusetts Genreal Hospital, Harvard Medical School, Charlestown, MA*
USA

1. Introduction

Optical Coherence Tomography is an imaging technique characterized by high spatial resolution and noninvasive subsurface detection[1]. OCT started as an interferometric technique utilizing the newly emerged low coherence or partial coherence light source and time-domain gating to achieve the depth resolution. With additional lateral scans, 2-D or 3-D tomographic images can be obtained. The instrumental development of OCT has experienced several phases. It goes from free space architectures to fiber-based systems, from intensity-based structural imaging to multiple functional extensions of polarization sensitive, Doppler, and spectroscopic OCT. Since the beginning of this century, a Fourier domain OCT infrastructure has been introduced that resulted in a new revolution in OCT technology[2, 3]. Not only was the new technology bringing a hundred times more sensitivity, it was also technically more convenient for the design of a higher speed scanning system structures. Nowadays, FD-OCT are implemented with either a spectrometer or a tunable laser design. Modern OCT is more accurately defined as a broadband rather than low-coherence interferometric technology. And the outcome is a true 3D imaging modality[4-9] with high data speed for real-time clinical diagnosis, free from the degradation of motion artifacts.

Bearing a two-decade history of fast pace research and development, OCT has established itself as a promising *in vivo* biomedical imaging modality. Constant efforts toward improving this imaging technology lead to more than 5000 journal publications. There is now a clear trend of extended interests towards the application side in addition to the technology development. Currently, the well established ophthalmic diagnostic application occupies about 50% of academic and industrial shares in OCT business[10-19]. Cardiovascular imaging[20-27] has become the next big thing when the coronary OCT products have seen FDA clearance in the United States. Besides the two types of applications, OCT holds promise in dermatological[8, 28-31], dental[32-43], small animal[44-46], development biology[47-49], and various endoscopic applications[50-55] such as for esophagus, colon, and ovarian imaging.

The focus of this chapter is on dental imaging. We will review the dental diagnostic approaches and discuss the clutching points where optical coherence tomography can seek contribution. The OCT technological prospective will be cut short in this chapter. A rich compilation of imaging figures will be present in such that readers with more application expertise may define the region of interests beyond the written text.

2. Traditional dental diagnosis and the limiting factors

Currently, the "gold standard" clinical diagnostic product for tooth diagnostics is dental radiography (X-ray). Although generally accepted by dental clinic, it has several imaging limitations, primarily, *the resolution and the contrast*. Dental X-ray has limited resolution. Dental X-ray images relatively smaller dental tissues compared to other applications such as chest X-ray and mammography. As a result, X-ray is not good at detecting from small tooth tissue even smaller lesions such as tiny precaries and cracks. Dental X-ray has limited imaging contrast. X-ray contrast arises from attenuation variation between different tissue composites. Human tooth consists of primarily enamel, dentin, and pulp which do not show strong X-ray contrast. Demineralization, as a major tooth decay indicator produces only subtle changes in image contrast that trained eye can tell. Believe it or not, standard diagnosis device would leave as much as 50 percent of tooth decay go undetected. To assess the tooth health, it is important to understand the microstructures, their mineralization level, and in particular the dynamic mineral exchanges within the dental tissues. High resolution imaging techniques such as AFM and TEM are used to investigate the microstructures of teeth. These studies however, can only perform under *ex vivo* scenario which is not able to clinically assess the status of the human dental health.

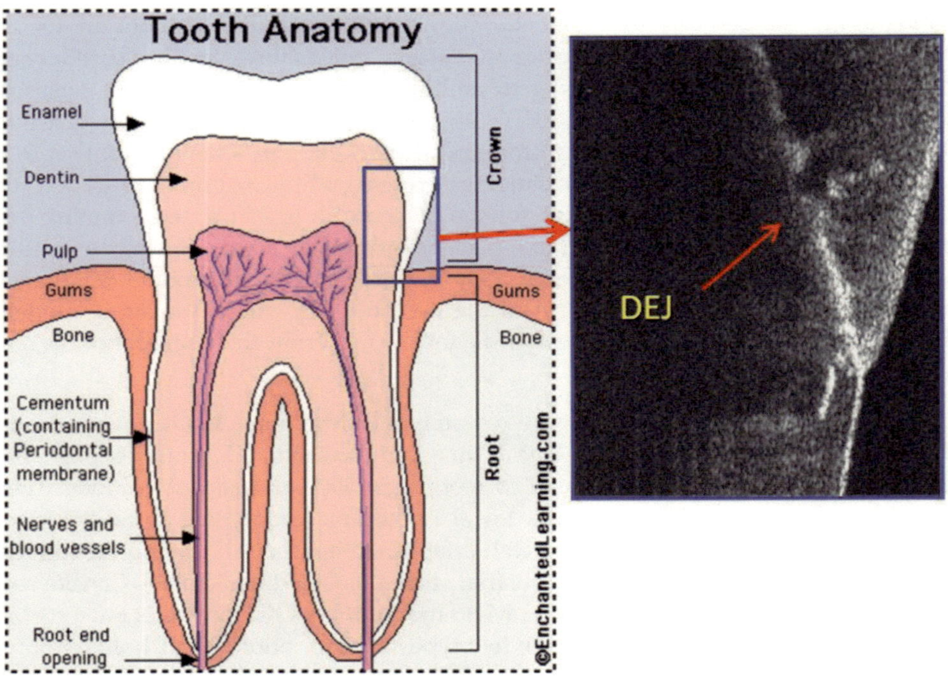

Fig. 1. The tooth anatomy. The primary components of a tooth are dentin and enamel. To the right side is an OCT B-scan (2D image), with which we can find the corresponding anatomic dental structure. This OCT image is oriented in such to get the general readers some salt on how to interpret the output of an OCT scan.

In particular, dental X-ray is not good at identify occlusal (the biting surface) cavities. As a projection method that overlaps the full volume along X-ray photon travel directions into one 2D image, the method fell short to detect occlusal cavities. Because the X-ray takes tooth scan from the side of the tooth, this orientation effectively hides the pit or valley cavities from the dentist's view. In the past, tooth cavities are primarily developed between teeth. As the use of fluoride became more widespread, the outer tooth became strengthened. Flossing also helps removing plaques and bacterial infections hiding between the gaps of teeth. Nowadays, it is actually the canyon-like topological chewing surface that cavity most likely to develop. Bacteria can accumulate especially around the sites of the pits and valleys, the weak spots where the plaques are relatively difficult to be brushed away. As health care keeps improving, early diagnosis becomes a favorite subject in dentistry. If we can spot tiny tooth decay in an early stage, rehabilitation procedures are possible to cure the lesion and before it goes to the wrong way.

3. What optical coherence tomography brings to the table

Dental OCT directly addresses the image quality issue with its intrinsic high resolution and contrast mechanism, which is useful to indentify tiny precaries and fissure lesions before their potential progression to serious dental decay. As a functional extension, polarization sensitive OCT is found to be especially interesting in dental imaging. It provides unique contrast beyond regular OCT's intensity contrast from the variation of tissue materials and boundaries. We will present data to show evidence that the cavity decay responses to the polarization states of the probing light.

OCT is now typically designed as a fiber system. Therefore a flexible handheld fiber-guided probe with light weight can be fabricated for clinical purpose. The probe will facilitate a small scanner head for doctors to directly aim at regions of interests of patient's teeth. Towards commercialization, OCT probe can sit near the dentist's tool-box just as other wired gadgets. OCT also has significant advantages due to its use of cheaper and much safer near infrared light rather than radioactive source for detection. Moreover, recent advance of OCT from time-domain to Fourier domain enhanced imaging sensitivity to another 100 times. The sensitivity advantage is transferred to high-speed dental imaging acquisition *in vivo*, which is an important prospective in dental clinic practice. When imaging a non-stationary target, i.e. a patient, high speed is required to reduce the motion smearing and thus retain the high resolution property of the imager. Meanwhile, shorter scan duration is necessary to reduce the discomfort of patients especially children. Current state of the art OCT scanning speed would enable a single scan of one tooth surface within a couple of seconds. With such an imaging paradigm, we have a true 3D dental scan to cover the full surface area of teeth. This opens options for more quantitative and comprehensive diagnostic approaches, for which we will be discussing in the later section.

3.1 Intensity based dental OCT

Intensity OCT images are mapped by the coherently mixed light fields between sample and reference arms where the detected signal is representing the amount of back scattered light from some certain depths of the tissue. Structural boundaries or regional optical scatterers bring different back scattering signal strength. Therefore intensity OCT primarily reveals the enfolded structural information of the imaging target. For soft tissues, OCT's penetration is usually 1-2 mm before the signal is attenuated to the noise floor. For dental tissue however, the light penetration can goes deeper to beyond 4 mm defined by optical path length in air.

This depth is achieved in our imaging system when a small numerical aperture was applied in the sample arm to increase the range of the depth of focus (DOF). The trade-off is a decrease of lateral resolution to larger than 20 micrometers. This depth range could cover the area of interests where tooth decay happens. The typical OCT resolution ranges from a few micrometers to more than ten micrometers, which is overkill to resolve a clinically significant tooth decay spot.

Figure 2 shows some typical dental OCT scans. With 256 gray scale mapping, the stronger signals are corresponding to whiter colors. The top air regions above the tooth surfaces are basically black because there is no back scattering light signal. Fig. 2A (premolar) and B (molar) are scans along the occlusal direction, meaning the scanner is pointing at the occlusal surface. In contrast to the projectile geometry of dental X-ray scans, where the images planes are perpendicular to the X-ray photon travel directions, the OCT B-scans are in the same planes of the near infrared optical photon probing trajectories. Therefore what we see from the black-white boundaries in Fig.2 A and B are in fact the topologies of the biting surfaces of the teeth. The whitish area pointed by two white arrows in Fig. 2 B likely could be signs of tooth decay.

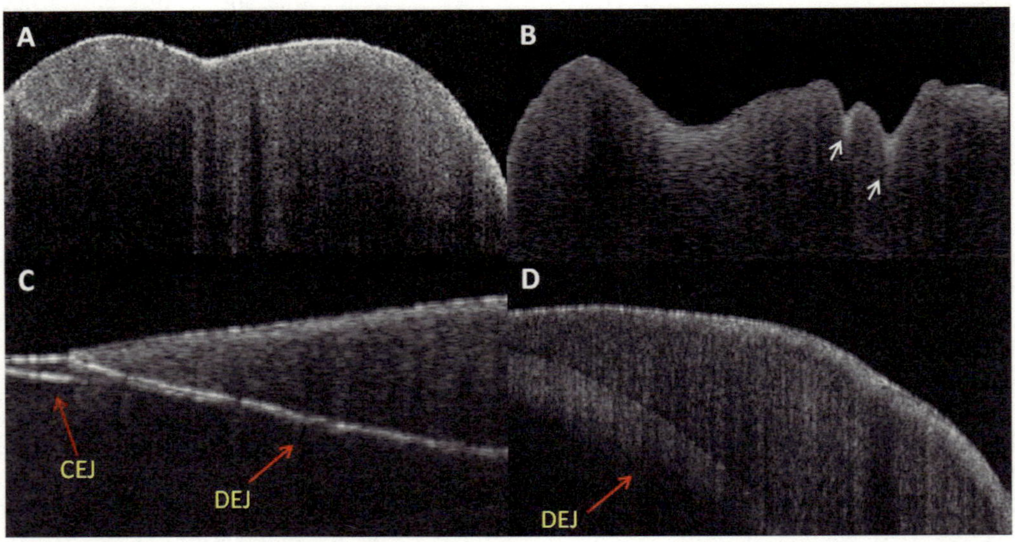

Fig. 2. Four typical intensity based OCT B-scans. A and B imaging from the occlusal direction of a premolar and molar tooth. C and D: scanning of teeth from the peripheral directions where the boundaries of dentin, enamel, and cementum can be seen. The four images are from three different systems. Therefore some system-dependent differences can be seen such as in contrast and noise levels. They are representative illustrations with different imaging scales.

The occlusal decay as mentioned earlier, is the most difficult to identify in X-ray diagnosis due to the projection of the full tooth thickness along lingual to facial direction. Even when a spurious tooth decay is spotted, it is also hard to determine the exact location of the lesion. OCT instead are capable of pinpointing the exact lesion sites. The two white arrows point to the pit areas, where bacterial infections are more likely to happen. Fig. 2C and D are scans from the side of teeth. Fig. 2C is more close to the root and Fig. 2D more close to the crown. The dentinoenamel junction (DEJ) and the cementoenamel junction (CEJ) are clearly visible in Fig. 2C as brighter boundaries. In Fig. 2D, the boundary can be roughly differentiated with the different imaging properties of dentin (weak) and enamel (strong) tissues. There is however not a specific white band associating with the junction. On the contrary, a dark line is indentified along the boundary area. The dark area in OCT indicates lacking of tissue scattering. In our dry dental hard tissue sample, it is most likely associated with an air gap. In fact, there appears to be some other less visible crack lines in the enamel. These microstructural features are difficult to be seen in X-ray due to the resolution and contrast limitations.

Early tooth decay, even at the surface of a tooth, may not be easy to be identified by a naked eye. Sometimes, the lesion could look whiter rather than browner associated with early demineralization. Up to this point, it is clear that OCT would have ample resolution to spot tiny lesions. OCT will also have the capability to locate the position of the lesions accurately. What important next, is thus to explore if there exists a clear contrast mechanism or marker to associate with the tooth decay, and especially in the early stage. This is by far still an ongoing research topic. From Fig.3, it appears the scattering intensity itself could potentially be a marker for the tooth decay. As can be seen from the referenced photo picture to the right side, the OCT B-scan goes across a lesion spot which most likely is caused by demineralization. The lesion spot shows significantly stronger signal intensity. This is coincident with the whitish spots at the pit areas of the Fig. 2B which likely are the lesion areas associated with decay too. There is also another decay marker discussed by Choo-Smith et al[56]. She has used OCT attenuation slope to characterize the healthiness of a tooth. It is possible that the two types of markers may originate from the same biophysical mechanism: that the demineralization process increases the light back scattering intensity into deeper imaging depth.

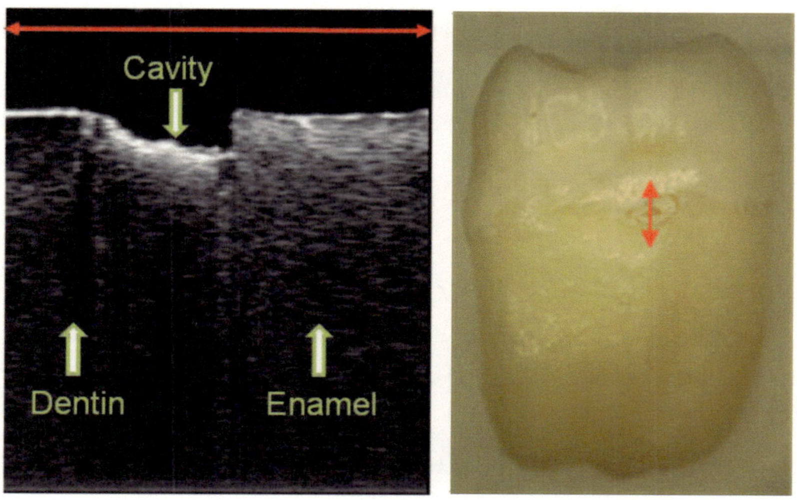

Fig. 3. An OCT B-scan frame from buccal orientation scanning across a hole about 1mm diameter on the surface near the cementoenamel junction line. We scanned across the lesion for about 4 mm in lateral length. The image depth is also about 4 mm. The scanning range is indicated with red arrows on the OCT image and the tooth photo. OCT image clearly shows stronger scattering from the lesion area.

3.2 Polarization-sensitive dental OCT

OCT is capable of coherence detection of polarization states from the backscattered signal. Dental tissue happens to be very sensitive to light polarization. Therefore more detection information can be obtained by polarization sensitive OCT (PS-OCT). Literatures have shown strong evidence that PS-OCT significantly enhances the detection power of OCT. In dental OCT, polarization is a metric parameter that may not be overlooked. It is because enamel and dentin as the primary components of human teeth, have shown interesting polarization effects. The effect can be used to evaluation the tooth structure. It is also because a polarization sensitive OCT imaging scheme is not deployed, the polarization effect could come back as strong polarization artifacts to distort the true structural information even in a regular intensity OCT.

Figure 4 shows the polarization sensitive system developed to produce the PS-OCT image results in this chapter. The polarization response can be calculated based on the Jone's matrix formalism. The complex light field is expressed as a vector of vertical and horizontal parts:

$$\mathbf{E} = \begin{pmatrix} \tilde{E}_V \\ \tilde{E}_H \end{pmatrix} \quad (1)$$

V and H indicate the two orthogonal polarization directions. , E_V and E_H are the detected field amplitude. The polarization effect of the sample to the light can be expressed in a general retarder form as

$$S(\phi,\theta) = \begin{pmatrix} \cos^2\theta + \sin^2\theta \cdot e^{-j2\phi} & \cos\theta \cdot \sin\theta \cdot (1 - e^{-j2\phi}) \\ \cos\theta \cdot \sin\theta \cdot (1 - e^{-j2\phi}) & \cos^2\theta \cdot e^{-j2\phi} + \sin^2\theta \end{pmatrix} \quad (2)$$

where ϕ is the average phase retardation angle (single trip of back scattered photon) and θ is the average fast axis orientation. Following this Jones matrix formalism, we have in the standard CP configuration:

$$\tilde{E}_V = A_V \exp[-(\Delta z/l)^2] \sin(\phi) \exp(-i\phi) \quad (3)$$

$$\tilde{E}_H = A_H \exp[-(\Delta z/l)^2] \cos(\phi) \exp[-I(\phi+2\theta-\pi)] \quad (4)$$

where Δz is the optical path difference and l is the SLD coherence length. Since the two channels are identical, constants A_V and A_H can be considered to be the same. The phase retardation ϕ can then be expressed by

$$\phi = \arctan(E_V/E_H) \quad (5)$$

The phase retardation values vary from 0 to 90 degree. The regular OCT image can be obtained by

$$E_{oct} = \mathrm{sqrt}(E_V^2 + E_H^2) \quad (6)$$

Detailed Jone's formalism calculation can be found from other papers[57, 58].

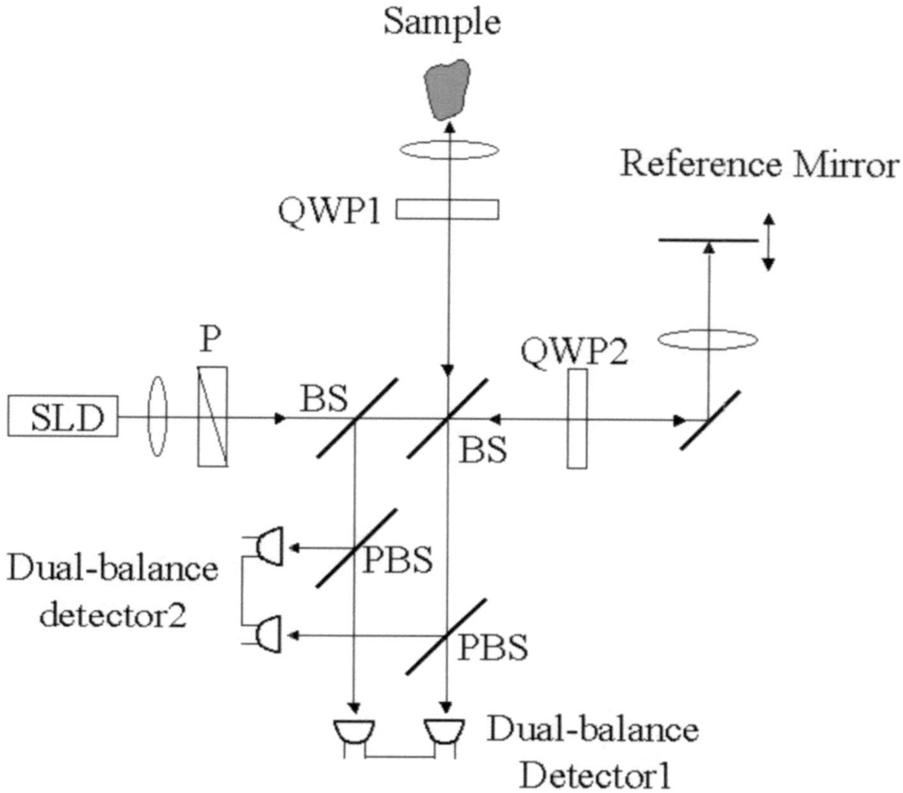

Fig. 4. Schematic of the PS-OCT system. SLD, superluminescent diode; P, polarizer; BS, beam splitter; PBS, polarizing beam splitters; QWP1,QWP2, quarter-wave plates; Galvo, galvanometer.

We'd like to point out that in PS-OCT two-channel detection is required. This increases the data volume and the complicity of data processing. There are subsequently more ways to representing the data. Figure 5 shows a generally accepted image construction standard that produces four sets of images. The four images map imaging parameters log(E_V), log(E_H), ϕ, and log(E_{oct}) accordingly. Fig.5A is the cross-polarization channel image. Fig. 5C is called PS-OCT image that maps a physical parameter of the phase retardation (0 to 90 degree angle). Fig. 5D is regular intensity OCT image. It will be approximate to the co-polarization or horizontal channel image in Fig. 5B, if the polarization effect is not strong.

Figure.5 shows the enamel structure and the well-delineated DEJ scanned from the facial aspect. The image size is 2.5mm in lateral and 3.6mm in depth (the depth in air, with no index modification). In Fig.5A, B, and D, DEJ can be identified as a white interface due to its strong reflection. The DEJ is differentiated as a line of texture pattern in phase retardation image shown in Fig. 5C. The penetration depth of dentin is generally found to be less than that of enamel. Images of enamel generally have richer information and deeper penetration, while images in dentin usually have a shallower depth profile. Two types of tissues can be clearly differentiated by their scattering properties.

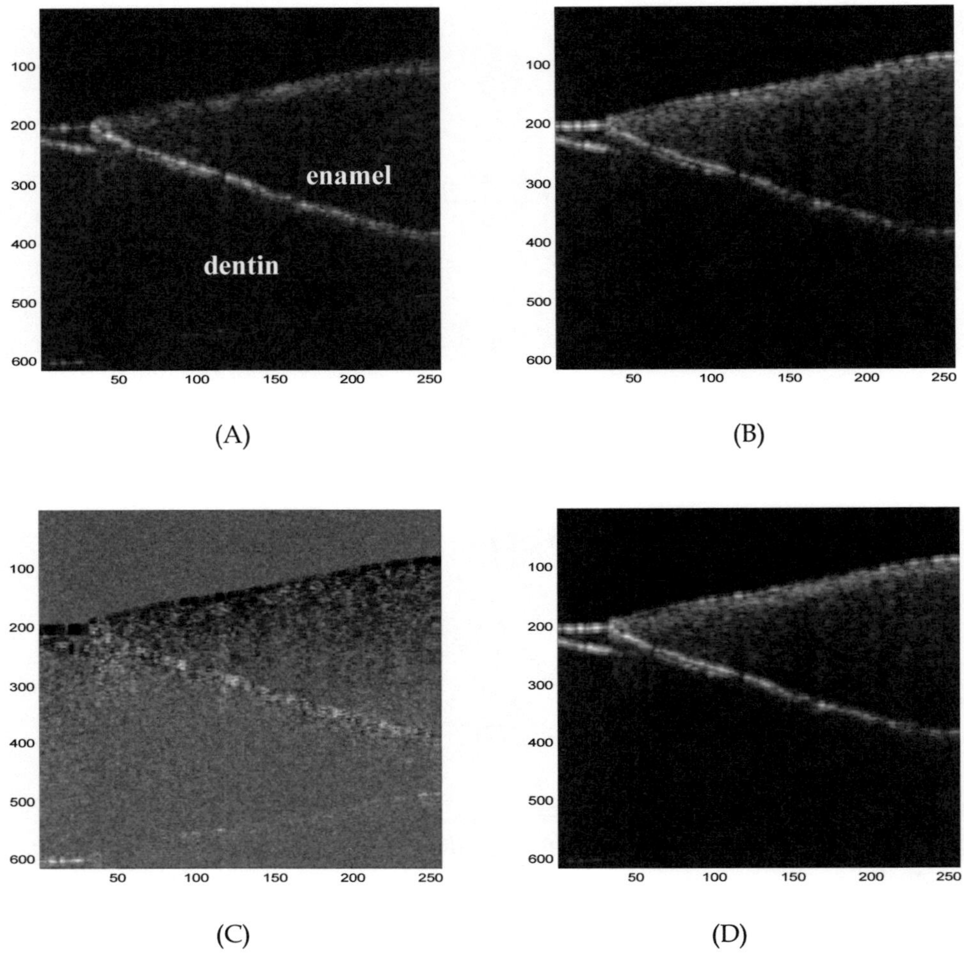

Fig. 5. (A), V-channel image. (B), H-channel image. (C), Polarization sensitive image by $\phi=\arctan(E_V/E_H)$. (D), Intensity image by $R=E_V^2+E_H^2$. The bright reflection band inside is the DEJ and towards surface on the left, the cementum boundary can be visualized too.

To measure the polarization sensitivity in dental matrix and its correlation to demineralization, Fried et al.[59] found to assess cross-polarization channel image are already satisfying. The PS-OCT images using the phase retardation brings more comprehensive information. It is well suited to evaluate the biophysical phenomenon of birefringence.

3.2.1 PS-OCT image birefringence in enamel

We prepared several excised human teeth that had no visible evidence of caries to study the dental structure. And several tooth samples with caries that can be visually identified in occlusal and interproximal regions were imaged to characterize carious lesion properties. The structural features of enamel were evaluated from the interproximal, facial, and occlusal aspects of the intact human teeth with and without visible caries evidence. For the assessment of dentin structural features, some teeth were also sectioned in a mesial to distal orientation and in a coronal orientation to image the underneath dentin tissue.

Figure 6 shows images from the interproximal (A) and occlusal aspects (B) of two toth sample. The global befringent properties of enamel arises from the regular orientation of the enamel rods. Enamel rods originate at the DEJ in a perpendicular orientation, after a short distance they turn in a plane horizontal to their long axis, first in one direction and then the other until they assume a straight aligment perpendicular to the surface. In longitudinal microscopic ground sections viewed with reflected light, this arrangement of the enamel rods gives rise to a light and dark pattern termed Hunter-Schreger bands. Our results indicate that Hunter-Schreger bands can be seen in PS-OCT of Figure 6A. This morphoplogy is consistent with that previosusly described in light microscopic images. It is interesting to note that the curvature of the horizontal black-and-white alternating band (the form birefrigent bands) aligns normally with the structure of the enamel rods, which implies a relationship of the form birefringence with the ordered spatial structures. The diameter of a single enamel rod is smallest at the DEJ and increases towards the surface. The average diameter of a single rod is about 4 μm while the PS-OCT limit is 5 μm /pixel. High resolution OCT should provide further definition to the study human enamel rod microstructure. Incremental growth lines of enamel (lines of Retzius) have been described in light microscoptic images of teeth. When viewed in coronal sections, the lines of Retizius are seen as parallel concentric circles similar to the growth rings on a tree, in longitudinal sections they appear obliqiue to the surface. The lines of Retizius are typically less prominent at the cervical aspect of the crowns. In PS-OCT images from the coronal aspect of enamel, we have observed alternate black-and-white bands that are consistent with the line of Retizius in most of the teeth imaged in this study. The form birefringence from the coronal aspect is generally stronger than that from the cervical aspect.

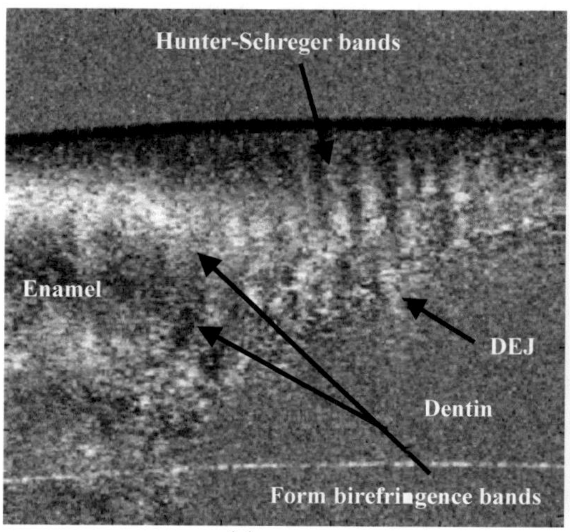

(a)

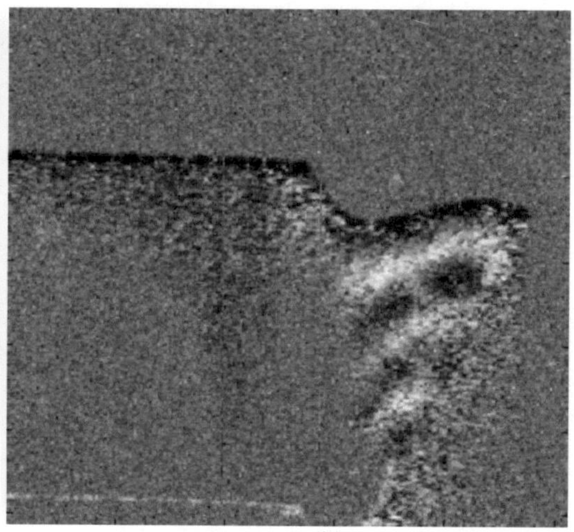

(b)

Fig. 6. The phase retardation image from the interproximal aspect. The horizontal black-and-white band structure is originated from the form birefringence. The image size is 2.6mm x 3.6mm (W x H).

Both dentin and enamel show local polarization-sensitive textures. These textural patterns are formed by PS particles about 20~100 micron in diameters. We put an emphasis on this feature because the textures reveal non-invasively rich information underneath the tooth surface. Systematic analysis of these textures such as particle size, polarization strength, orientation and distribution of the patterns etc. may correlate to the mineralization status of the teeth. As dental caries results from a gradual demineralization of enamel and underlying dentin, the mineralization level is an important indicator for the extent of the carious lesions.

Figure 7 shows images with occlusal and interproximal carious lesions. The carious site can be identified as phase retardation texture patern, which exhibit the strong local polarization sensitive scattering. This type of pattern was seen frequently around carious region. The carious lesions show richer texture information and higher contrast than non-caries site. The pattern is characterized by randomly distributed spots in black and white, which exhibit the strong local polarization sensitive scattering. Occlusal carious lesion is showed in the top figure of Fig. 7, and the caries area is emphasised in the rectangular area with a white arrow points toward the carious site. The site can be visually identified as a brown spot from the surface. The areas indicated by black arrows 1 and 2 show similar caries patterns but no caries can be visually identified at the corresponding surfaces. These areas may indicate the boundary of early caries progression that can not be directly identified by eyes yet. The white bands in area 3 and 4 indicate that the energy is preserved in V channel through a deep depth. These areas have textures made of spots with similar size as in caries site but the state of polarization tends to be maintained, i.e. white always appears white and black always appears black. This type of pattern was seen frequently around carious region. Similar features are found also when the images is taken from the interproximal aspect as see from the bottom image of Fig. 7.

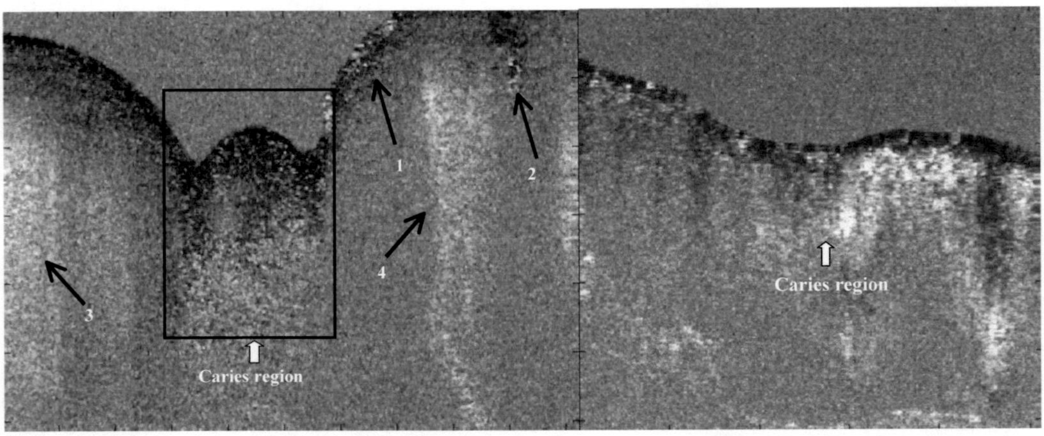

Fig. 7. The local polarization sensitive patterns in the phase retardation images of the tooth samples may closely relate to the mineral composition, which is an indicator of the carious affections. The upper image shows the occlusal carious lesion and the lower one images the lesion from the interproximal aspect as marked by white arrows.

Besides the imaging from the outer surface of the extracted tooth samples, we also imaged the interior aspect of sectioned teeth. In Fig. 8, we show two long PS-OCT scans about 1 cm in lateral length. The imaging depth is also 3.6 mm. The separation of dentin and enamel and there different polarization sensitive scattering properties are well delineated. In the bottom figure, the circled dark area may be associated with demineralization.

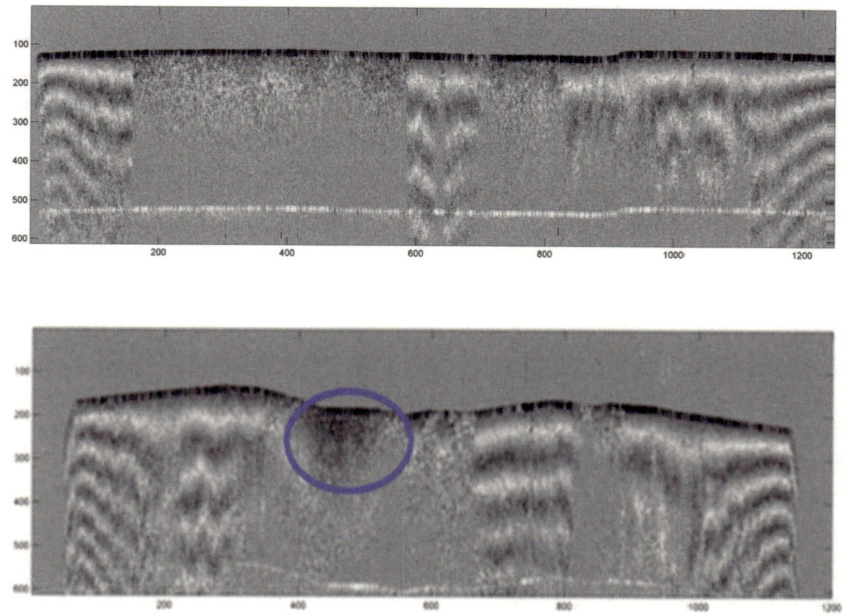

Fig. 8. Phase retardation image from the interior of sectioned tooth samples. The image size is about 10 mm x 3.6mm. The circled area from the bottom image reveals a dark spot, which may be associated with strong demineralization.

In summary, this section discussed the use of PS-OCT imaging to characterize dentin and enamel, and to study the special properties related to the structural orientation of enamel rods. We have performed imaging experiment for more than one hundred tooth samples of different age groups, healthy and carious, from human and animal. The results show that teeth are strong polarization-sensitive tissues. As a general comparison with the conventional intensity OCT, the PS-OCT images provide a unique contrast and could relate to functional information such as demineralization. The polarization detection capability should be regularly applied for OCT system to fully characterize the scattering information of dental tissues.

3.2.2 Polarization memory effect in dentin

Polarization memory describes a phenomenon whereby light retains its incident polarization state after it is back-scattered from a turbid medium [60]. When polarization memory effect (PME) is discussed, it is more convenient to define the two polarization channels by cross-polarization (x-pol) and co-polarization (co-pol) rather than physically the vertical and horizontal channels. In 3.2.1 section, the vertical channel is the x-pol channel, because this channel conventionally won't receive a big amount of photon signal unless there exists a significant polarization sensitive scattering mechanism in the tissue sample.

W will skip some lengthy maths and theory about PME for which readers can find from the authors' recent work [41, 42]. A simpler picture is PME happens when the back scattering circularly polarized light **remembers** the original helicity. As a result a significant amount of light power will be detected from the conventionally very weak x-pol channels. Because of the polarization memory, the light field energy is transferred from the co-pol channel to the x-pol channel and sometimes it results in signal strength reversal between the two channels. In this context, a cross-polarization discrimination (XPD) ratio is conveniently defined to tell us how much photon energy has leaked to the x-pol. Channel due the polarization effect of the tissue.

$$XPD(z) = 20 \log (E_{x\text{-pol}}(z) / E_{co\text{-pol}}(z)) \quad (7)$$

XPD and phase retardation angle have clear physics meanings for PME and birefringence, respectively. From the imaging prospective, the two terms give different mapping functions in PS-OCT. The XPD is defined to map the PS-OCT images in this section. Visually, it does not appear very different. The PS-OCT images in Fig. 9 for example looks much alike what we see in Fig. 8. XPD is however bears a clearer meaning in order characterizing and quantifying PME. PME is a relatively weak polarization effect and was found in dentin rather than in enamel. We will however, try to correlate the result with subtle demineralization process that is the sign of tooth decay.

To design this study, demineralization drug was used to create artificial cavities. 5 teeth were sectioned in an axial orientation. 37% phosphoric acid gel was placed on the sectioned dentin surface for 60 seconds and then washed away. This "acid conditioning of a dentin surface" produced micromorphological effects on the dentin surface, removing the organic material within the surface dentinal tubule orifices, as previously shown [29]. In other words after the gel was placed on the tooth, the surface dentin composed of tubules of mineral hydroxylapatite could lose a significant amount of organic material. Subsequently, OCT scans were taken across the enamel and the mantel dentin. The lesion region had a slight brownish hue which was helpful in steering the OCT beam through the target.

PME is seen in the averaged XPD lines of tooth samples for example in Fig. 9 A. The red line averages the drug affected region and the blue line averages the normal region. Before averaging, the XPD line was realigned along the dentin-air surface with an edge detection algorithm. According to the definition of XPD ratio in Eq. 7, when the blue line is larger than 0, it indicates a stronger x-pol channel singal strength than the co-pol channel, which usually is the dominating channel in signal strength. Therefore our result suggests that the normal dentin area, i.e. without demineralization drug treatment shows polarization memory. The result is a quick increase in x-pol channel signal strength as light travels inside the dentin as shown with the blue curves. The signal strength of x-pol channel exceeds the signal strength of co-pol channel as much as 80%. This is rarely happening unless a significant polarization effect is taken place. For the drug processed artificial cavity region, however, this significant memory effect disappears. The red curve appears to be gradually approach zero line when going into noise floor at deeper depth. Same effect is also seen in Fig. 9B. Only one sees the red curve rises above the zero line too, but at a deeper depth. This should be due to the limited progressing depth of the demineralization drug. The two black arrows point zero crossing points of the blue and the red curve at two different depth. It is interesting to see that after the second depth, the red XPD line seems to regain its polarization memory. The

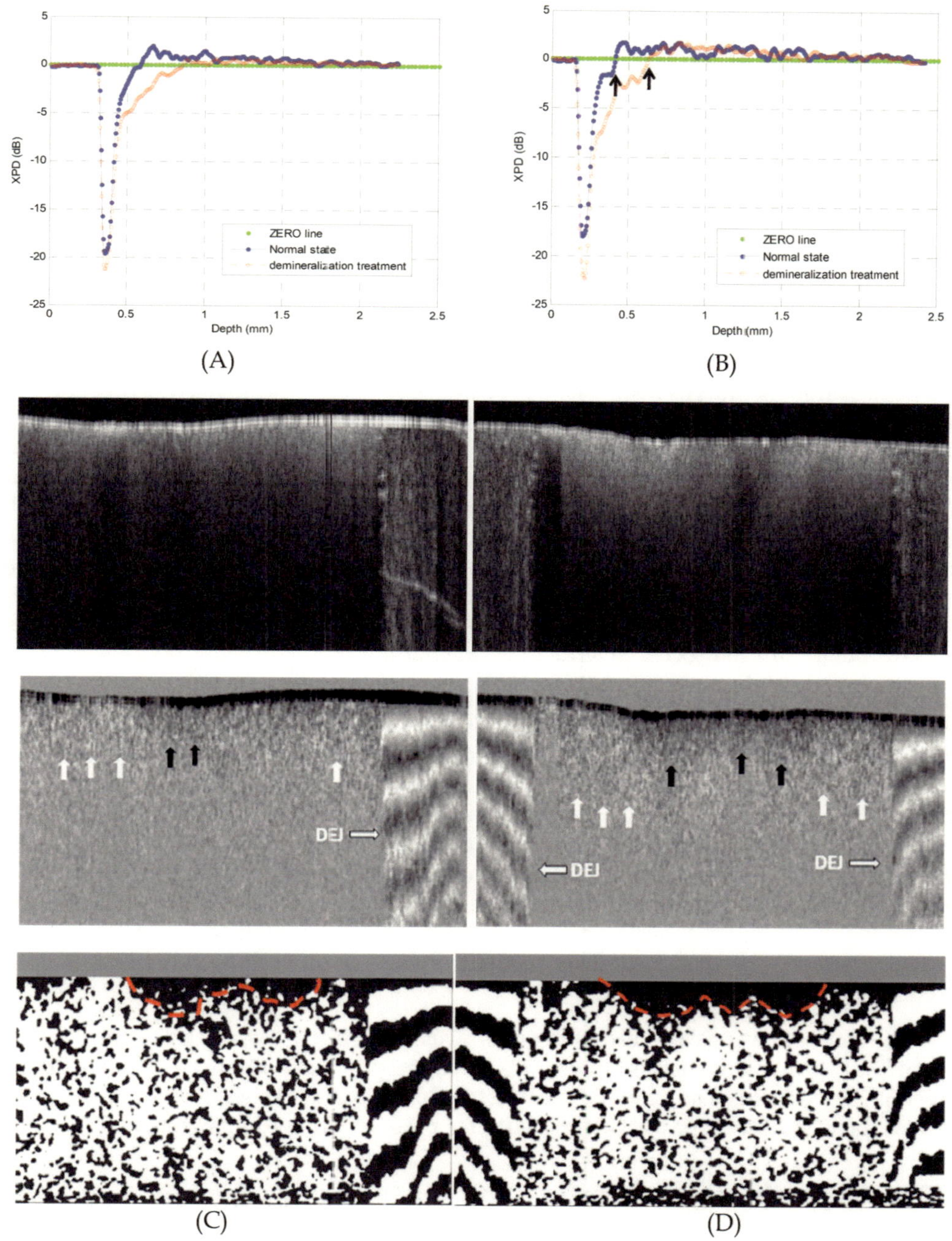

Fig. 9. Two tooth samples imaged after demineralization process. The image size is about 3.2x 8mm in air. (A) and (B) are the averaged XPD curves from treated (red) and intact (blue) area. (C) and (D) show the OCT intensity images (top), the PS-OCT images mapped by XPD lines(middle), and the binary images (bottom) with a better visualization of the progression of the demineralization treatment.

distance between the two arrows roughly indicates the progression of the demineralization treatment. Fig.9 C and D show the two corresponding OCT scans across both the dentin and the adjacent enamel. The regular intensity OCT images are shown at the top. The PS-OCT images mapped by XPD lines in the middle show the different imaging features of dentin and enamel due to the two different polarization behaviours: the alternate bright and dark bands on the right side of Fig. 9C and on both sides of Fig. 9D are typical features of birefringence in the enamel, while the dim single white band in the middle is a feature from PME in the dentin. DEJ, the junction between dentin and enamel identified as a vertical border clearly splits the two types of tissues which are much less separable in the intensity mapped OCT images. Birefringence is a well acknowledged effect in PS-OCT. PME is still new and will be examined more by future studies. Both effects could lead to useful medical applications. The middle parts of the PS-OCT images near the surface corresponded to where the phosphoric acid process was applied. These areas appear darker which imply that some polarization memory is lost. PME can be better estimated through averaging and other filtering processing with a penalty in spatial resolution. Furthermore, PME quantified by XPD ratio has a characteristic zero line which can serve as a sensitive benchmark for spatial demarcation of dematerialized and normal dentin tissue. The bottom images of Fig. 9 C and D are the processed binary images using zero XPD level as the threshold to enhance the contrast. It can be seen that the energy in cross-polarization channel exceeds that in co-polarization channel in most part of the dentin images except the dark areas near the middle of the dentin surface. Estimated spatial boundaries of acid progression are drawn in red dashed lines. A 5x5 medium filter and a 3x3 linear statistical de-speckle filter were used before the binary image process to reduce speckle noise.

In summary, we have discussed in this section a new type of polarization effect, PME that may help to diagnose decay in dentin tissues. As a follow-up future research work, it would be interesting to extend the study to the remineralization study to evaluate the efficacy of rehabilitation drugs. As a blind test, two tooth pastes with one plain (expected to do nothing) and the second containing for example, amorphous calcium phosphate that expected to put mineral back into the etched dentin can be used. PS-OCT using PME analysis may prove to be a useful *in vitro* method to evaluate the efficacy of drugs for repairing dental caries in addition to the potential application for the early caries detection. This remineralization and demineralization testing may be applied on extracted teeth repeatedly without the need to destroy them for investigation such as in the case of optical or electron microscopic imaging.

From the technology prospective, this study was performed with a less sensitive time-domain OCT. It would be helpful to use a 3D imaging protocol with more sensitive Fourier-domain OCT technology to study the changes before and after mineralization treatment. In this way, the tissue locations can be registered for more accurate comparison.

4. 3D and high dimensional imaging and multimodality registration

Fourier domain OCT (FD-OCT) with high speed and sensitivity makes it feasible for real-time 3D imaging. Towards the future development and application of OCT technology, 3D dental imaging enables registration of OCT to itself at different time points and therefore becomes 4D imaging modality. Moreover, once the 3D imaging structure is scanned, the OCT scans can be registering or fusing to other dental image modalities, for example, 3D micro CT scans.

Figure 10 shows the 3D imaging results of a molar tooth from the occlusal surface. The topology of tooth surface is clearly seen. The pit area is where a majority of caries affection occurs which is also hard to be detected by dental X-ray. The scan has a depth resolution about 10 μm in tissue assuming optical index of 1.38. The imaging volume consists of 60 frames (B-scans) each with 150 axial scan lines (A-line). With our scanner, image is acquired at a frame rate of 60 fps. Therefore the total time to acquire this 3D dataset is only one second. The lateral scanning area is about 10 mm x 10 mm basically covering the full surface area along the occlusal orientation. We also selected 3 typical B-scans to the left side of Fig.10. The imaging depth in air is about 3 mm. These B-scans reveals micron scale fine resolution of tooth structures, where the contrast is from optical scattering of small particles and interfaces.

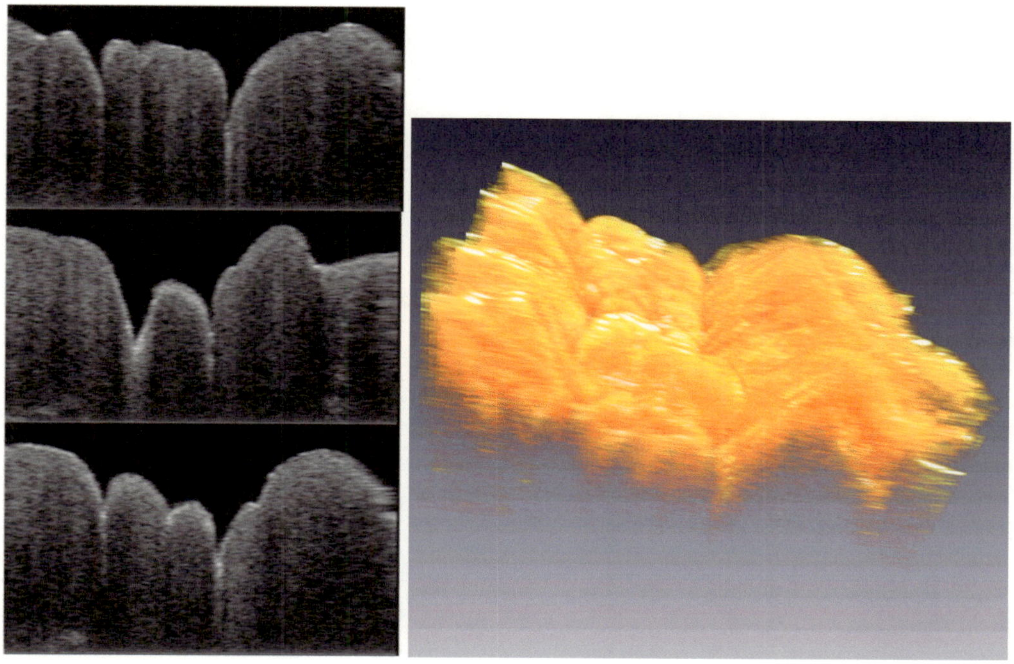

Fig. 10. Three dimentional volumetric imaging and three typical B-scan frames of a molar tooth ex vivo using FD-OCT.

3D imaging brings flexibility to view data from multiple angles such as regular tomographic B-scan frame, slow frame, and *en face* imaging similar to microscopy. 3D OCT can also generate projection image along multiple axes too. This is demonstrated in the bottom right images in Fig. 11, where a 3D rendering of acquired OCT data is overlaid with projections from fast axis and slow axis. We would also have maximal freedom to view projections along any arbitrary projectile directions. In the top left image of fig. 11, we intend to bring some comparisons between 3D OCT and X-ray, although this is not a strict sense apple-to-apple comparison, we could directly appreciate the enhanced resolution and contrast from OCT projections on top-left compared to the X-ray projection on right.3D imaging helps image registration of frame locations through correlations of the topological features to other detection such as photo picture or X-ray images. The red rectangles enclosed the OCT projectile imaging and X-ray projections are roughly matched in spatial location. Typically, dental expert will enhance the contrast of the X-ray image and look for a delicate trace of darker shade as an indication of tooth decay. This is a difficult metric that requires well trained eyes. The exact location of decay is uncertain. Many cavity lesions are left unnoticed. The OCT projection appeared to have better resolution and contrast. But future study may find that it may not be the OCT way to identify cavities. Likely scattering patterns in PS-OCT and intensity or slope changes in intensity OCT could prevail to be the better biomarkers to demark the lesion regions.

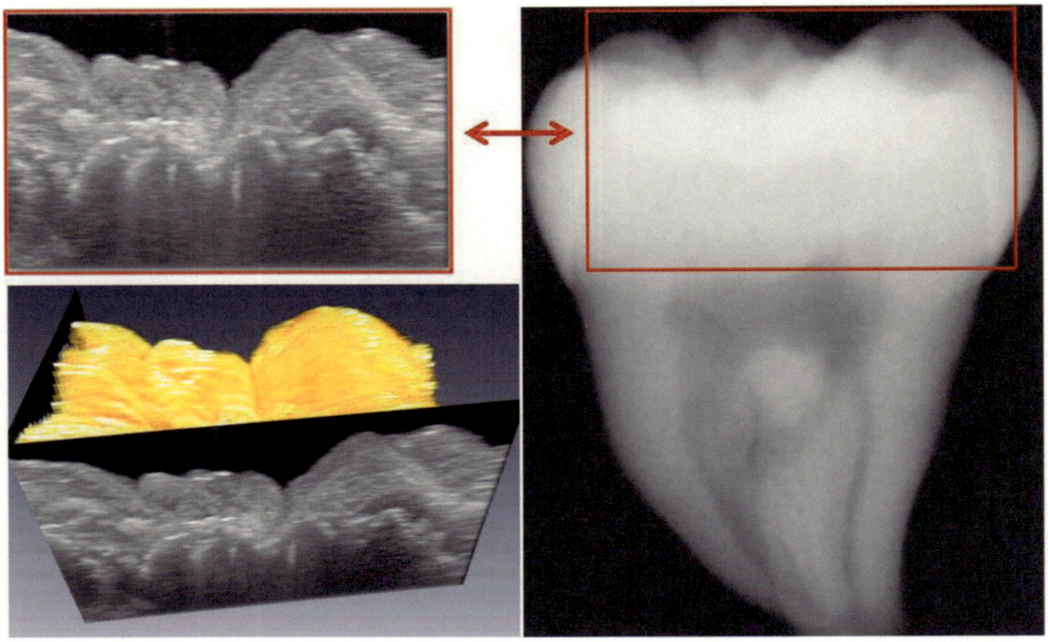

Fig. 11. Top left: OCT projection image roughly matched to the X-ray scan to the right. Bottom left: with 3D OCT, multiple projections can be assessed with a single dataset.

Figure 12 shows a another 3D scan from interproximal prospective. Beside a smoother tooth surface compared to occlusal orientation, it is notable we can clearly visualize boundary features of the dentin-enamel junction. 3D OCT enables a direct visual investigation of the two primary calcified components of tooth and their 2D boundary structure *in vivo*. In the top-left figure, we interleaved the DEJ topology from the tooth matrix. It appears to have a couple of holes which is also identified as discontinuities in the corresponding B-scans in the bottom pictures. We note that X-ray is much capable in finding interproximal tooth decay and it is actually more difficult for OCT to scan the tissue area in between the teeth. In this sense, conventional X-ray and new dental OCT imaging may benefit and complimentary from each other.

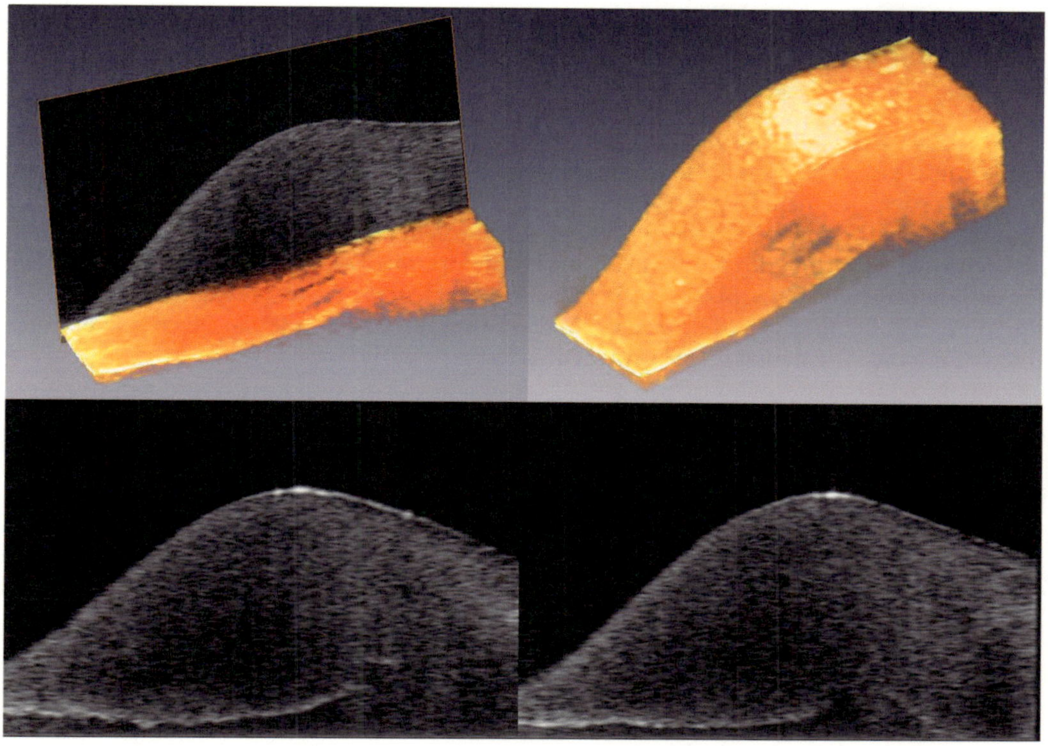

Fig. 12. A three dimensional OCT scan from the interproximal proscpective. It goes with the same scanning protocol as in Fig. 10. The top-left image removes some tissue to reveal the 2D DEJ topology. The top-right imagerenders the tooth surfaces. The bottom images are two sample frames of the OCT B-scans. 3D-OCT sometimes is called C-scan. A-scan, B-scan, and C-scan are borrowed from the existing ultrasound imaging terms.

5. Summary

The results of this study indicate that OCT and PS-OCT has the promising sensitivity to the physiologic and pathogenic changes of dentin and enamel unavailable by current diagnostic or imaging methods. It has the potential to be used for both dental research and clinic applications. As a relatively inexpensive and non-invasive system with high depth resolution, PS-OCT also has the capability of 3D imaging for caries detection. Additional studies that correlate the changes in PS-OCT ultrastructural features that occur in demineralization should provide important information regarding the usefulness of this technology for the clinical diagnoses of dental caries. Since the different texture patterns are most likely related to the mineral components within the tooth, it is interesting and promising to design dynamic processes with demineralization, remineralization and acid control to track the relation between mineralization level and PS-OCT features. The change of the texture patterns before and after treatment can be potentially monitored and compared. Dynamic experiments may prove to be a sensitive way to quantitatively assess the microstructural components in the tooth. It is a prior knowledge of these features and their relations with mineralization level that will provide verification of the diagnostic power of PS-OCT for caries and pre-carious lesions. Ultimately, clinical trials must be completed to study the sensitivity, specificity and the accuracy of OCT for dental caries diagnosis.

In the future, we expect that 3D-OCT with the polarization sensitivity will have the potential to become a powerful diagnostic tool in dental clinic. It is partially because OCT has several imaging properties including resolution, contrast, and image orientation that happens to be complimentary to some limitations of X-ray. Future clinic may see multiple-modality and co-registered imaging with X-ray, OCT, and other approaches such as fluorescent imaging for early lesion detections. 3D-OCT may also serve as a non-invasive research tools to study dynamic demineralization and remineralization process. The result can be compared with micro CT, an *in vitro* dental image standard.

6. Reference

[1] A. F. Fercher, W. Drexler, C. K. Hitzenberger and T. Lasser, "Optical coherence tomography-principles and applications," Reports on Progress in Physics 66(2), 239-303 (2003)

[2] M. Wojtkowski, R. Leitgeb, A. Kowalczyk and A. F. Fercher, "Fourier domain OCT imaging of the human eye in vivo," Proc. SPIE 4619(230-236 (2002)

[3] M. A. Choma, M. V. Sarunic, C. H. Yang and J. A. Izatt, "Sensitivity advantage of swept source and Fourier domain optical coherence tomography," Optics Express 11(18), 2183-2189 (2003)

[4] G. J. Tearney, B. E. Bouma and J. G. Fujimoto, "High-speed phase- and group-delay scanning with a grating-based phase control delay line," Optics Letters 22(23), 1811-1813 (1997)

[5] R. A. Leitgeb, L. Schmetterer, C. K. Hitzenberger, A. F. Fercher, F. Berisha, M. Wojtkowski and T. Bajraszewski, "Real-time measurement of in vitro flow by Fourier-domain color Doppler optical coherence tomography," Opt Lett 29(2), 171-173 (2004)

[6] R. Huber, K. Taira, M. Wojtkowski and J. G. Fujimoto, "Fourier Domain Mode Locked Lasers for OCT imaging at up to 290kHz sweep rates," in Optical Coherence Tomography and Coherence Techniques II W. Drexler, Ed., pp. 245-250, SPIE and OSA, Munich (2005).

[7] V. J. Srinivasan, M. Wojtkowski, A. J. Witkin, J. S. Duker, T. H. Ko, M. Carvalho, J. S. Schuman, A. Kowalczyk and J. G. Fujimoto, "High-definition and 3-dimensional imaging of macular pathologies with high-speed ultrahigh-resolution optical coherence tomography," Ophthalmology 113(11), 2054-2065 (2006)

[8] Y. Yasuno, T. Endo, S. Makita, G. Aoki, M. Itoh and T. Yatagai, "Three-dimensional line-field Fourier domain optical coherence tomography for in vivo dermatological investigation," Journal of biomedical optics 11(1), 7 (2006)

[9] Y. Park, T. J. Ahn, J. C. Kieffer and J. Azana, "Optical frequency domain reflectometry based on real-time Fourier transformation," Optics Express 15(8), 4597-4616 (2007)

[10] C. A. Puliafito, M. R. Hee, C. P. Lin, E. Reichel, J. S. Schuman, J. S. Duker, J. A. Izatt, E. A. Swanson and J. G. Fujimoto, "Imaging of macular diseases with optical coherence tomography," Ophthalmology 102(2), 217-229 (1995)

[11] W. Drexler, U. Morgner, R. K. Ghanta, F. X. Kartner, J. S. Schuman and J. G. Fujimoto, "Ultrahigh-resolution ophthalmic optical coherence tomography. [erratum appears in Nat Med 2001 May;7(5):636.]," Nature Medicine 7(4), 502-507 (2001)

[12] S. G. Schuman, E. Hertzmark, J. G. Fujimoto and J. S. Schuman, "Wavelength independence and interdevice variability of optical coherence tomography," Ophthal Surg Las Im 35(4), 316-320 (2004)

[13] V. J. Srinivasan, B. K. Monson, M. Wojtkowski, R. A. Bilonick, I. Gorczynska, R. Chen, J. S. Duker, J. S. Schuman and J. G. Fujimoto, "Characterization of outer retinal morphology with high-speed, ultrahigh-resolution optical coherence tomography," Investigative ophthalmology & visual science 49(4), 1571-1579 (2008)

[14] M. Pircher, B. Baumann, E. Gotzinger and C. K. Hitzenberger, "Retinal cone mosaic imaged with transverse scanning optical coherence tomography," Optics Letters 31(12), 1821-1823 (2006)

[15] E. Gotzinger, M. Pircher, W. Geitzenauer, C. Ahlers, B. Baumann, S. Michels, U. Schmidt-Erfurth and C. K. Hitzenberger, "Retinal pigment epithelium segmentation by polarization sensitive optical coherence tomography," Opt Express 16(21), 16410-16422 (2008)

[16] Y. Chen, D. M. de Bruin, C. Kerbage and J. F. de Boer, "Spectrally balanced detection for optical frequency domain imaging," Optics Express 15(25), 16390-16399 (2007)

[17] J. Ho, A. J. Witkin, J. Liu, Y. Chen, J. G. Fujimoto, J. S. Schuman and J. S. Duker, "Documentation of intraretinal retinal pigment epithelium migration via high-speed ultrahigh-resolution optical coherence tomography," Ophthalmology 118(4), 687-693

[18] Y. Chen, L. N. Vuong, J. Liu, J. Ho, V. J. Srinivasan, I. Gorczynska, A. J. Witkin, J. S. Duker, J. Schuman and J. G. Fujimoto, "Three-dimensional ultrahigh resolution optical coherence tomography imaging of age-related macular degeneration," Opt Express 17(5), 4046-4060 (2009)

[19] V. J. Srinivasan, Y. Chen, J. S. Duker and J. G. Fujimoto, "In vivo functional imaging of intrinsic scattering changes in the human retina with high-speed ultrahigh resolution OCT," Opt Express 17(5), 3861-3877 (2009)

[20] S. Chia, O. C. Raffel, M. Takano, G. J. Tearney, B. E. Bouma and I. K. Jang, "In-vivo comparison of coronary plaque characteristics using optical coherence tomography in women vs. men with acute coronary syndrome," Coronary Artery Disease 18(6), 423-427 (2007)

[21] M. Kawasaki, B. E. Bouma, J. Bressner, S. L. Houser, S. K. Nadkarni, B. D. MacNeill, I. K. Jang, H. Fujiwara and G. J. Tearney, "Diagnostic accuracy of optical coherence tomography and integrated backscatter intravascular ultrasound images for tissue characterization of human coronary plaques," Journal of the American College of Cardiology 48(1), 81-88 (2006)

[22] B. E. Bouma, G. J. Tearney, H. Yabushita, M. Shishkov, C. R. Kauffman, D. D. Gauthier, B. D. MacNeill, S. L. Houser, H. T. Aretz, E. F. Halpern and I. K. Jang, "Evaluation of intracoronary stenting by intravascular optical coherence tomography," Heart 89(3), 317-320 (2003)

[23] T. Kubo, T. Imanishi, S. Takarada, A. Kuroi, S. Ueno, T. Yamano, T. Tanimoto, Y. Matsuo, T. Masho, H. Kitabata, K. Tsuda, Y. Tomobuchi and T. Akasaka, "Assessment of culprit lesion morphology in acute myocardial infarction - Ability

of optical coherence tomography compared with intravascular ultrasound and coronary angioscopy," Journal of the American College of Cardiology 50(10), 933-939 (2007)

[24] T. Sawada, J. Shite, T. Shinke, S. Watanabe, H. Otake, D. Matsumoto, Y. Imuro, D. Ogasawara, O. L. Paredes and M. Yokoyama, "Persistent malapposition after implantation of sirolimus-eluting stent into intramural coronary hematoma - Optical coherence tomography observations," Circulation Journal 70(11), 1515-1519 (2006)

[25] T. Kume, T. Akasaka, T. Kawamoto, N. Watanabe, E. Toyota, Y. Neishi, R. Sukmawan, Y. Sadahira and K. Yoshida, "Assessment of coronary arterial plaque by optical coherence tomography," American Journal of Cardiology 97(8), 1172-1175 (2006)

[26] M. E. Brezinski, "Optical coherence tomography for identifying unstable coronary plaque," International Journal of Cardiology 107(2), 154-165 (2006)

[27] G. J. Tearney, I. K. Jang, D. H. Kang, H. T. Aretz, S. L. Houser, T. J. Brady, K. Schlendorf, M. Shishkov and B. E. Bouma, "Porcine coronary imaging in vivo by optical coherence tomography," Acta cardiologica 55(4), 233-237 (2000)

[28] J. Weissman, T. Hancewicz and P. Kaplan, "Optical coherence tomography of skin for measurement of epidermal thickness by shapelet-based image analysis," Optics Express 12(23), (2004)

[29] M. C. Pierce, J. Strasswimmer, B. H. Park, B. Cense and J. F. de Boer, "Birefringence measurements in human skin using polarization-sensitive optical coherence tomography," Journal of biomedical optics 9(2), 287-291 (2004)

[30] Y. H. Zhao, Z. P. Chen, C. Saxer, S. H. Xiang, J. F. de Boer and J. S. Nelson, "Phase-resolved optical coherence tomography and optical Doppler tomography for imaging blood flow in human skin with fast scanning speed and high velocity sensitivity," Optics Letters 25(2), 114-116 (2000)

[31] J. Welzel, E. Lankenau, R. Birngruber and R. Engelhardt, "Optical coherence tomography of the skin," Current problems in dermatology 26(27-37 (1998)

[32] A. Baumgartner, S. Dichtl, C. K. Hitzenberger, H. Sattmann, B. Robl, A. Moritz, A. F. Fercher and W. Sperr, "Polarization-sensitive optical coherence tomography of dental structures," Caries research 34(1), 59-69 (2000)

[33] B. W. Colston, Jr., M. J. Everett, U. S. Sathyam, L. B. DaSilva and L. L. Otis, "Imaging of the oral cavity using optical coherence tomography," Monographs in oral science 17(32-55 (2000)

[34] L. L. Otis, B. W. Colston, Jr., M. J. Everett and H. Nathel, "Dental optical coherence tomography: a comparison of two in vitro systems," Dento maxillo facial radiology 29(2), 85-89 (2000)

[35] L. L. Otis, M. J. Everett, U. S. Sathyam and B. W. Colston, Jr., "Optical coherence tomography: a new imaging technology for dentistry," The Journal of the American Dental Association 131(4), 511-514 (2000)

[36] D. Fried, J. Xie, S. Shafi, J. D. B. Featherstone, T. M. Breunig and L. Charles, "Imaging caries lesions and lesion progression with polarization sensitive optical coherence tomography," Journal of biomedical optics 7(4), 618-627 (2002)

[37] L. L. Otis, R. I. al-Sadhan, J. Meiers and D. Redford-Badwal, "Identification of occlusal sealants using optical coherence tomography," The Journal of clinical dentistry 14(1), 7-10 (2003)

[38] A. C.-T. Ko, L.-P. Choo-Smith, M. Hewko, L. Leonardi, M. G. Sowa, C. C. S. Dong, P. Williams and B. Cleghorn, "Ex vivo detection and characterization of early dental caries by optical coherence tomography and Raman spectroscopy," Journal of biomedical optics 10(3), 31118-31111 (2005)
[39] R. S. Jones, C. L. Darling, J. D. B. Featherstone and D. Fried, "Remineralization of in vitro dental caries assessed with polarization-sensitive optical coherence tomography," Journal of biomedical optics 11(1), 9 (2006)
[40] R. S. Jones, C. L. Darling, J. D. B. Featherstone and D. Fried, "Imaging artificial caries on the occlusal surfaces with polarization-sensitive optical coherence tomography," Caries Research 40(2), 81-89 (2006)
[41] Y. L. Chen, L. Otis and Q. Zhu, "Polarization Memory Effect in Optical Coherence Tomography and Dental Imaging Application," Journal of biomedical optics 16((2011)
[42] Y. Chen, L. Otis and Q. Zhu, "Polarization memory effect in the polarization-sensitive optical coherence tomography system," Proc. SPIE 6429(6429K), 1-5 (2007)
[43] Y. Chen, L. Otis, D. Piao and Q. Zhu, "Characterization of dentin, enamel, and carious lesions by a polarization-sensitive optical coherence tomography system," Appl Optics 44(11), 2041-2048 (2005)
[44] K. Hosseini, A. I. Kholodnykh, I. Y. Petrova, R. O. Esenaliev, F. Hendrikse and M. Motamedi, "Monitoring of rabbit cornea response to dehydration stress by optical coherence tomography," Investigative ophthalmology & visual science 45(8), 2555-2562 (2004)
[45] A. Popp, M. Wendel, L. Knels, T. Koch and E. Koch, "Imaging of the three-dimensional alveolar structure and the alveolar mechanics of a ventilated and perfused isolated rabbit lung with Fourier domain optical coherence tomography," Journal of biomedical optics 11(1), 9 (2006)
[46] D. Piao, M. M. Sadeghi, J. Zhang, Y. Chen, A. J. Sinusas and Q. Zhu, "Hybrid positron detection and optical coherence tomography system: design, calibration, and experimental validation with rabbit atherosclerotic models," Journal of biomedical optics 10(4), 44010 (2005)
[47] S. A. Boppart, M. E. Brezinski, B. E. Bouma, G. J. Tearney and J. G. Fujimoto, "Investigation of developing embryonic morphology using optical coherence tomography," Developmental biology 177(1), 54-63 (1996)
[48] M. W. Jenkins, D. C. Adler, M. Gargesha, R. Huber, F. Rothenberg, J. Belding, M. Watanabe, D. L. Wilson, J. G. Fujimoto and A. M. Rollins, "Ultrahigh-speed optical coherence tomography imaging and visualization of the embryonic avian heart using a buffered Fourier Domain Mode Locked laser," Optics Express 15(10), 6251-6267 (2007)
[49] W. Luo, D. L. Marks, T. S. Ralston and S. A. Boppart, "Three-dimensional optical coherence tomography of the embryonic murine cardiovascular system," Journal of biomedical optics 11(2), 8 (2006)
[50] J. P. Su, J. Zhang, L. F. Yu and Z. P. Chen, "In vivo three-dimensional microelectromechanical endoscopic swept source optical coherence tomography," Optics Express 15(16), 10390-10396 (2007)

[51] Z. Yaqoob, J. G. Wu, E. J. McDowell, X. Heng and C. H. Yang, "Methods and application areas of endoscopic optical coherence tomography," Journal of biomedical optics 11(6), 19 (2006)

[52] D. Daniltchenko, M. Sachs, E. Lankenau, F. Koenig, G. Huettmann, D. Schnorr, S. Al-Shukri and S. Loening, "Optical coherence tomography of the urinary bladder: The potential of a high-resolution visual investigation technique for endoscopic diagnostics," Optics and Spectroscopy 101(1), 40-45 (2006)

[53] H. Mashimo, S. Desai, M. Pedrosa, M. Wagh, Y. Chen, P. Herz, P. L. Hsiung, A. Aguirre, A. Koski, J. Schmitt and J. G. Fujimoto, "Ultrahigh resolution endoscopic optical coherence tomography: a novel technology for gastrointestinal imaging," Gastroenterology 128(4), A251-A251 (2005)

[54] Y. Chen, P. R. Herz, P.-L. Hsiung, A. D. Aguirre, K. Schneider, J. G. Fujimoto, H. Mashimo, S. Desai, M. Pedrosa, J. M. Schmitt and A. Koski, "Ultrahigh resolution endoscopic optical coherence tomography for gastrointestinal imaging," pp. 4-10, International Society for Optical Engineering, Bellingham, WA 98227-0010, United States, San Jose, CA, United States (2005).

[55] G. J. Tearney, M. E. Brezinski, B. E. Bouma, S. A. Boppart, C. Pitvis, J. F. Southern and J. G. Fujimoto, "In vivo endoscopic optical biopsy with optical coherence tomography," Science 276(5321), 2037-2039 (1997)

[56] D. P. Popescu, M. G. Sowa, M. D. Hewko and L. P. Choo-Smith, "Assessment of early demineralization in teeth using the signal attenuation in optical coherence tomography images," Journal of biomedical optics 13(5), 054053 (2008)

[57] B. H. Park, M. C. Pierce, B. Cense and J. F. de Boer, "Jones matrix analysis for a polarization-sensitive optical coherence tomography system using fiber-optic components," Optics Letters 29(21), 2512-2514 (2004)

[58] J. F. de Boer and T. E. Milner, "Review of polarization sensitive optical coherence tomography and Stokes vector determination," Journal of biomedical optics 7(3), 359-371 (2002)

[59] D. Fried, J. Xie, S. Shafi, J. D. Featherstone, T. M. Breunig and C. Le, "Imaging caries lesions and lesion progression with polarization sensitive optical coherence tomography," Journal of biomedical optics 7(4), 618-627 (2002)

[60] F. C. MacKintosh, J. X. Zhu, D. J. Pine and D. A. Weitz, "Polarization memory of multiply scattered light," Physical review 40(13), 9342-9345 (1989)

13

Using Optical Coherence Tomography to Characterize the Crack Morphology of Ceramic Glaze and Jade

M.-L. Yang, A.M. Winkler, J. Klein, A. Wall and J.K. Barton
Tamkang University, Taipei, Taiwan

1. Introduction

The utilization of optical coherence tomography (OCT) in artworks' examination for the past several years has confirmed its feasibility (Elias et al., 2010; Targowski, 2008). The results not only aid authentication of museum collections, but also provide crucial information for understanding artworks' manufacturing technology and use history, as well as for continuing preservation. To display certain characteristics of ceramic glaze and jade materials, such as components assemblage, bubbles distribution, glaze-layer structure, cracks morphology and alteration phenomenon, OCT is an ideal tool. In previous research, the bubble distribution and components assemblage within Chinese glaze samples has been discussed (Yang et al., 2011, 2009), and the alteration of archaic jade has also been examined (Liang et al., 2008; Yang et al., 2004). In addition, with specific algorithm programs, the researcher is also able to obtain quantitative data, such as the bubble size and number in a glaze or intensities of texture vector in a jade material (Klein et al., 2011; Chang et al., 2010).

In the present chapter, various cracks' morphology in Chinese glaze and jade samples are described and characterized using OCT systems. Cracks are common in brittle materials, such as traditional glass, ceramics, or even tougher semi-gem or rock. In general, they are regarded as defective in artistic or industrial products. However, certain cracks were endowed with an artistic or cultural attribute or significance because of their special morphology and uniquely formed patterns. Moreover, they were surmised to be intentionally created, such as Chinese Song Dynasty (AD 960-1279) Ru and Guan wares. They were made by contemporary imperial potters and possessed a high density and diversity of crack patterns. Therefore, determining morphology and characteristics of cracks in glaze and jade artifacts would not only contribute to scientific ceramics and jade research, but also benefit art history study.

2. OCT systems and samples properties

Cracks in jade or glaze, translucent or somewhat transparent materials, can be viewed by the naked eye or observed on the surface of the artifact under a microscope at low magnification. Then, for accurate examination of their structure, the destructive thin section method, or scanning electron fractography, has been used for the past several decades (Friedman et al., 1972; Coppola & Bradt, 1972). However, the present OCT systems not only provide a non-destructive, rapid technique for presenting crack morphology in a two-dimension or even three-dimension image in cross section, and also yield abundant information about the relationship between cracks and local components.

2.1 Three OCT systems

Three different OCT systems were utilized for this study, in order to meet different research objectives. The systems have varying wavelengths, resolution and sensitivity to features in the glaze and jade samples. The chosen system presents the optimal image resolution of crack and their matrix. The first OCT system was a commercial system equipped with a handheld probe, a Thorlabs Spectral Radar OCT system (THORLABS, 2011). This system uses a central wavelength of 930-nm and a spectrum width of nearly 100-nm as its light source, resulting in an image resolution in axial resolution approximately 6.0-μm and the lateral resolution approximately 9.0-μm. This system presents a clear crack structure in complicated microstructure glaze samples.

The second OCT system was custom built (Winkler et al., 2010). The light source is a superluminescent diode (Superlum Broadlighter, Moscow, Russia) with an 890-nm center wavelength and a 150-nm bandwidth that results in an image resolution better than 3.0-μm axial and 5-μm lateral, in glaze or jade. This system provides the most optimal crack structure images for most jade (nephrite) samples in a depth of over 1-mm.

The third system was also custom built. It is a focus-tracking OCT system. Its light source (Superlum Broadlighter 855) features 100-nm in bandwidth with a center wavelength of 855-nm, that, when coupled with a moderate numerical aperture objective, permits a 4-5.0-μm isotropic imaging resolution. The benefit of this system is that it optimally maintains lateral resolution at all depths within a sample having a refractive index of ~1.4 (Yang et al., 2011). For the present research, to image sealed cracks located in a deeper position from the sample's surface, this system is a powerful tool.

2.2 Glaze material and crack types

Three primary phases (components): homogeneous glass phase, crystallization phase, and liquid-liquid phase separation, with a few un-melted quartz or residuals particles, are usually contained in traditional Chinese glazes in a multi-phase assemblage or single phase dominant states. However, for the feldspar glaze used in Chinese celadon, the crystallization phase is usually formed by anorthite ($CaO \cdot Al_2O_3 \cdot 2SiO_2$) and wollastonite (or pseudowollastonite $CaO \cdot SiO_2$) (Yang et al., 2009; Kingery et al., 1976).

These phases (components) are displayed in nuanced gray scale in the OCT image based on the relative difference of their individual refractive index (n) as the homogeneous glass n = 1.5, then, wollastonite $n_\alpha = 1.616 - 1.640$, $n_\beta = 1.628 - 1.650$, $n_\gamma = 1.631 - 1.653$, anorthite $n_\alpha = 1.577$, $n_\beta = 1.585$, $n_\gamma = 1.590$ and quartz $n_\omega = 1.544$, $n_\varepsilon = 1.553$. At times, a few iron oxides are formed in the glaze, such as hematite (Fe_2O_3, $n_\omega = 3.22$, $n_\varepsilon = 2.94$). In addition, the liquid-liquid phase separation is in a somewhat different refractive index from the homogeneous glass phase (Simmons, 1977). The relevant optical properties and OCT image expression of these components within Chinese glaze was introduced in a previous publication (Yang et al., 2009).

Two classes of cracks occurring in glaze are usually mentioned: one caused by thermal shock when the ceramic product is removed from the kiln; the other caused by moisture on porcelain or pottery bodies during storage or use (Shaw, 1971; Norton, 1952; Schurecht & Fuller, 1931). The latter is also called 'delayed crazing.' Actually, the former is the primary crazing on all glazed ceramics. In the past, some researchers categorized crack morphology into a few types based on surface viewing (Faber et al., 1981; Schurecht & Pole, 1932; Schurecht & Fuller, 1931; Gao, 1591). However, viewing the cross section from the surface to the interior glaze or body seems to simplify all crack morphology types to a single one, a 'T' structure with various inclining angles in 'I', that represent the crack path basically in a vertical direction from the surface of the glaze, and '—' representing the horizontal direction of the surface. In addition, we kept all samples in a horizontal position during scanning.

Crack presentation in an OCT image should theoretically be a bright (white), linear structure, because it is actually a narrow gap (air) or a boundary between two displaced faces. However, the brightness of the crack line partly depends on local components and texture. In addition to the thermal stress within a glaze, the glaze's features, such as components' species, micro-structure, even bubbles' distribution, impurity grains' size, among others, also influence crack morphology (Seaton & Dutta, 1974; Coppola & Bradt, 1972; Hasselman, 1969; Coble & Kingery, 1955). Three different features of celadon glaze samples are examined to describe the variation in crack structure. The glaze samples' descriptions are listed in Table 1.

2.3 Jade material and crack types

Two primary minerals, nephrite and jadeite are used as jade material in China. The former was always highly valued by the ancient Chinese, and used for fashioning ritual and ceremonial objects or even utility tools in the very early stage, the Neolithic period (5000-2000 BCE). In contrast, the latter was used very late, around the middle of the eighteenth century (Palmer, 1967; Whitlock & Ehrmann, 1949). Nephrite possesses considerable toughness and strength because of its compact fibrous crystalline structure, permitting considerable mechanic stress during the fashioning or mining process (Bradt et al., 1973).

According to ancient Chinese texts, cracks in jade materials were usually described by various terms based on visible features, such as *'liu(綹),' 'wen(璺)'* or *'dian(玷)'* (Gao, 1591; Li, 1925), but, respectively, they were not defined clearly. However, based on cross section viewing in OCT images, two basic types of crack in jade materials are the linear structure open to the air, usually with brown corrosion (iron oxidation) along its path, and the cloudy clustering structure sealed off from the surface in a deeper position inside the jade material.

However, because of its compact crystalline structure and a refractive index n=1.606-1.632, a pure nephrite's matrix is displayed in OCT image to be very simple and even light gray scale (Yang et al., 2004). Then, regardless of the linear or clustering structure cracks in jade (nephrite), because most cracks propagate along the boundary of the grains in a jade material, the crack path is revealed somewhat irregularly or zigzag. Four jade (nephrite) samples are examined, as described in Table 1.

sample #	thickness/mm	material	date	form	provenance
glaze-1	~0.7	feldspar glaze	10-13th century	shard	Hangzhou, Zhejiang
glaze-2	~0.7	feldspar glaze	10-13th century	shard	Hangzhou, Zhejiang
glaze-3	~0.5	feldspar glaze	10th century	shard	Chinglianssu, Henan
jade-1	0.2-0.25	nephrite	~2500 BCE	huang-arch	Gansu
jade-2	0.5-0.6	nephrite	~2500 BCE	adze (broken)	Shaanxi
jade-3*	~0.4	nephrite	~2500 BCE	huang-arch	Gansu
jade-4**	-	nephrite	-	natural pebble	Xinjiang

*jade-3 in the author's original samples collection number is jade-12.
**jade-4 in the author's original samples collection number is jade-7.

Table 1. Samples' descriptions.

3. Characterizing crack morphology in glaze

The three crucial characteristics of crack morphology in the glaze, its opening on the surface, structure and terminal tip in the matrix, and its relationship with local components, are discussed below.

3.1 Cracks in a homogeneous glass phase dominant glaze

Figure 1a presents a crack in a homogeneous glass phase dominant glaze, sample glaze-1, with several bubbles (pairing bright dots). The crack morphology is a typical 'T' structure in cross section. A small chip reveals its opening on the surface of the glaze. In the OCT image, with an increased scanning depth, the crack resembles an upside down cone hanging from the surface, explaining the scattering signals' gradual weakening by crack surrounding components. However, along the crack path, two larger impurity grains are revealed. The upper one is surmised to influence the crack's continuing direction, and the lower one to terminate this crack.

Three cracks are presented in Figure 1b. The right crack is large with two chips at its opening. This crack displays a typical 'T' structure with a slight incline to the right. The tip of crack seems to terminate at an impurity grain (lower arrow) just below the tip. The 'T' structure crack is similar to the crack in a modern blown glass fragment (Figure 2). Thus, a reasonable conclusion seems to be that in a homogeneous glass phase dominant glaze, a crack usually propagates in a typical 'T' structure with a slight incline.

In addition, in Figure 1b, on the left, next to the large right crack, two thin crack lines are displayed. One is long, propagating at an inclining angle of around 30 degrees to the left, and terminating in the interface area between the glaze and body. The other is short and probably terminated at the long crack gap. However, the openings of the two thin cracks are not revealed clearly on the surface.

The image in Figure 1c clearly presents two cracks and another vague crack behind the left crack. The right one is almost a typical 'T' structure with a slight incline to the right, terminating at an impurity grain just below its tip. No chip is revealed at its opening on the

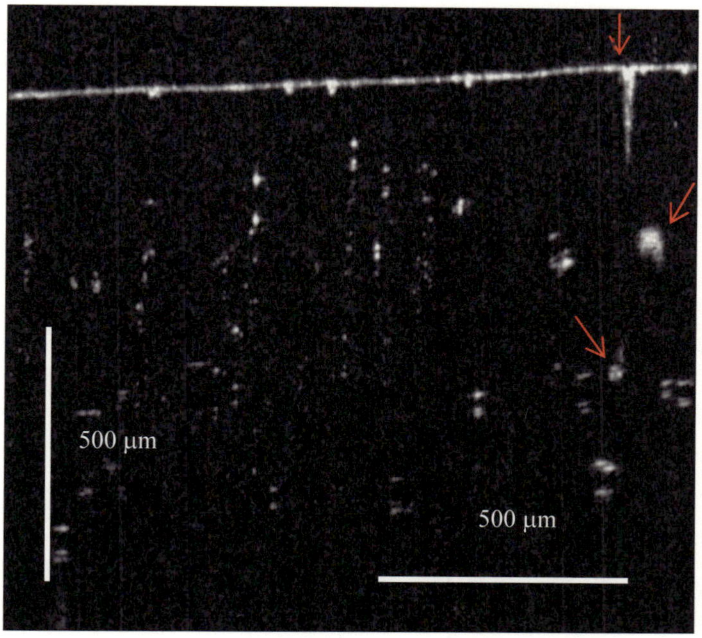

Fig. 1a. A typical 'T' structure crack is presented in the sample glaze-1 (upper arrow). A chip reveals its opening on the surface, and below the tip of crack two impurities grains (middle and lower arrows) probably governed its path. (image acquired by 930-nm system).

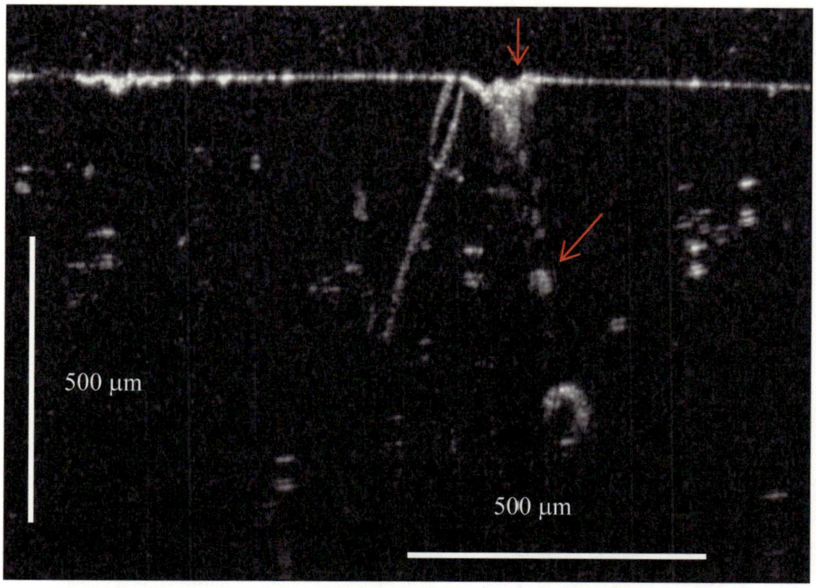

Fig. 1b. The right arrow points to a large 'T' structure crack with a slight incline to the right. Two big chips are at its opening, and the crack is probably terminated at an impurity grain (lower arrow). The left two cracks, one long and the other short are almost parallel and incline to the left at around 30 degrees. (image acquired by 930-nm system).

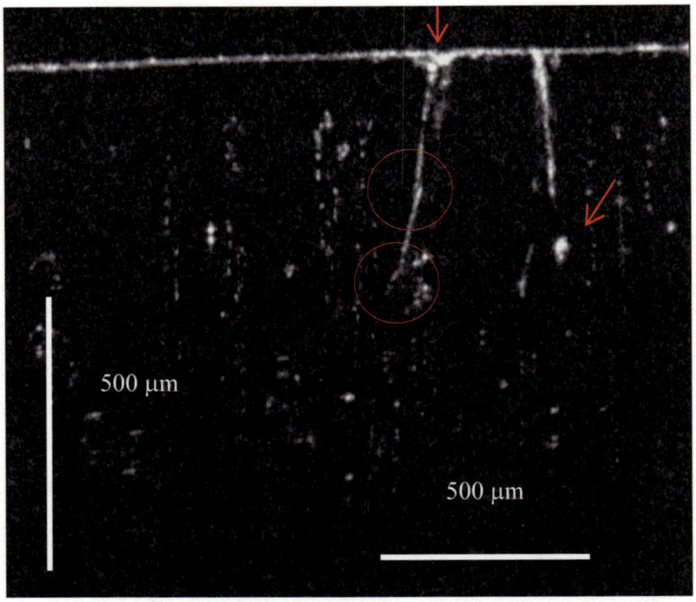

Fig. 1c. The right crack is almost a typical 'T' structure with a slight incline to the right, and terminates at an impurity grain just below its tip (lower arrow). The left crack seems to transfer its path at two positions (circles). In addition, a vague crack is revealed behind the left crack. (image acquired by 930-nm system).

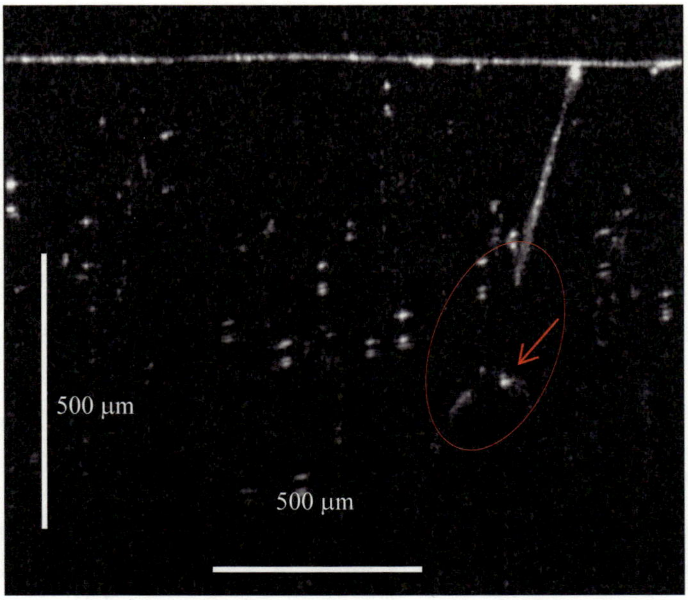

Fig. 1d. A crack inclines to the left at around 30 degrees. This crack probably transferred its path at a position (circle) further to the left as it encountered an impurity grain (arrow). (image acquired by 930-nm system).

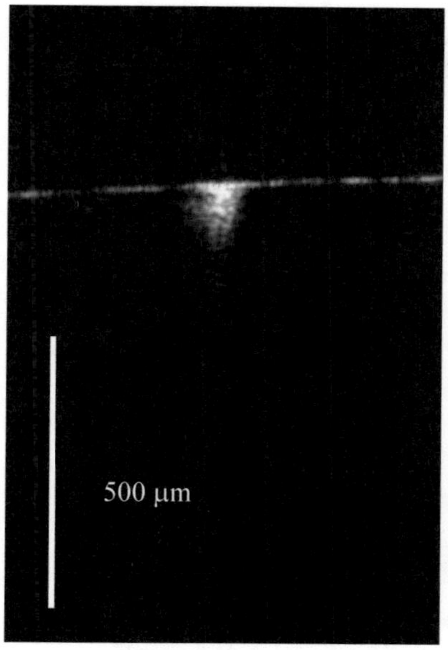

Fig. 2. A typical 'T' structure crack in a homogeneous blown glass fragment. (image acquired by 930-nm system).

surface. In contrast, the left one displays its opening chip and path that inclines somewhat to the left. However, its path transfers at two positions (upper and lower circles), around 0.3-mm and 0.5-mm in depth from the surface.

A crack in Figure 1d is similar to the left crack structure in Figure 1c. This crack probably diverged from the original path more to the left at the interface area between the glaze and body, around 0.7-mm in depth from the surface, as the crack encountered an impurity grain (arrow). Then, it continued to propagate into the body where it diminished. The opening is not open to the air.

3.2 Cracks in a multi-phase inhomogeneous glaze

Figure 3a presents a somewhat complicated phases' assemblage in the sample glaze-2. The black portion and various gray scale portions entangled and assembled into a multi-phase inhomogeneous glaze texture with several bubbles. Two cracks are presented in this image. The right one is large with a broad chip at the opening on the surface, and is characterized as a typical 'T' structure crack. The left crack's path is not clearly revealed at this scanning position, but its chip at the opening is clearly revealed. However, a large impurity grain (lower arrow) surrounding it probably governed this crack's path.

Figure 3b presents three cracks in a somewhat tight space. The central one is a 'T' structure crack with a slight incline to the left. The left one (left arrow) propagated its path into two sides in almost same inclining angle, around 60 degrees. It appears to be apparent that this crack propagated in a shallower position from the surface of the glaze. The right one (right arrow) is not displayed clearly at this scanning position. However, its structure seems similar to the left crack.

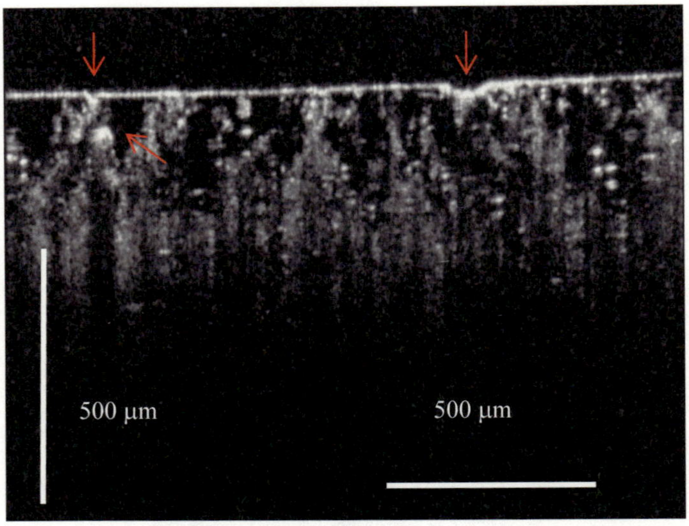

Fig. 3a. The right crack is a typical 'T' structure with big chip at its opening on the surface. The left crack path is not clearly presented at this scanning position, but the chip of its opening (left upper arrow) is clearly revealed. The impurity grain (lower arrow) probably influenced this crack path. (image acquired by 930-nm system)

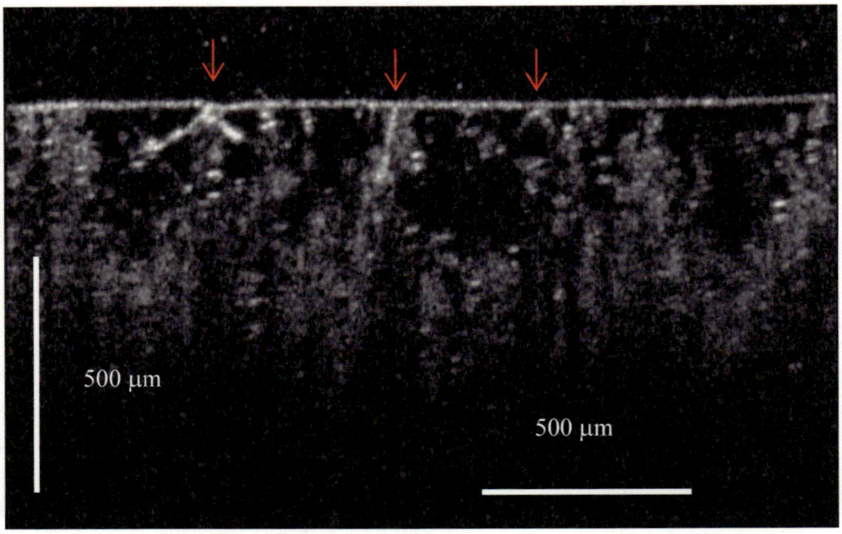

Fig. 3b. The left crack separated into left and right paths. A large inclining angle, around 60 degrees, propagated the crack path in a shallower position from the surface. The central crack is a typical 'T' structure with a slight incline to the left. The right crack is not clearly visualized at this scanning position. (image acquired by 930-nm system)

A crack that propagates in a shallower position from the surface creates a specific visual effect. Figure 4 displays several cracks in a tight space with a nuanced visual effect in the microphotograph of the sample glaze-3. However, the primary distinction among these cracks lies in their inclining angles. It appears to be apparent that the larger the inclining angle, the shallower the crack propagates. It causes a cloudy visual effect in the texture of the crack's range. In contrast, the smaller the inclining angle, the deeper the crack propagates almost vertically penetrating to the interior glaze and usually without changing the original visual effect in the local texture.

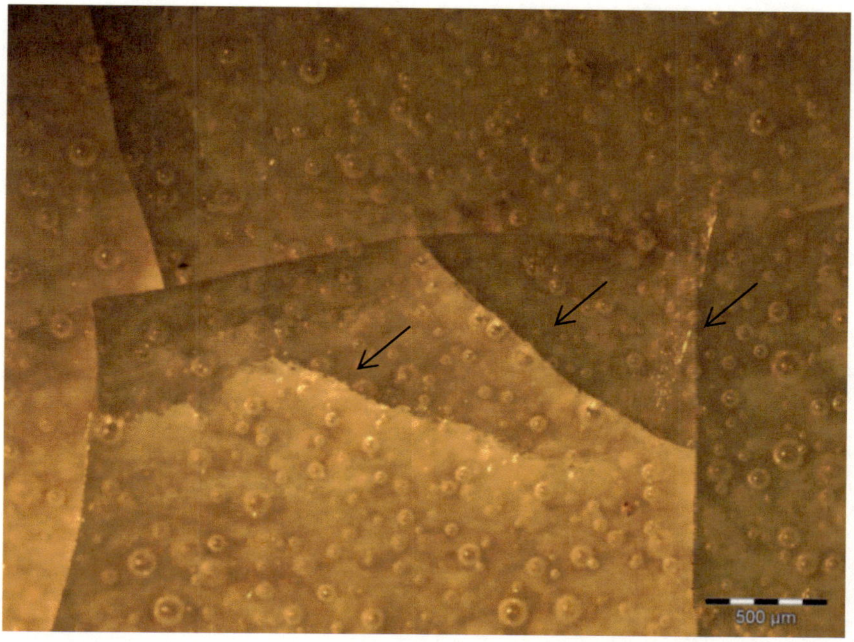

Fig. 4. The microphotograph of the sample glaze-3 presents several cracks in the tight space. Three arrows point to three different visual effect cracks. The lower crack (left arrow) presents cloudy texture, whereas the right crack (right arrow) is close to original translucent glaze quality.

Comparing with the glaze-2, the sample glaze-3 is a more structural multi-phase inhomogeneous glaze with a richer gray portion. According to our previous research on glaze-3, it consists of homogeneous glass phase, crystallization phase (anorthite and pseudowollastonite) and liquid-liquid phase separation (Yang et al., 2009). Two cracks are presented in images in Figure 4a (including Figure 4a-1 and 4a-2). The right crack is characterized as a 'T' structure with an inclining angle around 30 degrees and terminated at a bubble (Figure 4a-2; lower arrow). The chip of its opening is revealed on the surface. However, the left crack seems to somewhat bend its path slightly to the left.

Figure 4b displays a very shallow crack which propagated its path in an almost horizontal direction to the right, and terminated at a bubble. This shallow crack appears in a disconnected path based on the OCT image. It meets the lower crack (Figure 4; left arrow) in the microphotograph that exhibits a considerable cloudy visual effect in this crack range.

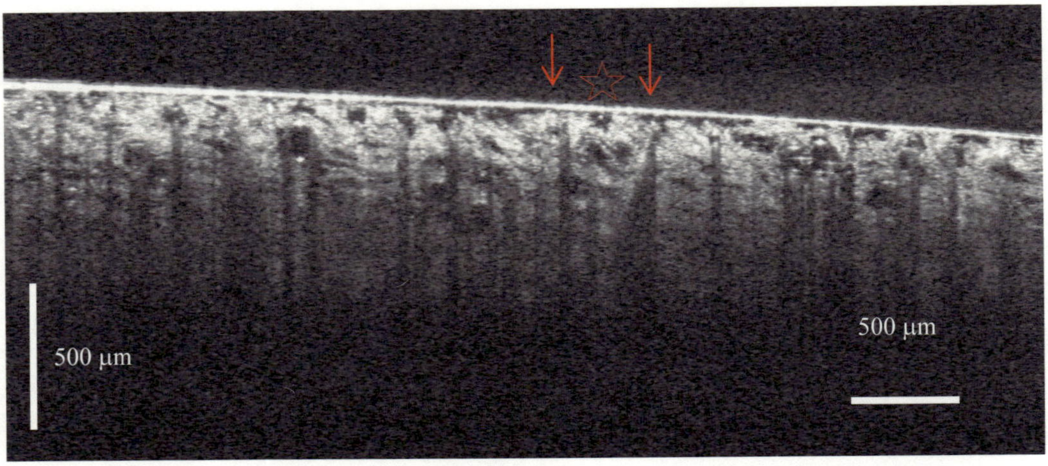

Fig. 4a. A multi-phase inhomogeneous glaze is in tight compact structure, and two cracks are revealed (two arrows; the star is a landmark in the sample glaze-3). (image acquired by 890-nm system).

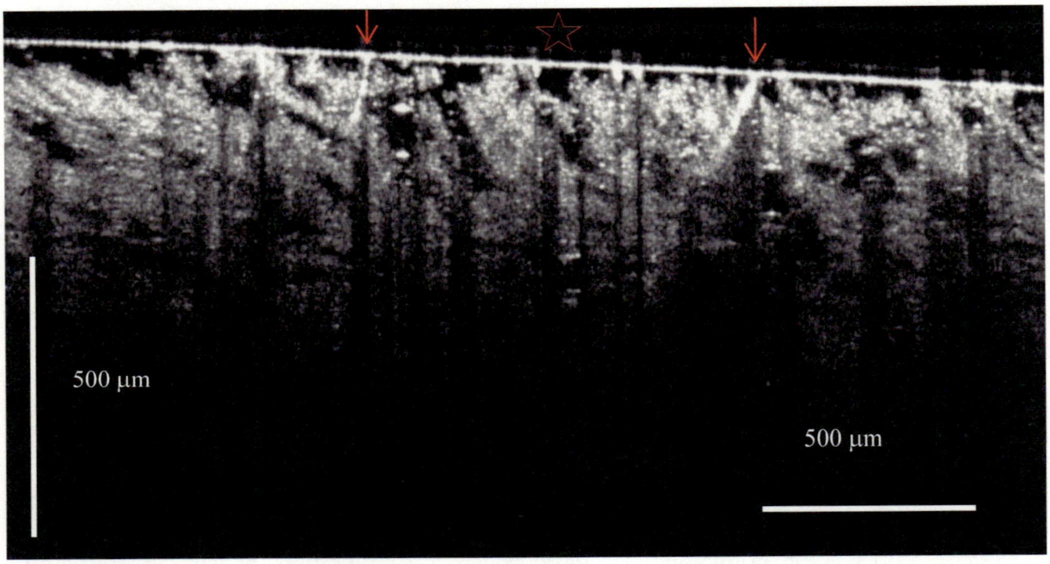

Fig. 4a-1. The right crack is apparently inclining to the left around 45 degrees, whereas the left inclines slight to the left. The former reveals a partially clear chip at its opening. (image acquired by 930-nm system).

3.3 Discussion of the characteristics of crack morphology in glaze

For a homogeneous glass dominant glaze, the characteristics of crack morphology are concluded as: (1) some cracks are not open to the air; (2) crack structure is basically presented in a 'T' structure with a slight incline; (3) most cracks are terminated at larger impurity grain or bubble located just below the tip of the crack; and, (4) some cracks probably diverge from their original path when they encounter grain impurities.

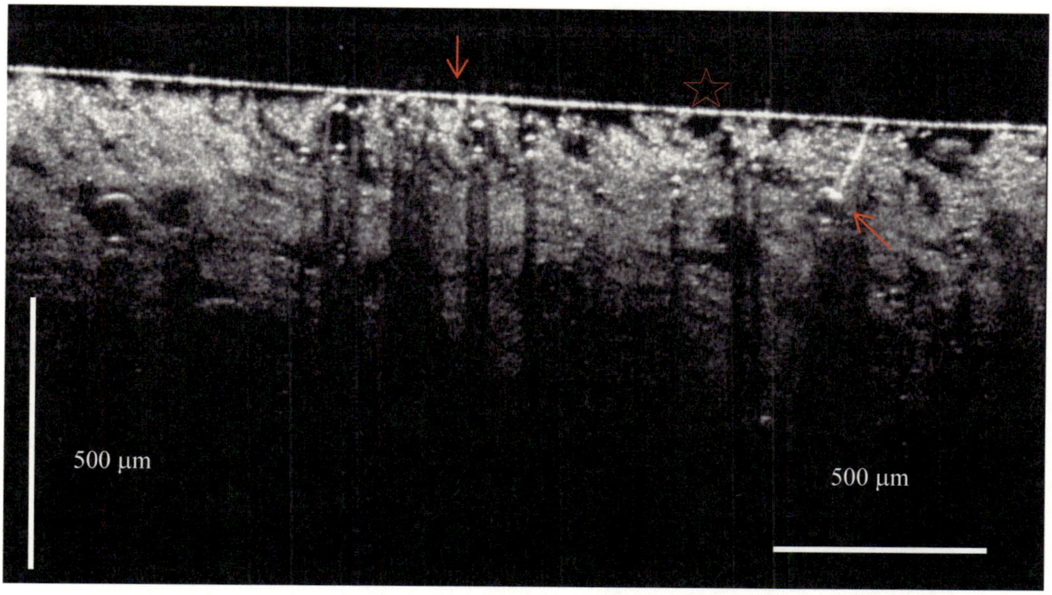

Fig. 4a-2. The right crack is terminated at a bubble. The left crack is not clearly revealed at this scanning position (image acquired by 930-nm system).

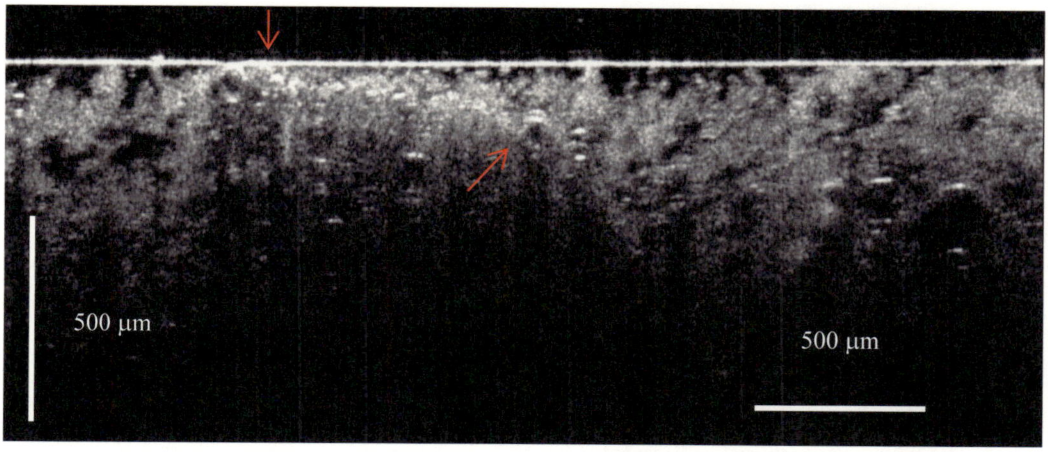

Fig. 4b. A crack appears in very shallow position from the surface that propagated in disconnected and horizontal path, and terminated at a bubble. (image acquired by 930-nm system).

Most of the characteristics of cracks in a multi-phase inhomogeneous glaze are the same as those in the homogeneous glass dominant glaze. However, because the inclining angle variation is richer and more nuanced in the former, it appears to create a higher diversity and higher density of crack patterns. Moreover, it also achieves a subtle visual effect in the texture of the crack range.

4. Characterizing crack morphology in jade

Compared with the considerable diversity of gray scale in the OCT images of a multi-phase inhomogeneous glaze, in addition to lacking bubbles, the jade's OCT images are quite simple and even. As formerly mentioned, the two basic types of crack in jade are clustering and linear structure.

4.1 Clustering structure crack in jade

Figure 5 is a microphotograph of the sample jade-1, presenting several clustering cracks in the cloudy clusters, most of them sealed below the surface in various depths, whereas a few micro-cracks are open to the air in a few bright sparks within the circle. Figure 5a presents two clustering structure cracks in the image. The left one reveals that it consisted of many micro-cracks and propagated into a considerable volume. The right one is not clearly presenting its clustering structure at this scanning position, but it reveals a few chips on the surface, and damage to the texture of the local matrix.

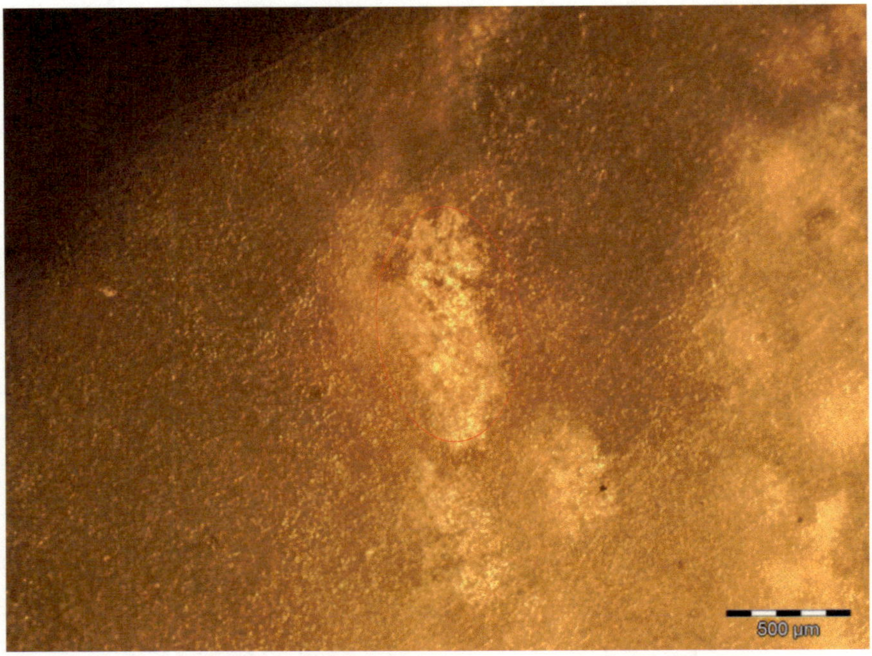

Fig. 5. The microphotograph of the sample jade-1 presents several cloudy clustering cracks sealed below the glaze surface. A few micro-cracks are open to the air (in bright sparks within the circle) in this cluster.

In fact, in terms of the OCT image, it appears to be apparent that the clustering crack is structured in an orderly fashion by an initial fractured (damaged) core and several gradually propagated micro-cracks from the core along the grain boundaries to form a considerable volume of crack body. Some branching cracks in skirts of the crack body are continuing to grow, and they sometimes joined with other branching cracks of the other crack body. Such structured clustering crack can be viewed in Figure 5a, Figure 6, and

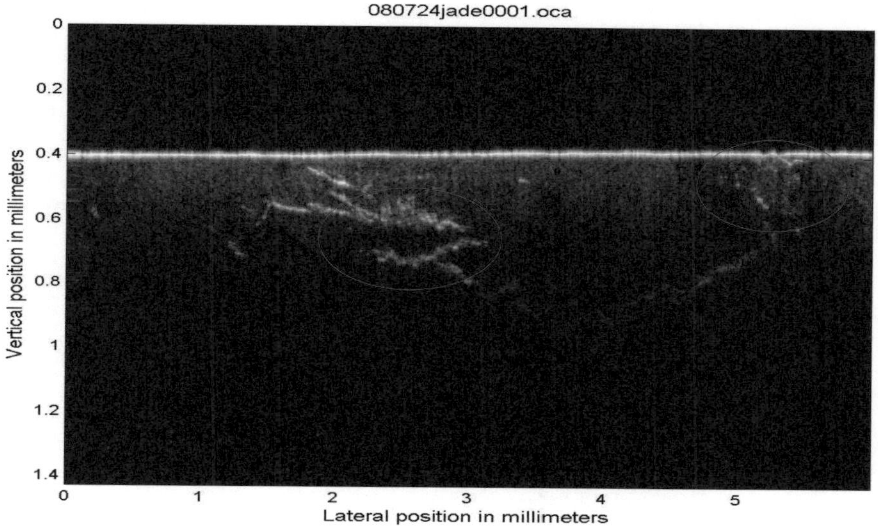

Fig. 5a. Two clustering structure cracks are presented in the image. A clustering crack usually consists of a crack body (circles) with some branching cracks that probably join other branching cracks of another crack body. The left crack presents a typical clustering structure crack in a considerable volume. The right one reveals some chips (open to the air) on the glaze surface. (image acquired by 890-nm system).

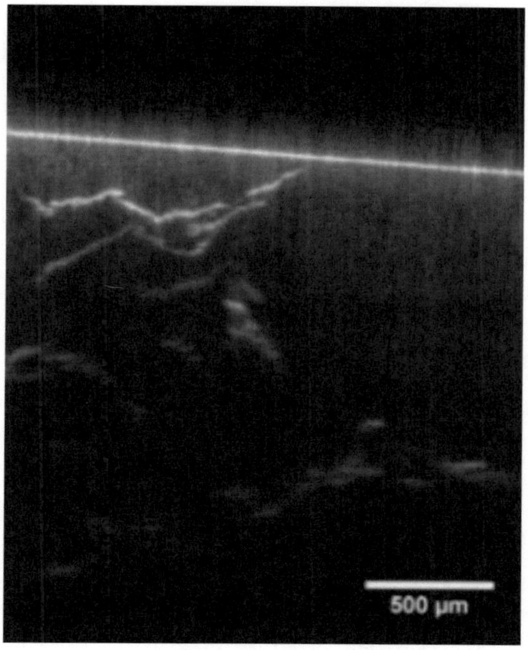

Fig. 5b. Several clustering structure cracks are presented in a tight space in the sample jade-1. (image acquired by 855-nm, focus-tracking system).

Figure 7b (circles). Moreover, when branching cracks join together among crack bodies, they should create a more complicated macrostructure in a jade material, as displayed in Figure 5b and 7a.

In contrast with Figure 5a and Figure 6, Figure 7 presents an uneven gray scale in the OCT image that implies the jade material, sample jade-3, contained several impurities. However, clustering structure cracks of various sizes are sealed in a deeper position below the surface of the sample. These complicated clustering structure cracks are exhibited more clearly in Figure 7a.

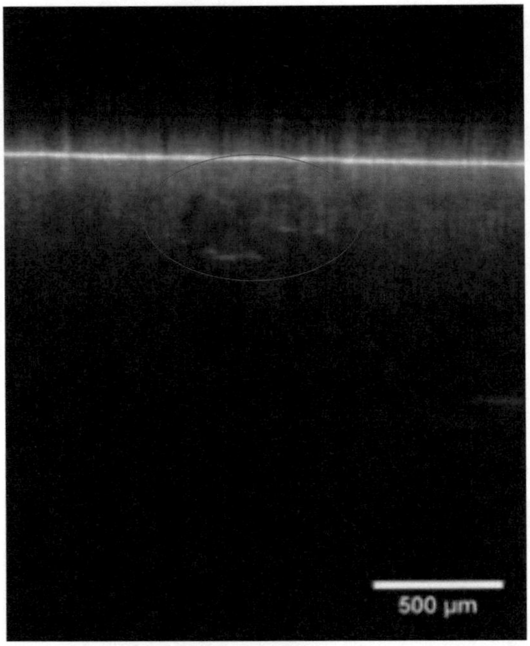

Fig. 5c. Some damage to the texture of local matrix is presented in the image of the sample jade-1. (image acquired by focus-tracking system).

4.2 Linear structure crack in jade

Figure 8 presents an extremely pure nephrite matrix of the sample jade-4 in an even and light gray scale. A 'U' shape crack is displayed in the image. Chips at the openings of this crack are revealed on the surface. This crack propagated its path in zigzag form. Figure 8-1 presents the same crack growing in an almost horizontal direction with the surface of this jade. However, the terminal tip of this crack isn't clearly revealed.

Figure 7b displays three cracks in the sample glaze-3. The left two are not open to the air, whereas the right one is open to the air with a couple of chips on the surface. However, based on the OCT images, the linear structure cracks in jade-3 and jade-4 appear to be broader and brighter than the former glaze cracks due to iron oxides deposits caused by corrosion along the crack gap in these jade samples.

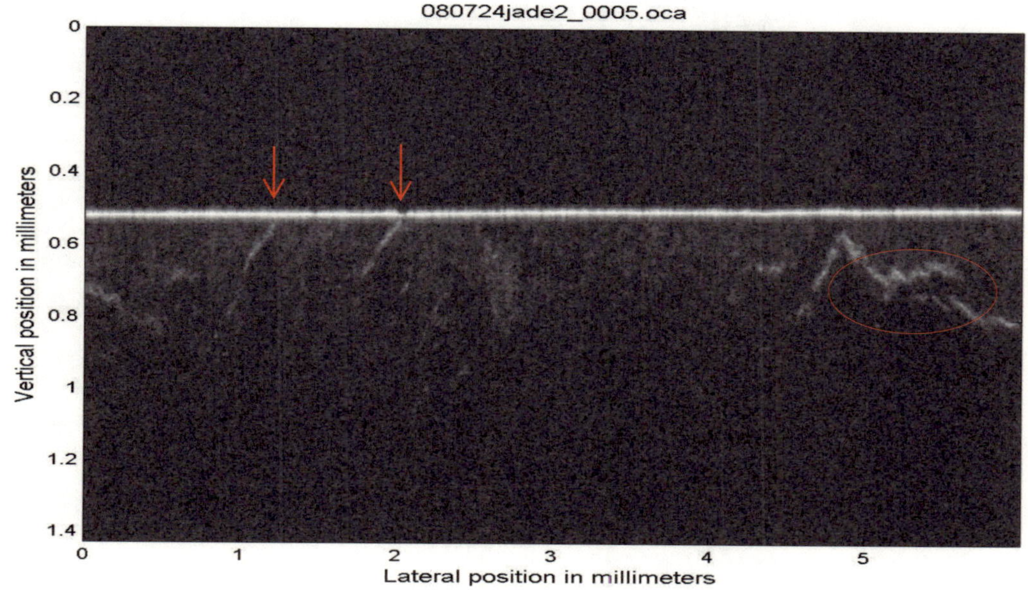

Fig. 6. A clustering structure crack is displayed on the right of the image of the sample jade-2. The circle marks the same structure crack as the one in the left circle of Figure 5a. The left arrows points to two thin linear cracks. (image acquired by 890-nm system).

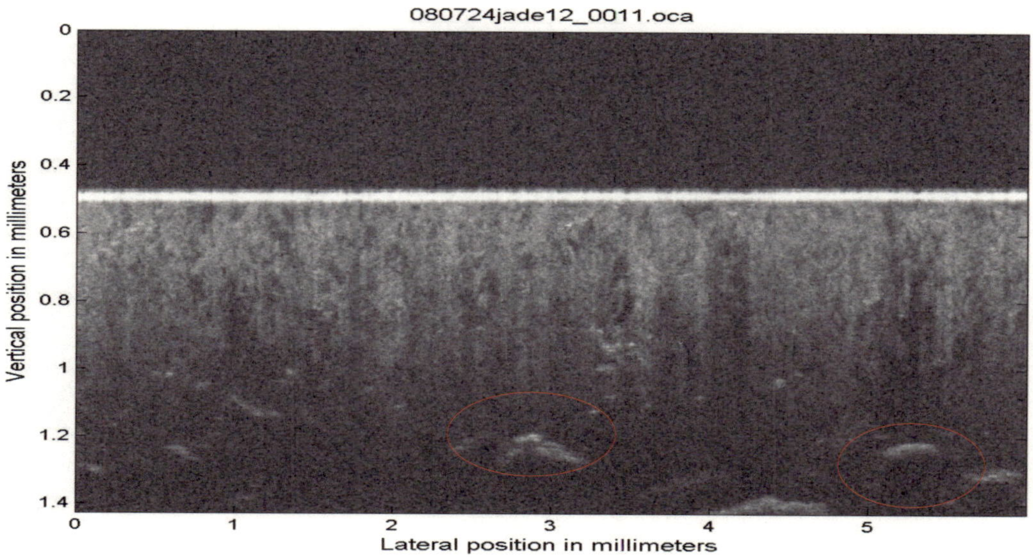

Fig. 7. Several sealed clustering structure cracks (circles) are presented in the image of sample jade-3. However, the jade matrix seems to contain rich impurities (the bright and black nodules). (image acquired by 890-nm system).

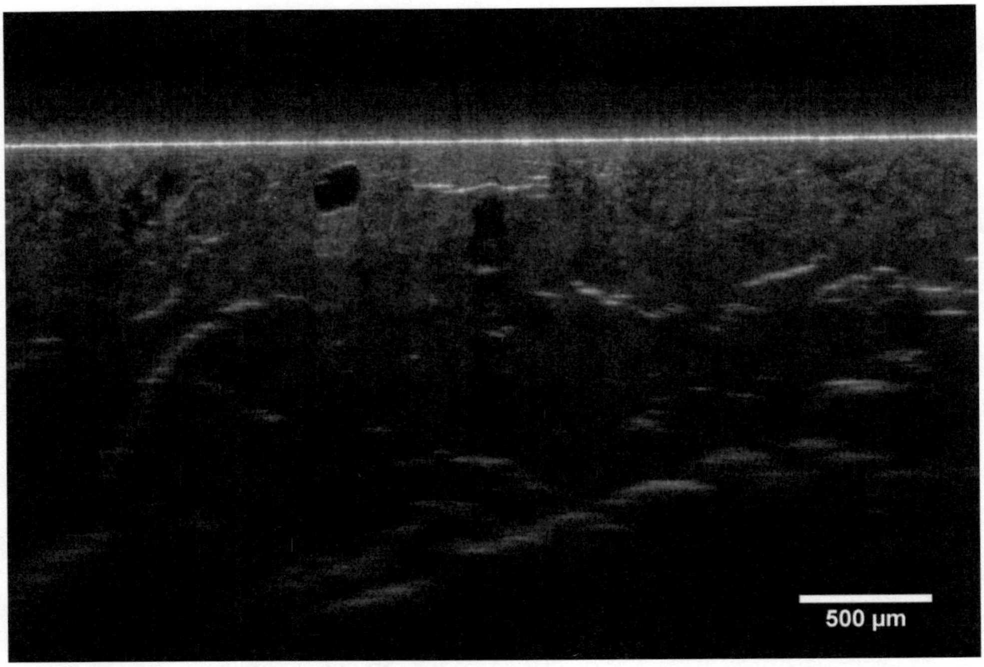

Fig. 7a. A detailed image presents considerably confused clustering and linear structure cracks with rich impurities in the sample jade-3. The imaging depth is over 2-mm in the sample. (image acquired by 855-nm, focus-tracking system).

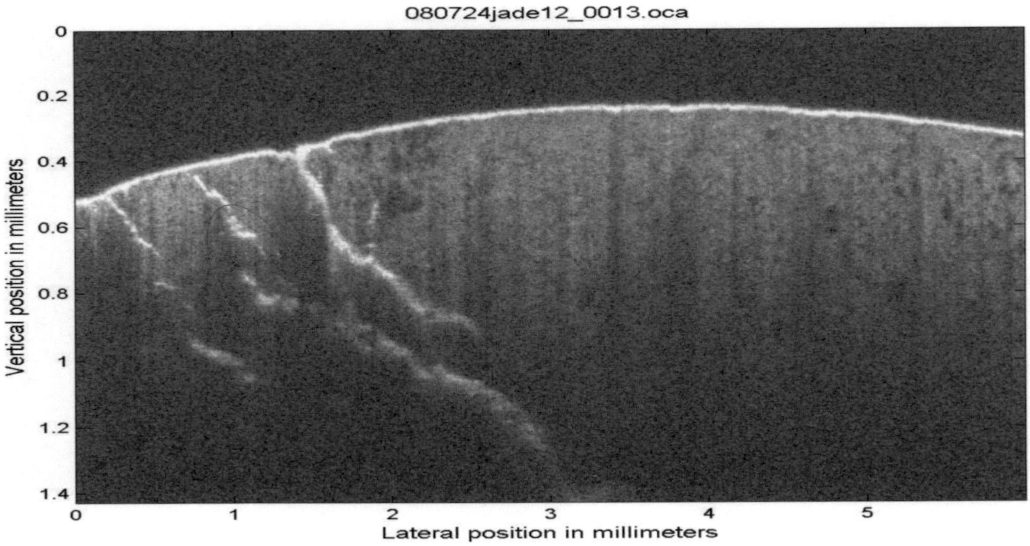

Fig. 7b. Three cracks are presented in the image of jade-3. The right one seems to be a linear structure. The other two are clustering structure cracks. The circle marks off a probable crack body of the clustering structure crack. (image acquired by 890-nm system)

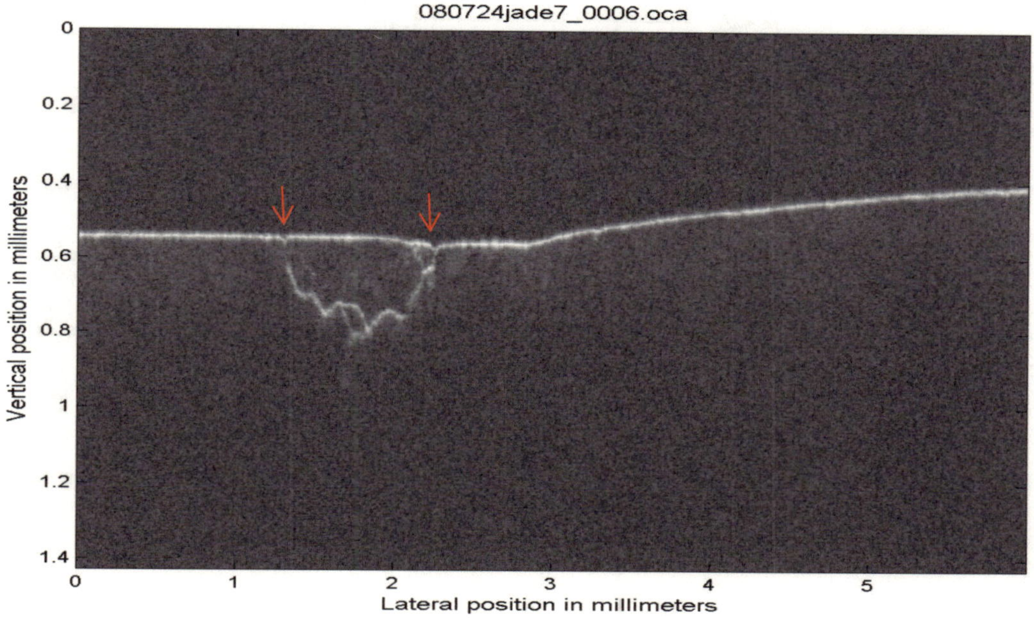

Fig. 8. A linear structure crack is presented in the image of the jade (nephrite) pebble. Some chips are revealed on the pebble's surface (arrows). The crack path propagated in zigzag form. (image acquired by 890-nm system).

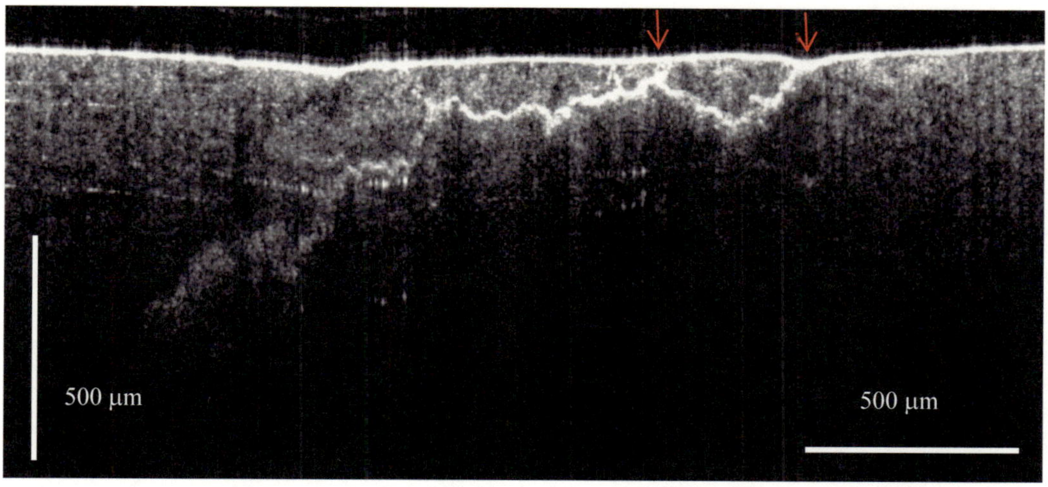

Fig. 8-1. Due to corrosion (iron oxidation) along the crack gap, the irregular or zigzag path appears to be brighter in the OCT image. The terminal tip of the crack is not clear. Two arrows indicate the same openings presented in Fig. 8. (image acquired by 930-nm system).

In addition, some thin and short linear cracks are presented in Figure 6. Two very thin cracks (left two arrows) are similar to 'T' structure crack in the glaze samples with an inclining angle of around 45 degrees. The right one reveals its opening in a small chip on the surface, whereas the left one is not open to the air. The thinness and shortness of the two cracks seem to imply the driving force for continued crack propagation in them is weak.

4.3 Discussion of the characteristics of crack morphology in jade

The characteristics of the clustering structure crack in the jade material are likely to be summarized as: (1) its basic structure is a crack body formed by many micro-cracks in clusters, with some branching cracks in skirts of the crack body; (2) some branching cracks have joined together among crack bodies to form a complicated and considerable macrostructure network; (3) most cracks are not open to the air; and (4) no clear terminal tip is revealed.

In fact, most clustering structure cracks are initiated by damage to the local texture of the jade matrix. Sometimes the damage did not expand or deteriorate in the material, and it remained for a lengthy period, as displayed in Figure 5c (circle). However, once the micro-cracks begin propagating from the damage site, the crack develops along the grain boundaries in the jade. Therefore, regardless of whether the crack has a clustering structure or linear structure, unlike most glazes' smooth path, the jades' crack path is usually in irregular or zigzag form.

However, for some thin and short cracks, such as those in Figure 6, there may be a logical interpretation. Because the sample jade-2 (Figure 6) was used by ancient peoples as a tool (Yang, 2003), these thin cracks are probably due to that function. Under an imposed stress by the force of a human arm for routine work in a non-metal ancient society, small and thin cracks were propagated within the material, as presented in the image.

5. Conclusion

The focus-tracking system is a forceful tool for imaging deeper microstructure in jade or glaze materials, with over 2-mm of depth visualized. For exploring the sealed cracks inside jade material, it is suitable. In contrast, the 890-nm system presents a detail structure of cracks in a shallower position from the surface of the sample. However, the 930-nm system should be the most effective tool to highlight the crack structure within a multi-phase inhomogeneous glaze material. With a handheld probe, a portable tool, it can be applied directly to the surface of an artifact or artwork and to rapidly acquire appropriate images. However, scanning at different positions of a crack probably obtains different information related to the same crack. It enhances the advanced 3-dimension imaging to obtain more complete information related to the cracks.

In terms of OCT demonstrating crack morphology of glaze and jade materials, it not only reveals the basic structure characteristics, but also provides quantitative research about crack variation, such as the inclining angles from the typical 'T' structure or the depth of crack. Moreover, it is also likely to offer a more scientific classification of crack in ceramic or jade materials. Although crack in brittle materials is always a difficult issue to clarify, especially the mechanism of crazing related to the thermal stress and thermal shock (Andersson & Rowcliffe, 1996; Bertsch et al., 1974; Hasselman, 1969; Clarke et al., 1966), establishing the structure of crack and the relationship between crack and local components would make an important contribution to advanced scientific research.

In addition, the present result also contributes to art history study, especially in verifying certain Chinese historical records. For instance, according to ancient Chinese texts, some Southern Song (AD 1127-1279) Guan wares were dyed using eel blood to make the crack line is dark brown (Gao, 1591). However, based on the present research, several cracks are not open to the air, thus, the dyed eel blood legend seems to become more fancifully. Moreover, with regard to specific endowed artistic attributes of crack patterns in glaze, the research also provides a logical and scientific interpretation for their unique and subtle visual effect.

6. Acknowledgment

The author thanks Prof. Vandiver for providing a Ru shard sample (the present glaze-3) and Ms. Carol Elliott for her English editing suggestions.

7. References

Andersson, Tomas & Rowcliffe, David J. (1996). Indentation thermal shock test for ceramics. *Journal of the American Ceramic Society*, 79, 6, pp. 1509-1514, ISSN 0002-7820

Bertsch, B. E.; Larson, D. R. & Hasselman, D. P. H. (1974). Effect of crack density on strength loss of polycrystalline Al_2O_3 subjected to severe thermal shock. *Journal of the American Ceramic Society – Discussions and Notes*, 57, 5, pp. 235-236, ISSN 0002-7820

Bradt, Richard C.; Newnham, Robert E. & Biggers, J. V. (1973). The toughness of jade. *American Mineralogist*, 58, 7 & 8, pp. 727-732, ISSN 0003-004X

Chang, Shoude; Mao, Youxin; Chang, Guangming & Flueraru, Costel. (2010). Optical Coherence Tomography used for jade industry. *Proc. of SPIE*, 7855 785514, pp. 1-9, ISSN 1996-756X (web)

Clarke, F. J. P.; Tattersall, H. G. & Tappin, G. (1966). Toughness of ceramics and their work of fracture. *Proceedings of the British Ceramic Society*, 6, pp. 163-172, ISSN 0524-5141

Coble, R. L. & Kingery, W. D. (1955). Effect of porosity on thermal stress fracture. *Journal of the American Ceramic Society*, 38, 1, pp. 33-37, ISSN 0002-7820

Coppola, J. A. & Bradt, R. C. (1972). Measurement of fracture surface energy of SiC. *Journal of the American Ceramic Society*, 55, 9, pp. 455-460, ISSN 0002-7820

Elias, Mady; Magnain, Caroline & Frigerio, Jean Marc. (2010). Contribution of surface state characterization to studies of works of art. *Applied Optics*, 49, 11, pp. 2151-2160, ISSN 1559-128X

Faber, K. T.; Huang, M. D. & Evans, A. G. (1981). Quantitative studies of thermal shock in ceramics based on a novel test technique. *Journal of the American Ceramic Society*, 64, 5, pp. 296-301, ISSN 0002-7820

Friedman, M.; Handid, J. & Alani, G. (1972). Fracture-surface energy of rocks. *International Journal of Rock Mechanics and Mining Sciences*, 9, pp. 757-766, ISSN 0020-7624

Gao, Lian. (1591). *Ya Shang Zhai Zun Sheng Ba Jian (雅尚齋遵生八牋)*, Shu Mu Wen Xian Chu Ban She, ISBN 7-5013-0586-2, Beijing.

Hasselman, D. P. H. (1969). Griffith criterion and thermal shock resistance of single-phase versus multiphase brittle ceramics. *Journal of the American Ceramic Society – Discussions and Notes*, 52, 5, pp. 288-289, ISSN 0002-7820

Hasselman, D. P. H. (1969). Unified theory of thermal shock fracture initiation and crack propagation in brittle ceramics. *Journal of the American Ceramic Society*, 52, 11, pp. 600-604, ISSN 0002-7820

Kingery, W. D.; Bowen, H. K. & Uhlmann, D. R. (1976). *Introduction to Ceramics (Second Edition)*, p. 550, John Wiley & Sons, ISBN 0471478601, New York.

Klein, Justin; Winkler, Amy M.; Yang, M.-L.; Tumlinson, Alex & Barton, Jennifer K. (2011). Quantitative bubble imaging in ceramic glazes using a custom algorithm and focus-tracking optical coherence tomography. (forthcoming)

Li, Fenggong. (1925). *Yu Ya (玉雅)*, in *Gu Yu Kao Shi Jian Shang Cong Bian*, pp. 941-1046, Shu Mu Wen Xian Chu Ban She, ISBN 7-5013-0962-0, Beijing.

Liang, Haida; Peric, Borislava; Hughes, Michael; Podoleanu, Adrian; Spring, Marika & Roehrs, Stefan. (2008). Optical Coherence Tomography in archaeological and conservation science - a new emerging field. *Proc. of SPIE*, 7139 713915, pp. 1-9, ISSN 1996-756X (web)

Norton, F. H. (1952). *Elements of Ceramics*, Addison-Wesley, Cambridge.

Palmer, J. P. (1967). *Jade*, pp. 13-19, Spring Books, London.

Schurecht, H. G. & Fuller, D. H. (1931). Some effects of thermal shock in causing crazing of glazed ceramic ware. *Journal of the American Ceramic Society*, 14, 8, pp. 565-571, ISSN 0002-7820

Schurecht, H. G. & Pole, G. R. (1932). Some special types of crazing. *Journal of the American Ceramic Society*, 15, 11, pp. 632-637, ISSN 0002-7820

Seaton, C. C. & Dutta, S. K. (1974). Effect of grain size on crack propagation in thermally shocked B_4C. *Journal of the American Ceramic Society – Discussions and Notes*, 57, 5, pp. 228-229, ISSN 0002-7820

Shaw, Kenneth. (1971). *Ceramic Glazes*, pp. 128-129, Elsevier Publishing Company Limited, ISBN 0444201076, Amsterdam.

Simmons, Joseph. (1977). Refractive index and density changes in a phase-separated Borosilicate glass. *Journal of Non-Crystalline Solids*, 24, pp. 77-88, ISSN 0022-3093

Targowski, Piotr. (2008). Publications, In: *Optical Coherence Tomography for Examination of Objects of Art*, August 1, 2011, Available from: http://www.oct4art.eu/

THORLABS. (2011). Spectral Radar OCT system. *Microscopy and laser imaging*, August 1, 2011, Available from: http://www.thorlabs.com/catalogPages/595.pdf

Whitlock, Herbert P. & Ehrmann, Martin L. (1949). *The Story of Jade*, Sheridan House, New York.

Winkler, A. M.; Rice, P. F.; Drezek, R. A & Barton, J. K. (2010). Quantitative tool for rapid disease mapping using optical coherence tomography images of azoxymethane treated mouse colon. *Journal of Biomedical Optics*, 15, 4, 041512, ISSN 1083-3668

Yang, M.-L.; Winkler, Amy M.; Klein, Justin & Barton, Jennifer K. (2012). Using Optical Coherence Tomography to characterize thick-glaze structure: Chinese Southern Song Guan glaze case study. *Studies in Conservation*, 57, 1, ISSN 0039-3630 (publishing)

Yang, M.-L.; Winkler, Amy M.; Barton, Jennifer K. & Vandiver, Pamela B. (2009). Using Optical Coherence Tomography to examine the subsurface morphology of Chinese glazes. *Archaeometry* 51, 5, pp. 808-821, ISSN 0003-813X

Yang, M.-L.; Lu, C.-W.; Hsu, I.-J. & Yang, C. C. (2004). The use of Optical Coherence Tomography for monitoring the subsurface morphologies of archaic jades. *Archaeometry*, 46, 2, pp. 171-182, ISSN 0003-813X

Yang, Mei-Li. (2003). *The Story of Stone Tools: Special Exhibition of Stone Artifacts Donated by Lin Yao-chen*, the National Palace Museum, ISBN 957-562-448-3, Teipei.